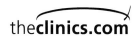
the**clinics**.com

MEDICAL CLINICS
OF NORTH AMERICA

Acute Myocardial Infarction

GUEST EDITORS
Mandeep Singh, MD, MPH
David R. Holmes, Jr., MD, FACC, FSCAI

July 2007 • Volume 91 • Number 4

SAUNDERS

An Imprint of Elsevier, Inc.
PHILADELPHIA LONDON TORONTO MONTREAL SYDNEY TOKYO

W.B. SAUNDERS COMPANY
A Division of Elsevier Inc.

1600 John F. Kennedy Boulevard • Suite 1800 • Philadelphia, Pennsylvania 19103-2899

http://www.theclinics.com

MEDICAL CLINICS OF NORTH AMERICA   Volume 91, Number
July 2007   ISSN 0025-712
Editor: Rachel Glover   ISBN-13: 978-1-4160-4333-
    ISBN-10: 1-4160-4333-

Medical Clinics of North America (ISSN 0025-7125) is published bimonthly by W.B. Saunders, 360 Park Avenu South, New York, NY 10010-1710. Business and editorial offices: 1600 John F. Kennedy Boulevard, Suite 180 Philadelphia, PA 19103-2899. Accounting and circulation offices: 6277 Sea Harbor Drive, Orlando, FL 3288. 4800. Periodicals postage paid at New York, NY, and additional mailing offices. Subscription prices are US 157 per year for US individuals, USD 273 per year for US institutions, USD 81 per year for US students, US 200 per year for Canadian individuals, USD 347 per year for Canadian institutions, USD 119 per year f Canadian students, USD 227 per year for international individuals, USD 347 per year for international instit tions and USD 119 per year for international students. To receive student/resident rate, orders must be accon panied by name of affiliated institution, date of term, and the *signature* of program/residency coordinator (institution letterhead. Orders will be billed at individual rate until proof of status is received. Foreign air spee delivery is included in all *Clinics* subscription prices. All prices are subject to change without notic POSTMASTER: Send address changes to *Medical Clinics of North America*, Elsevier Periodicals Customer Se vice, 6277 Sea Harbor Drive, Orlando, FL 32887-4800. **Customer Service: 1-800-654-2452 (US). From outsic of the USA, call (+1) 407-345-1000. E-mail: hhspcs@harcourt.com.**

Reprints. For copies of 100 or more, of articles in this publication, please contact the Commercial Reprin Department, Elsevier Inc., 360 Park Avenue South, New York, New York 10010-1710. Tel.: (+1) (212) 63. 3813; Fax: (+1) (212) 462-1935; E-mail: reprints@elsevier.com.

Medical Clinics of North America is also published in Spanish by McGraw-Hill Interamericana Editores S. A P.O. Box 5-237, 06500 Mexico, D.F., Mexico.

Medical Clinics of North America is covered in *Index Medicus, Current Contents, ASCA, Excerpta Medic Science Citation Index,* and *ISI/BIOMED.*

Printed in the United States of America.

GOAL STATEMENT

The goal of *Medical Clinics of North America* is to keep practicing physicians up to date with current clinical practice by providing timely articles reviewing the state of the art in patient care.

ACCREDITATION

The *Medical Clinics of North America* is planned and implemented in accordance with the Essential Areas and Policies of the Accreditation Council for Continuing Medical Education (ACCME) through the joint sponsorship of the University of Virginia School of Medicine and Elsevier. The University of Virginia School of Medicine is accredited by the ACCME to provide continuing medical education for physicians.

The University of Virginia School of Medicine designates this educational activity for a maximum of 90 *AMA PRA Category 1 Credits™*. Physicians should only claim credit commensurate with the extent of their participation in the activity.

The American Medical Association has determined that physicians not licensed in the US who participate in this CME activity are eligible for *AMA PRA Category 1 Credits™*.

Credit can be earned by reading the text material, taking the CME examination online at http://www.theclinics.com/home/cme, and completing the evaluation. After taking the test, you will be required to review any and all incorrect answers. Following completion of the test and evaluation, your credit will be awarded and you may print your certificate.

FACULTY DISCLOSURE/CONFLICT OF INTEREST

The University of Virginia School of Medicine, as an ACCME accredited provider, endorses and strives to comply with the Accreditation Council for Continuing Medical Education (ACCME) Standards of Commercial Support, Commonwealth of Virginia statutes, University of Virginia policies and procedures, and associated federal and private regulations and guidelines on the need for disclosure and monitoring of proprietary and financial interests that may affect the scientific integrity and balance of content delivered in continuing medical education activities under our auspices.

The University of Virginia School of Medicine requires that all CME activities accredited through this institution be developed independently and be scientifically rigorous, balanced and objective in the presentation/discussion of its content, theories and practices.

All authors/editors participating in an accredited CME activity are expected to disclose to the readers relevant financial relationships with commercial entities occurring within the past 12 months (such as grants or research support, employee, consultant, stock holder, member of speakers bureau, etc.). The University of Virginia School of Medicine will employ appropriate mechanisms to resolve potential conflicts of interest to maintain the standards of fair and balanced education to the reader. Questions about specific strategies can be directed to the Office of Continuing Medical Education, University of Virginia School of Medicine, Charlottesville, Virginia.

The authors/editors listed below have identified no professional or financial affiliations for themselves or their spouse/partner:
Eve D. Aymong, MD, MSc, FRCPC; Christopher E. Buller, MD, FRCPC, FACC; Allen P. Burke, MD; Rachel Glover (Acquisitions Editor); Mario Gössl, MD; Rajiv Gulati, MD, PhD; Richard J. Gumina, MD, PhD, David Hasdai, MD; Heike Hildebrandt; David R. Holmes, Jr., MD, FACC, FSCAI (Guest Editor); Zaza Iakobishvili, MD, PhD; Wissam A. Jaber, MD; Thomas J. Kiernan, MD, MRCPI; Amir Lerman, MD; Lilach O. Lerman, MD, PhD; Calin V. Maniu, MD; Dallit Mannheim, MD; Monica L. Olson, BS; Krishnan Ramanathan, MB, ChB, FRACP, FRCPC; Véronique L. Roger, MD, MPH; Amy K. Saenger, PhD; Kanwar P. Singh, MD; Mandeep Singh, MD (Guest Editor); Stephen E. Van Horn, Jr., MD; Daniele Versari, MD; and, Renu Virmani, MD.

The authors/editors listed below identified the following professional or financial affiliations for themselves or their spouse/partner:
Bernard J. Gersh, MB, ChB, Dphil is on the advisory committee/board of Astra Zeneca, Bristol Myers Squibb, Abbott Laboratories, Boston Scientific Corporation, Amorcyte Inc., and Cardiovascular Therapeuties.
Robert A. Harrington, MD is the director of DCRI, and has extensive relationships with industry. A detailed report may be found at http://www.dcri.duke.edu/research/coi.jsp.
Allen S. Jaffe, MD is a consultant for: Dade-Behring, Beckman-Coulter, Ortho Diagnostics, Pfizer, Bayer, GSK, and Siemens.
Robert D. Simari, MD is a patent holder for Anexon.

Disclosure of Discussion of non-FDA approved uses for pharmaceutical products and/or medical devices:
The University of Virginia School of Medicine, as an ACCME provider, requires that all faculty presenters identify and disclose any "off label" uses for pharmaceutical and medical device products. The University of Virginia School of Medicine recommends that each physician fully review all the available data on new products or procedures prior to instituting them with patients.

TO ENROLL

To enroll in the Medical Clinics of North America Continuing Medical Education program, call customer service at 1-800-654-2452 or visit us online at http://www.theclinics.com/home/cme. The CME program is available to subscribers for an additional fee of USD 205.

FORTHCOMING ISSUES

September 2007
Nanomedicine
Chiming Wei, MD, PhD, *Guest Editor*

November 2007
Metabolic Syndrome
Robert T. Yanagisawa, MD, and
Derek LeRoith, MD, PhD, *Guest Editors*

January 2008
Atrial Fibrillation
R.K. Thakur, MD and Andrea Natale, MD,
Guest Editors

RECENT ISSUES

May 2007
Bariatric Surgery Primer for the Internist
Nilesh A. Patel, MD and Lisa S. Koche, MD,
Guest Editors

March 2007
Pain Management, Part II
Howard S. Smith, MD, *Guest Editor*

January 2007
Pain Management, Part I
Howard S. Smith, MD, *Guest Editor*

November 2006
Antimicrobial Therapy
Burke A. Cunha, MD, MACP, *Guest Editor*

THE CLINICS ARE NOW AVAILABLE ONLINE!

Access your subscription at:
http://www.theclinics.com

GUEST EDITORS

MANDEEP SINGH, MD, MPH, Division of Cardiovascular Diseases and Internal Medicine, Mayo Clinic College of Medicine; and Division of Biostatistics, Mayo Clinic College of Medicine, Rochester, Minnesota

DAVID R. HOLMES, Jr., MD, FACC, FSCAI, Mayo Clinic, Cardiovascular Diseases and Internal Medicine, Rochester, Minnesota

CONTRIBUTORS

EVE D. AYMONG, MD, MSc, FRCPC, Clinical Assistant Professor of Medicine, Division of Cardiology, University of British Columbia, Vancouver, British Columbia, Canada

CHRISTOPHER E. BULLER, MD, FRCPC, FACC, Professor of Medicine; Head, Division of Cardiology, University of British Columbia, Vancouver, British Columbia, Canada

ALLEN P. BURKE, MD, Associate Medical Director, CVPath Institute, Gaithersburg, Maryland

BERNARD J. GERSH, MB, ChB, Dphil, Division of Cardiovascular Diseases, Mayo Clinic, Rochester, Minnesota

MARIO GÖSSL, MD, Division of Cardiovascular Diseases, Mayo Clinic, Rochester, Minnesota

RAJIV GULATI, MD, PhD, Assistant Professor of Medicine, Division of Cardiovascular Diseases and Internal Medicine, Mayo Clinic College of Medicine, Rochester, Minnesota

RICHARD J. GUMINA, MD, PhD, Assistant Professor of Medicine, Cardiovascular Medicine, The Ohio State University Medical Center, Columbus, Ohio

ROBERT A. HARRINGTON, MD, Professor of Medicine, Duke University Medical Center; Director, Duke Clinical Research Institute, Durham, North Carolina

DAVID HASDAI, MD, Associate Professor of Cardiology and Director, Intensive Cardiac Care Unit, Department of Cardiology, Rabin Medical Center, Beilinson Campus, Petah Tikva, Israel; and Sackler Faculty of Medicine, Tel Aviv University, Tel Aviv, Israel

HEIKE HILDEBRANDT, Division of Cardiovascular Diseases, Mayo Clinic, Rochester, Minnesota

DAVID R. HOLMES, Jr., MD, FACC, FSCAI, Mayo Clinic, Cardiovascular Diseases and Internal Medicine, Rochester, Minnesota

ZAZA IAKOBISHVILI, MD, PhD, Staff Physician, Intensive Cardiac Care Unit, Department of Cardiology, Rabin Medical Center, Beilinson Campus, Petah Tikva, Israel; and Sackler Faculty of Medicine, Tel Aviv University, Tel Aviv, Israel

WISSAM A. JABER, MD, Division of Cardiovascular Diseases, Mayo Clinic, Rochester, Minnesota

ALLAN S. JAFFE, MD, Department of Laboratory Medicine and Pathology; Cardiovascular Division, Mayo Clinic, Rochester, Minnesota

THOMAS J. KIERNAN, MD, MRCPI, Division of Cardiovascular Diseases, Mayo Clinic, Rochester, Minnesota

LILACH O. LERMAN, MD, PhD, Division of Nephrology and Hypertension, Mayo Clinic, Rochester, Minnesota

AMIR LERMAN, MD, Division of Cardiovascular Diseases, Mayo Clinic, Rochester, Minnesota

CALIN V. MANIU, MD, Assistant Professor of Medicine, Division of Cardiology, Medical University of South Carolina, Charleston, South Carolina

DALLIT MANNHEIM, MD, Division of Cardiovascular Diseases, Mayo Clinic, Rochester, Minnesota

MONICA L. OLSON, BS, Division of Cardiovascular Diseases, Mayo Clinic, Rochester, Minnesota

KRISHNAN RAMANATHAN, MB, ChB, FRACP, FRCPC, Clinical Assistant Professor of Medicine, Division of Cardiology, University of British Columbia, Vancouver, British Columbia, Canada

VÉRONIQUE L. ROGER, MD, MPH, Division of Cardiovascular Diseases, Department of Internal Medicine and Department of Health Sciences Research, Mayo Clinic College of Medicine, Rochester Minnesota

AMY K. SAENGER, PhD, Department of Laboratory Medicine and Pathology, Mayo Clinic, Rochester, Minnesota

ROBERT D. SIMARI, MD, Professor of Medicine, Division of Cardiovascular Diseases and Internal Medicine, Mayo Clinic College of Medicine, Rochester, Minnesota

KANWAR P. SINGH, MD, Assistant Professor of Medicine, Pat and Jim Calhoun Cardiovascular Center, University of Connecticut, Farmington, Connecticut

MANDEEP SINGH, MD, MPH, Division of Cardiovascular Diseases and Internal Medicine, Mayo Clinic College of Medicine; and Division of Biostatistics, Mayo Clinic College of Medicine, Rochester, Minnesota

STEPHEN E. VAN HORN, Jr., MD, Cardiology Fellow, Division of Cardiology, Medical University of South Carolina, Charleston, South Carolina

DANIELE VERSARI, MD, Division of Cardiovascular Diseases, Mayo Clinic, Rochester, Minnesota

RENU VIRMANI, MD, Director, CVPath Institute, Gaithersburg, Maryland

CONTENTS

before the event, experts widely accept that the morphology, composition, and degree of inflammation of a coronary atherosclerotic plaque is more important than the degree of luminal stenosis. Two depicting examples are the concentric, calcified lesion that shows significant luminal stenosis but is stable because of the stabilizing clasp of calcification. In contrast, a smaller but inflamed thin fibrous cap atheroma with a big lipid/necrotic core may rupture and cause an immediate fatal coronary occlusion.

medical therapy and the use of drug-eluting stents in the catheterization laboratory. Research efforts are also focusing on the implementation of streamlined transfer systems from community centers to tertiary care centers, akin to systems used in the trauma model. Furthermore, experience with the performance of primary PCI at community centers without onsite surgical backup is growing. This article summarizes data regarding the current state, challenges, and future directions of primary PCI for STEMI, emphasizing adherence to current American College of Cardiology/American Heart Association guidelines.

The Use of Biomarkers for the Evaluation and Treatment of Patients with Acute Coronary Syndromes

Amy K. Saenger and Allan S. Jaffe

The advent of inexpensive, highly accurate, and predictive markers of myocardial injury, inflammation, and hemodynamic stability has revolutionized the evaluation and treatment of patients who have acute coronary syndromes (ACSs). These blood biomarkers require small sample volumes, can be run expeditiously, and provide important information concerning the diagnosis, risk stratification, and treatment of these patients. To understand the use of these markers, one must have some knowledge about what elevations in these markers imply, how they have to be collected and measured to provide reliable information, when to suspect analytic confounds, and what the key values are that impart the diagnostic, prognostic, and therapeutic information. This article discusses these issues, emphasizing what clinicians must know for optimal test use, and then addresses the practical use of these markers in patients who have ACS.

Management of non–ST-Segment Elevation Myocardial Infarction

Stephen E. Van Horn, Jr., and Calin V. Maniu

Non–ST-segment elevation myocardial infarction (NSTEMI) is a major cause of cardiovascular morbidity and mortality in the United States. It represents the highest risk category of non–ST-segment elevation acute coronary syndromes (NSTEACS), for which timely diagnosis and appropriate therapy are paramount to improve outcomes. Evidence-based treatment, with combination of antiplatelet and anticoagulant therapy, and with serious consideration of early coronary angiography and revascularization along with anti-ischemic medical therapy, is the mainstay of management for NSTEMI. Aggressive risk-factor control after the acute event is imperative for secondary prevention of cardiovascular events. Applying in practice the American College of Cardiology/American Heart Association (ACC/AHA) guideline recommendations results in improved outcomes.

men, and is the topic of much medical literature. Recently, multiple therapies have emerged to save lives after acute myocardial infarction (AMI), backed by well-conducted studies; however, appropriate implementation of therapy guidelines is less than optimal. Recent efforts have focused on improving the quality of care (QC) after AMI in order to improve outcomes. This article illustrates how outcome after AMI is related to QC, describes the underuse of evidence-based therapies, and discusses factors associated with poor guideline adherence. It also reviews current quality improvement projects, and some available means to measure and optimize the QC for patients with AMI.

Med Clin N Am 91 (2007) xv–xvi

THE MEDICAL
CLINICS
OF NORTH AMERICA

Preface

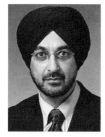 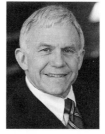

Mandeep Singh, MD, MPH   David R. Holmes, Jr., MD, FACC, FSCAI
Guest Editors

The knowledge base about acute myocardial infarction continues to accrue rapidly with information on pathophysiology, epidemiology, reperfusion therapy, and adjunctive treatment strategies. Given the fact that coronary artery disease is the leading cause of morbidity and mortality in the Western World, multiple studies have focused on these issues. In a relatively short time, we have progressed from the development of coronary care units to lytic therapy to percutaneous coronary intervention. These advances have markedly decreased mortality in patients who have this specific condition.

However, more substantial investigation is required in areas such as (1) patient education strategies for earlier recognition of symptoms which would facilitate earlier and more effective therapy, (2) ways to maximize myocardial flow rather than just epicardial flow very early in the disease progression, (3) improving myocardial salvage with either pharmacologic or mechanical adjunctive approaches, (4) secondary prevention after the initial event, including the need for testing and treatment with multiple antiplatelet strategies, (5) ways to define and deliver optimal care in patients who have acute myocardial infarction, and (6) new approaches to myocardial cell regeneration therapy.

Approaches to these areas will define the future of the treatment of acute myocardial infarction. This issue of *Medical Clinics of North America*

doi:10.1016/j.mcna.2007.04.002   *medical.theclinics.com*

explores these areas and defines what works, what has not worked, and what may work in the future.

Mandeep Singh, MD, MPH
David R. Holmes, Jr., MD, FACC, FSCAI
*Mayo Clinic, 200 First Street
SW, Rochester, MN 55905, USA*

E-mail addresses: Singh.Mandeep@mayo.edu (M. Singh);
holmes.david@mayo.edu (D.R. Holmes)

ELSEVIER
SAUNDERS

THE MEDICAL
CLINICS
OF NORTH AMERICA

Med Clin N Am 91 (2007) 537–552

Epidemiology of Myocardial Infarction

Véronique L. Roger, MD, MPH

*Division of Cardiovascular Diseases, Department of Internal Medicine and Department
of Health Sciences Research, Mayo Clinic College of Medicine, 200 First Street SW,
Rochester, MN 55905, USA*

Scope of the problem

Epidemiology can be defined as "the study of the distribution and determinants of health-related events in specified populations, and the applications of this study to control health problems" [1].

Coronary heart disease (CHD) is the number one cause of death in the Western world and as such constitutes an immense public health problem [2]. Although CHD mortality declined in the last four decades in the United States as life expectancy increased (http://www.cdc.gov/nchs), the use of age-adjusted rates to describe the CHD mortality obscures the fact that the decline largely represents the postponement of CHD deaths until older age. The burden of CHD is thus increasing in parallel with the increase in life expectancy [3,4]. As more people live with heart disease, the burden of prevalent disease with its assorted comorbid complications is increasing. The matter of identifying people who have heart disease, measuring the incidence of disease and its outcome and how these may have changed over time becomes essential as multifaceted approaches to reduce the burden of disease, including drug discovery, clinical trials, and policies, have shaped the practice of cardiology for decades and will likely continue to do so in the future. In this context, myocardial infarction occupies a central role in the assessment of the burden of heart disease.

Herein, we address the occurrence of myocardial infarction across populations, place, and time and examine how the epidemiology of myocardial infarction relates to the broader framework of cardiovascular population and clinical sciences.

Supported in part by grants from the National Institutes of Health (RO1 HL 59205, K24 HL 68765).

E-mail address: roger.veronique@mayo.edu

Methodology

In contrast to the magnitude of the burden of heart disease, there is no nationally representative surveillance approach for heart disease. The Centers for Disease Control and Prevention conducts nationally representative surveys on hospital discharges, ambulatory medical care, risk factors, and population characteristics, and the Agency for Healthcare Research and Quality collects information on medical expenditures and hospital inpatient samples. Death certificate data are collected by state health departments and gathered by Centers for Disease Control and Prevention, and the Centers for Medicare and Medicaid Services collect data pertaining to Medicare hospital reimbursements. These systems are not designed to be linked, however, and thus can only provide a partial assessment of the morbidity and mortality related to heart disease.

Measuring the occurrence of myocardial infarction in diverse populations and settings requires that several conditions be met. These include the availability of a defined population, which is indispensable to generate incidence rates, and the reliance on a valid definition that actually measures the intended event. This definition should be amenable to standardization to enable reliable data collection and comparisons across studies. Finally, the components of this definition should be relatively immune to temporal changes so that time trends in the occurrence of myocardial infarction can be appraised. Despite their apparent simplicity, these conditions are rarely met. The commonly used approaches to assess the burden of myocardial infarction along with their respective advantages and disadvantages are reviewed in this article.

The *National Hospital Discharge Survey* samples hospital discharges using codes from the International Classification of Disease (ICD) [5]. These are event-based, not person-based, and thus allow for multiple hospitalizations for the same individual to be counted. The diagnoses are not validated using standardized criteria, such that myocardial infarction may reflect different entities across hospitals depending on care delivery patterns, which in turn depend on insurance coverage, medical practice habits, and so forth [6].

Further, National Hospital Discharge Survey data do not differentiate between first and subsequent admission for a given condition and thus cannot measure incidence. Finally, documented shifts in hospital discharge diagnoses after the introduction of the Diagnosis-Related Groups payment system hinders the validity of these sources for epidemiology research [7–9]. Although hospital discharge data provide important insights into the burden of disease, which are important for resource allocation, policy making, and analysis of health care delivery, they cannot provide information on the true epidemiology of myocardial infarction.

Community surveillance can be envisioned as a comprehensive multifaceted approach designed to track heart disease at the community level. It has proven feasible and less costly than a cohort study [10]. Typical indicators tracked in community surveillance of heart disease include deaths, myocardial infarction incidence and outcomes, and less frequently heart failure incidence and outcomes.

Because it is conducted within a defined population, community surveillance enables measuring attack rates for myocardial infarction and, in some cases, incidence rates. In the absence of a national surveillance system for heart disease, community surveillance is essential to precisely monitor heart disease trends. These programs share several common key features. They are retrospective by design and typically rely on dismissal diagnosis using codes of the ICD for case finding. Once potential cases are identified, they are subjected to rigorous validation procedures using standardized diagnostic approaches, most often incorporating coding of the electrocardiographic findings with the Minnesota code [11], which can be accomplished manually or electronically [12]. The main characteristics of heart disease community surveillance programs are reviewed here.

The *Minnesota Heart Survey* (MHS) has been monitoring hospitalized patients who have myocardial infarction along with CHD deaths among residents of the Minneapolis–St. Paul metropolitan area since the 1970s. It relies on a standardized definition for myocardial infarction that combines cardiac pain, biomarkers, and Minnesota coding of the electrocardiogram [13] and has in place rigorous quality assurance and quality control measures.

The surveillance component of the *Atherosclerosis Risk in Communities* (ARIC) study was originally designed to evaluate CHD incidence differences by race and by geographic location; however, it has adequate power to assess trends [14,15]. ARIC relies on a standardized definition for myocardial infarction that combines cardiac pain, biomarkers, and Minnesota coding of the electrocardiogram. Like the Minnesota Heart Survey, ARIC has in place rigorous quality assurance methodology [14]. Initially, ARIC had an upper age limit of 74 years that has since been extended to include a growing segment of the aging United States population.

The *Olmsted County Study* is conducted under the auspices of the Rochester Epidemiology Project, which has a longstanding tradition of monitoring disease occurrence and outcomes of many chronic diseases [16–18]. Heart disease surveillance within the population of Olmsted County examined myocardial infarctions and cardiac deaths since 1979. The study uses standardized epidemiologic diagnostic criteria for myocardial infarction similar to those of the ARIC study, including Minnesota coding of the electrocardiogram, and has in place rigorous quality control measures [19]. The Olmsted County Study has no upper age limit and has access to outpatient and inpatient data, which are essential to evaluate long-term outcomes after myocardial infarction given the current shift from inpatient care settings.

The *Worcester Heart Attack Study* is a multihospital community study that focuses on trends in the incidence and mortality of hospitalized patients who have myocardial infarction in all age groups [20,21]. It relies on a standardized definition of myocardial infarction combining chest pain, biomarkers, and electrocardiogram data without Minnesota coding of the electrocardiogram.

The *Framingham Heart Study* is a prospective study of cardiovascular disease and its determinants among a sample of residents of the town of Framingham, Massachusetts. As a population-based cohort focusing on risk factors for the development of heart disease, it has generated transformational discoveries that have shaped the practice of cardiology for more than half a century. Longitudinal trends in disease occurrence and outcomes, including myocardial infarction, have also been evaluated in the Framingham Heart Study under the auspices of the Framingham Cardiovascular Disease Survey [22,23]. The Framingham Cardiovascular Disease Survey defined myocardial infarction as a combination of symptoms, electrocardiographic, and enzyme changes.

The *Corpus Christi Heart Project* was designed to focus on the comparison of disease burden and outcome between Mexican Americans and whites [24,25]. To define myocardial infarction, the Corpus Christi Heart Project relied on a standardized definition of myocardial infarction combining cardiac pain, biomarkers, and electrocardiogram data with Minnesota coding of the electrocardiogram.

The World Health Organization *MONICA* (Multinational MONItoring of trends and determinants in CArdiovascular disease) Project was established in the early 1980s to monitor trends in cardiovascular diseases and to relate these to risk factor changes [26]. It was set up to explain the diverse trends in cardiovascular disease mortality observed from the 1970s. There were 32 MONICA centers in 21 countries. The population monitored included 10 million men and women aged 25–64 years. The diagnosis of myocardial infarction integrates cardiac pain, Minnesota code of the electrocardiograms, and biomarker levels (http://www4.ktl.fi/publications/monica/manual) [27,28]. The breadth of populations covered by MONICA is unique and the data exceptionally rich. To interpret MONICA data, however, it is essential to remember that the upper age limit of 64 years does not account for a large segment of the population in whom coronary events and myocardial infarctions occur.

FINAMI is a population-based myocardial infarction registry initiated as part of the FINMONICA study and was originally the Finnish contribution to the MONICA Project [29]. FINAMI evaluates all events compatible with myocardial infarction or coronary heart disease death among residents of several geographic areas in Finland. These areas are mostly urban, and in 1995 there were 82,849 men and 87,360 women aged 35 to 64 years living in the FINAMI areas. The FINAMI registry ensures complete capture and ascertainment of all coronary events and relies on a standardized definition of myocardial infarction combining cardiac pain, biomarkers, and electrocardiogram data with Minnesota coding of the electrocardiogram [30].

Finally, *myocardial infarction registries* are currently active, including, in particular, the National Registry of Myocardial Infarction (NRMI) and the Global Registry of Acute Coronary Events (GRACE). Sponsored by Genentech, Inc. NRMI is a large observational study of acute myocardial infarction (http://www.nrmi.org/nrmi; web site last accessed 09-01-2006). Since 1990, NRMI has collected data on more than 2 million patients in the United States with a central focus on care delivery and short-term outcomes. NRMI is a voluntary, industry-sponsored registry that cannot measure incidence rates in populations. GRACE is a multinational observational study of management and outcomes of acute coronary syndromes [31]. It uses a cluster design involving sites in the United States, Brazil, Europe, Argentina, and Australia. The diversity of the populations and attending patterns of practice is a unique feature of GRACE, yet like NRMI its main focus is on the delivery of care. As such, these important registries and other smaller similar studies provide essential data for outcomes research, particularly as it relates to health care delivery. It cannot by design provide information on incidence rates and cannot measure the true population burden of myocardial infarction and how it may have changed over time, however.

In summary, several well-established studies conduct surveillance of heart disease using the appropriate methodology within defined populations to provide data on the epidemiology of myocardial infarction. These studies have included myocardial infarction as one of their central measures and use well-validated criteria anchored within solid quality assurance that rely on three central elements: cardiac pain, electrocardiographic analysis, and biomarker changes. Each of the aforementioned surveillance programs has a slightly different appraisal of this important public health problem and thus provides complementary information. Although some studies, such as ARIC and Corpus Christ Heart Study, have been designed to enable analysis of diverse ethnic groups others have more limited ethnic diversity. Because no study by itself could ever be representative of all ethnic groups, this further supports the need for a national surveillance approach for myocardial infarction and coronary disease, which is currently lacking. The lack of a national surveillance approach hinders the understanding of heart disease and reduces the ability to accurately treat it and prevent it.

Incidence of myocardial infarction

Selected results pertaining to the incidence of myocardial infarction and how it changed over time are presented in Table 1. These results call for several comments.

In the ARIC [32] study, no overall change was detected in the incidence of hospitalized myocardial infarction between 1987 and 1994. There were divergences in the trends by race and sex with an alarming increase in myocardial infarction among black women. In the MHS, between 1985 and

Table 1
Incidence of myocardial infarction in selected community studies

Study	Time period	Incidence[a] (per 100,000)	Temporal trends in incidence	Comment
ARIC [32]	1987–1994	Women: 190 Men: 410	Stable or increasing	Ages 35–74
Minnesota Heart Survey [34]	1985–1997	—	Decline	Ages 35–74
Olmsted County Study [36,37]	1979–1998	Overall 205	Stable overall; age/sex-specific diverging trends	No upper age limit
Worcester Heart Attack Study [35]	1975–1995	Overall 244	Increase in earlier years followed by decline and plateau	No upper age limit
Corpus Christi Study [25]	1988–1992	MA Women: 354 NHW Women: 224 MA Men: 486 NHW Men: 346	—	Ages 25–74

Abbreviations: MA, Mexican American; NHW, non-Hispanic white.
[a] Rates are age-adjusted and the numbers presented pertain to the first years of each study that include a large time span.

1995, the rates of hospitalization for acute myocardial infarction declined [33,34]. In MHS and ARIC, published data do not include people older than age 74 and are thus not accounting for a growing segment of the population.

In the Worcester Heart Attack Study, analyses spanning a 20-year period until 1995 indicated qualitatively flat trends in incidence from the mid 1980s to the mid 1990s [35]. The trends between1975 and 1988 underscored the importance of examining age- and sex-specific patterns in addition to overall rates. Larger declines in myocardial infarction incidence were noted among elderly individuals along with an increase in incidence among some, but not all, age groups in women.

In Olmsted County, there was little change in the incidence of hospitalized patients who had myocardial infarction between 1979 and 1998. Important age- and sex-specific patterns were noted as trends diverged with an increase in myocardial infarction incidence in women and the elderly [36,37]. In the Olmsted County Study, like in the Worcester Heart Attack Study, the absence of an upper age limit enables the detection of age- and sex-specific disease patterns that denote a shift in the burden of myocardial infarction toward women and the elderly. These findings have important clinical and public health implications.

Data from the Framingham Heart Study, which pertain to earlier time periods since the inception of the cohort, indicated that the incidence of myocardial infarction and other manifestations of coronary disease declined over a 20-year period starting in the 1950s [38].

The Corpus Christi Study reported important data comparing and contrasting the incidence of myocardial infarction in Mexican American and non-Hispanic white men and women indicating that the incidence of myocardial infarction was greater among Mexican Americans than non-Hispanic whites for both men and women [25].

The diversity of the populations included in MONICA precludes summarizing its rich data in one aggregate measure amenable to inclusion in Table 1. MONICA reported seminal data illustrating a wide variation in the incidence of myocardial infarction and other coronary events across populations [27,28].

Case fatality rate after myocardial infarction

Selected results pertaining to the case fatality rate after myocardial infarction and how it changed over time are presented in Table 2 [36,39]. Several points should be underscored to enable appropriate interpretation of these results. First, the ARIC and MHS studies do not reflect the disproportionate burden of death after myocardial infarction that occurs in the elderly because their published results do not include people older than age 74. Second, the Worcester Heart Attack Study has reported on in-hospital mortality, which is problematic over the 20-year time span of their study given the marked reduction on the duration of hospital stay that occurred during that time period. The 28-day case fatality is a better metric to appraise the change in mortality after acute myocardial infarction within the context of changing practice in hospitalization duration. These important considerations notwithstanding, all studies have reported a favorable decline in early

Table 2
Case fatality rates of myocardial infarction in selected community surveillance studies

Study	Time period	Case fatality rate[a]	Temporal trends	Comment
ARIC [31]	1987–1994	Men 9% Women 11%	Mortality declined over time	28-day mortality
Minnesota Heart Survey [33]	1985–1997	Men 13% Women 16%	Mortality declined over time	28-day mortality
Olmsted County Study [35]	1979–1994	12%	Mortality declined over time only in younger persons	28-day mortality
Worcester Heart Attack Study [38]	1975–1995	18%	Mortality declined over time	In-hospital deaths

[a] Numbers are age-adjusted and pertain to the first year of the study period.

mortality after acute myocardial infarction among younger individuals with a persistently high case-fatality rate among the elderly. The mortality of acute myocardial infarction in community surveillance studies remains high and is consistently higher than that reported in clinical trials, reflective of the bias ensuing from the rigorous selection process necessary for the internal validity of clinical trials [40]. Although clinical trials are the only valid approach to test the efficacy of a novel treatment, the data from community surveillance reflect the effectiveness of these new treatments once implemented in clinical practice, thereby underscoring how complementary the two approaches are.

Severity of myocardial infarction

Epidemiologic studies offer the possibility of examining whether the severity of acute myocardial infarction differs according to time, place, and person. Some of the aforementioned surveillance programs have primarily evaluated if the severity of myocardial infarction declined over time.

Although epidemiology studies constitute the only environment in which this question can be addressed given the need for a reference population and for rigorous definition and criteria, evaluating the severity of myocardial infarction is challenging for multiple reasons [41].

First, the time between the onset of symptoms and the presentation to medical care can affect each indicator of severity (Killip class, biomarkers, electrocardiographic findings) such that time trends in time to presentation can affect any association between time and infarction severity. Second, some indicators can be affected by treatment. Although Killip class and ST-segment elevation reflect the characteristics of the infarction during the first 24 hours and are unlikely to be affected by treatment, peak creatine kinase (CK) and Q-waves conversely may be impacted by treatment, particularly reperfusion. Third, the interpretation of the changes in Killip class requires knowledge in the trends in out-of-hospital coronary disease deaths, because a decline in such deaths may result in larger numbers of people admitted to the hospital who would have died out of hospital. This observation, in turn, may impact the relationship between Killip class and time by modifying the case mix of hospitalized infarctions. Finally, accurate determination of the severity of infarction through biomarker measurement is affected by the timing and frequency of the biomarker measurements such that the recorded values may not accurately reflect the true peak.

Overall, among studies that included all age groups, the frequency of cardiogenic shock declined some over time, although the magnitude of the decline was attenuated after age adjustment [42–44].

The frequency of ST-segment elevation at presentation and the occurrence of Q waves decreased over time in the Olmsted County Study [42,43]. In the ARIC study, the frequency of these indicators increased (ST segment elevation) or remained stable (Q waves) [45]. It is conceivable that differences in age distributions between studies contribute to this discrepancy. Notwithstanding these possible explanations, these findings underscore the importance of continuous monitoring of such trends across time and age groups.

Peak CK values declined in the ARIC and in the Olmsted County studies [45,46]. These values are influenced by reperfusion therapy, the use of which increased during the surveillance period for both studies. The decline in peak CK was observed among all patients in Olmsted County irrespective of reperfusion therapy, such that it can be viewed as a pertinent indicator of myocardial infarction severity [46].

Altogether, within the methodologic caveats mentioned, the data from published studies converge to suggest a decline in the severity of myocardial infarction over time.

The new definition of myocardial infarction

In 2000, the American College of Cardiology and the European Society of Cardiology published a consensus document redefining myocardial infarction [47]. The new definition combined increase and decrease of biochemical markers of myocardial necrosis with any of the following conditions: ischemic symptoms, ECG changes, and coronary intervention. The recommended biochemical markers are the troponins (T or I), which have gradually replaced CK and CK–myocardial band (CK-MB) in clinical practice since the mid 1990s. These changes stem largely from reports on the prognostic value of troponin indicating that troponin provided prognostic information incremental to previously available clinical factors [48–50].

Troponin is more specific than CK/CK-MB for the diagnosis of myocardial infarction in the setting of associated skeletal muscle damage or injury, including surgery. Of critical importance to clinicians and epidemiologists, the troponins have higher sensitivity that allows for the detection of small amounts of myocardial necrosis, which would have gone undetected by CK-MB. Proponents of the new definition recognized that the change in myocardial infarction criteria, particularly as they rely highly on more sensitive biochemical markers, "will confuse efforts to follow trends in disease rates and outcomes" [47]. The implications of changing the criteria for the diagnosis of myocardial infarction, however, reach far beyond their impact on the study of the epidemiology of myocardial infarction and the discontinuity in the trends that this change will unavoidably introduce. The new definition can be expected to increase the number of myocardial infarctions and shift the clinical spectrum of the disease. For example, patients previously diagnosed with unstable angina will now be classified as myocardial infarction because of detectable troponin levels despite normal CK-MB. Altogether, the new criteria generated considerable controversy on their appropriateness and their degree of reliance on troponin [51–56].

The controversy notwithstanding, because of the profound consequences of a diagnosis of myocardial infarction on patient care, disease trends, and use of health care resources, it is of critical importance for clinicians and public health to critically evaluate the impact of the new criteria on incidence, case mix, and outcome. Anticipating these concerns, the proponents of the new definition had recommended that the established definition of myocardial infarction be "retained by specific epidemiological centers" [47]. This recommendation is challenging, however, for most surveillance programs rely on multiple hospitals and health care systems for case finding. Unless CK-MB and cardiac troponins are measured simultaneously in the same patients in a population-based setting, the shifts in incidence, case mix, and outcomes resulting from the change in criteria cannot be accurately measured. The simultaneous measurements of the two biomarkers and the determination of the impact of the changes in myocardial infarction diagnosis require active surveillance with an approach that applies simultaneously the CK and troponin-based criteria to all patients who have acute coronary syndrome in a given population, irrespective of the clinical practice patterns. The enunciation of these prerequisites underscores the complexity of designing such a study.

Studies that examined the impact of troponin on the diagnosis of myocardial infarction used mostly convenience samples from case series and often single values of troponin [16,57–60]. All documented increases in the number of myocardial infarctions, but the estimates of the magnitude of the increase varied widely from 23% [16,61] to 195% [59]. The interpretation of these data is complex because the type of biomarker (troponin T versus I), the assays, and the cut-points differed across studies, as did the reference criteria used. These important methodologic limitations [12,62–64] hinder the inference from these data. Finally, all studies used single values of troponin and thus did not evaluate the increment in the number of infarctions related to increase and decrease in troponin values, the recommended approach in the new definition [47].

In the FINAMI study, [65] the impact of troponin was addressed by examining the trends in coronary disease events in Finland over a decade (1993 to 2002). Among people aged 35 to 74 years, the incidence of the first coronary event declined by 2% per year in men and 1% per year in women. The decline was statistically significant in men but not in women. Among people aged 75 or older, the incidence of first coronary events did not change. The authors applied coefficients derived from a large number of infarctions with simultaneous determination of troponin and enzymatic markers to correct for the use of troponin. Correcting for the effect of troponin resulted in unmasking a larger decline in the incidence of first coronary events in both sexes and all age groups. These key findings thus directly validate the concern stemming from the redefinition of myocardial infarction by documenting that the change in the biomarker indeed "confuses" the interpretation of temporal trends in coronary disease [47].

In the Olmsted County Study, active (otherwise termed prospective) surveillance was implemented to examine the impact of the redefinition of myocardial infarction in the community [66]. The data demonstrate that the prospective and rigorous application of the new criteria relying on dynamic changes in troponin values results in a 68% increase in the number of infarctions compared with the number of infarctions that would have been detected using previously used criteria relying on the biomarkers CK and its MB fraction. The use of single troponin values provides different results than the criteria relying on increase and decrease. The increments in the number of infarctions, importantly, are always large even with conservative cut-points and likely to increase as limits of normal of the troponin assays are lowered. Further, this study also underscored the frequency of potentially spurious elevation of troponin [60,67] in clinical practice [66].

Interpretation of the changes in the epidemiology of myocardial infarction

Studying the trends in the incidence and outcome of myocardial infarction and of coronary disease mortality provides crucial insights into the determinants of heart disease that are essential to its treatment and prevention. For example, a decline in coronary mortality with stable incidence trends most likely reflects the impact of secondary prevention and medical care, whereas declining incidence of disease would point to primary prevention as the main driver of mortality trends. Within this framework, it is important to recognize that the trends in the incidence and outcome of coronary disease are complex, likely multifactorial, and evolve over time.

Altogether, from the early to mid 1980s until the mid to late 1990s within the context of a decline in coronary disease mortality, the incidence of myocardial infarction declined little (even increasing in certain groups) while case fatality improved. This finding suggests that medical care played a major role in the genesis of the decline of coronary deaths. This observation resonates with the dramatic changes in the treatment of acute coronary disease that has marked this time period and suggests that the changes in treatment approaches have been translated to the community resulting in important survival benefits. During this time period, by contrast, the impact of primary prevention as measured by the incidence of myocardial infarction seems more modest, contrasting with its impact in earlier years marked by a reduction in the incidence of myocardial infarction [38]. This finding demonstrates that the determinants of coronary mortality are multifactorial and that the respective responsibilities of changing incidence and reduced fatalities change over time. As the respective role of these two theoretic determinants varies across person, time, and place, continued surveillance is essential to detect changes in the trends and their determinants and to evaluate the effectiveness of clinical and public health strategies to combat coronary disease [32,68,69].

Epidemiology and clinical practice

Traditional studies of the epidemiology of myocardial infarction have focused on infarction and have seldom reported on the clinical entity of acute coronary syndromes, with or without biomarker elevation. Part of the reason for this resides in the need for a standardized definition in epidemiology and the relative ease of standardizing the definition of myocardial infarction, contrasting with the more challenging task of defining acute coronary syndromes from an epidemiologic point of view particularly in forms without biomarker elevation and with transient or absent electrocardiographic changes. Over the years, epidemiologic studies did not account for a large segment of the burden of nonfatal coronary disease, namely acute coronary syndromes, that do not meet validated infarction criteria. The redefinition of myocardial infarction has underscored this important issue, thereby challenging epidemiologists to incorporate acute coronary syndromes in the surveillance of coronary disease. Studies that have evaluated the implications of the redefinition of myocardial infarctions illustrate that reliance on one biomarker or the other alters the categorization between types of acute coronary syndromes [65,66]. Advocates of the widespread use of troponin have argued that acute coronary syndromes represent a continuum of disease, a concept familiar to clinicians, and that any increase in cardiac biomarkers has prognostic implications. Although the implications of the shift across types of acute coronary syndromes may arguably be modest from a clinical and pathophysiologic point of view, the consequences of a diagnosis of myocardial infarction for employment, health insurance, evaluation of health care delivery, epidemiology, and public health are enormous.

For this reason, operational definitions of acute coronary syndromes have been proposed that include a purposeful effort to categorize such events while also specifically identifying myocardial infarctions that would have met criteria using the previous enzymatic biomarkers [70]. This approach would enable health care providers to relate the newly defined myocardial infarctions to the previous classification [70]. As the new myocardial infarction criteria generate continued reflection and discussion, more data on their clinical and epidemiologic implications are clearly needed. This underscores the need to broaden the approach to coronary disease surveillance to include acute coronary syndromes rather than focusing primarily on myocardial infarction as traditionally defined. This inclusion is critical to understanding the trends that will be measured over the next decade marked by the change in biomarkers and to accurately evaluate the burden of heart disease.

References

[1] Last JM. Dictionary of epidemiology. New York: Oxford University Press; 2000.

[2] Writing Group Members, Thom T, Haase N, et al. Heart disease and stroke statistics—2006 update. A report from the American Heart Association Statistics Committee and Stroke Statistics Subcommittee, 10.1161/CIRCULATIONAHA.105.171600. Circulation 2006.

[3] Bishop E. Heart disease may actually be rising; researchers claim deaths are now being delayed to a later age group. Wall Str J 1996; pB3(W) pB6(E) col 1 (11 col in).

[4] Gerber Y, Jacobsen SJ, Killian J, et al. Impact of participation bias in a population-based study of myocardial infarction in Olmsted County, Minnesota, 2002 to 2004. Circulation 2006; 13:e827.

[5] Gillum RF. Acute myocardial infarction in the United States, 1970–1983. Am Heart J 1987; 113(3):804–11.

[6] Feinleib M, Lentzner H, Collins J, et al. Regional variations in coronary heart disease mortality and morbidity. In: Luepker Ha, editor. Trends in coronary heart disease mortality: Oxford University Press; 1988. p. 31–53.

[7] Assaf AR, Lapane KL, McKenney JL, et al. Possible influence of the prospective payment system on the assignment of discharge diagnoses for coronary heart disease. N Engl J Med 1993;329(13):931–5.

[8] Jollis JG, Ancukiewicz M, DeLong ER, et al. Discordance of databases designed for claims payment versus clinical information systems. Implications for outcomes research. Ann Intern Med 1993;119(8):844–50.

[9] Psaty BM, Boineau R, Kuller LH, et al. The potential costs of upcoding for heart failure in the United States. Am J Cardiol 1999;84(1):108–9, A109.

[10] Gillum RF. Community surveillance for cardiovascular disease: methods, problems, applications—a review. J Chronic Disease 1978;31:87–94.

[11] Prineas R, Crow R, Blackburn H. The Minnesota code manual of electrocardiographic findings. Littleton (MA): John Wright-PSG, Inc.; 1982.

[12] Kors JA, Crow RS, Hannan PJ, et al. Comparison of computer-assigned Minnesota codes with the visual standard method for new coronary heart disease events. Am J Epidemiol 2000;151(8):790–7.

[13] Gillum RF, Fortmann SP, Prineas RJ, et al. International diagnostic criteria for acute myocardial infarction and acute stroke. Am Heart J 1984;108(1):150–8.

[14] White AD, Folsom AR, Chambless LE, et al. Community surveillance of coronary heart disease in the Atherosclerosis Risk in Communities (ARIC) Study: methods and initial two years' experience. J Clin Epidemiol 1996;49(2):223–33.

[15] The ARIC Investigators. The Atherosclerosis Risk in Communities (ARIC) Study: design and objectives. Am J Epidemiol 1989;129:687–702.

[16] Melton LJ 3rd. History of the Rochester Epidemiology Project. Mayo Clin Proc 1996;71(3): 266–74.

[17] Melton LJ 3rd. Selection bias in the referral of patients and the natural history of surgical conditions. Mayo Clin Proc 1985;60(12):880–5.

[18] Kurland LT, Elveback LR, Nobrega FT. Population studies in Rochester and Olmsted County, Minnesota, 1900–1968. In: Kessler IT, Levin ML, editors. The community as an epidemiologic laboratory; a casebook of community studies. Baltimore (MD): Johns Hopkins Press; 1970. p. 47–70.

[19] Roger VL, Killian J, Henkel M, et al. Coronary disease surveillance in Olmsted County objectives and methodology. J Clin Epidemiol 2002;55(6):593–601.

[20] Goldberg RJ, Gore JM, Alpert JS, et al. Recent changes in attack and survival rates of acute myocardial infarction (1975 through 1981). The Worcester heart attack study. JAMA 1986; 255(20):2774–9.

[21] Goldberg RJ, Gorak EJ, Yarzebski J, et al. A communitywide perspective of sex differences and temporal trends in the incidence and survival rates after acute myocardial

infarction and out-of-hospital deaths caused by coronary heart disease. Circulation 1993; 87(6):1947–53.

[22] Gillum RF, Feinleib M, Margolis JR, et al. Community surveillance for cardiovascular disease: the Framingham cardiovascular disease survey. Some methodological problems in the community study of cardiovascular disease. J Chronic Dis 1976;29(5):289–99.

[23] Margolis JR, Gillum RF, Feinleib M, et al. Community surveillance for coronary heart disease: the Framingham Cardiovascular Disease survey. Comparisons with the Framingham Heart Study and previous short-term studies. Am J Cardiol 1976;37(1):61–7.

[24] Nichaman MZ, Wear ML, Goff DC Jr, et al. Hospitalization rates for myocardial infarction among Mexican-Americans and non-Hispanic whites. The Corpus Christi Heart Project. Ann Epidemiol 1993;3(1):42–8.

[25] Goff DC, Nichaman MZ, Chan W, et al. Greater incidence of hospitalized myocardial infarction among Mexican Americans than non-Hispanic whites. The Corpus Christi Heart Project, 1988–1992. Circulation 1997;95(6):1433–40.

[26] The World Health Organization MONICA Project (monitoring trends and determinants in cardiovascular disease): a major international collaboration. WHO MONICA Project Principal Investigators. J Clin Epidemiol 1988;41(2):105–14.

[27] Tunstall-Pedoe H, Kuulasmaa K, Mahonen M, et al. Contribution of trends in survival and coronary-event rates to changes in coronary heart disease mortality: 10-year results from 37 WHO MONICA project populations. Monitoring trends and determinants in cardiovascular disease [see comments]. Lancet 1999;353(9164):1547–57.

[28] Tunstall-Pedoe H, Kuulasmaa K, Amouyel P, et al. Myocardial infarction and coronary deaths in the World Health Organization MONICA Project. Registration procedures, event rates, and case-fatality rates in 38 populations from 21 countries in four continents. Circulation 1994;90(1):583–612.

[29] Mahonen M, Salomaa V, Torppa J, et al. The validity of the routine mortality statistics on coronary heart disease in Finland: comparison with the FINMONICA MI register data for the years 1983–1992. Finnish multinational MONItoring of trends and determinants in CArdiovascular disease. J Clin Epidemiol 1999;52(2):157–66.

[30] Salomaa V, Ketonen M, Koukkunen H, et al. Trends in coronary events in Finland during 1983–1997. The FINAMI study. Eur Heart J 2003;24(4):311–9.

[31] Rationale and design of the GRACE (Global Registry of Acute Coronary Events) Project: a multinational registry of patients hospitalized with acute coronary syndromes. Am Heart J 2001;141(2):190–9.

[32] Rosamond WD, Chambless LE, Folsom AR, et al. Trends in the incidence of myocardial infarction and in mortality due to coronary heart disease. N Engl J Med 1998;339:861–7.

[33] McGovern PG, Pankow JS, Shahar E, et al. Recent trends in acute coronary heart disease—mortality, morbidity, medical care, and risk factors. The Minnesota Heart Survey Investigators. N Engl J Med 1996;334(14):884–90.

[34] McGovern PG, Jacobs DR Jr, Shahar E, et al. Trends in acute coronary heart disease mortality, morbidity, and medical care from 1985 through 1997: the Minnesota heart survey. Circulation 2001;104(1):19–24.

[35] Goldberg RJ, Yarzebski J, Lessard D, et al. A two-decades (1975 to 1995) long experience in the incidence, in-hospital and long-term case-fatality rates of acute myocardial infarction: a community-wide perspective. J Am Coll Cardiol 1999;33(6):1533–9.

[36] Roger VL, Jacobsen SJ, Weston SA, et al. Trends in the incidence and survival of patients with hospitalized myocardial infarction, Olmsted County, Minnesota, 1979 to 1994. Ann Intern Med 2002;136(5):341–8.

[37] Arciero TJ, Jacobsen SJ, Reeder GS, et al. Temporal trends in the incidence of coronary disease. Am J Med 2004;117(4):228–33.

[38] Sytkowski PA, D'Agostino RB, Belanger A, et al. Sex and time trends in cardiovascular disease incidence and mortality: the Framingham Heart Study, 1950–1989. Am J Epidemiol 1996;143(4):338–50.

[39] Goldberg RJ, Konstam MA. Assessing the population burden from heart failure: need for sentinel population-based surveillance systems. Arch Intern Med 1999;159(1):15–7.

[40] Lindsted KD, Fraser Ge, Steinkohl M, et al. Healthy volunteer effect in a cohort study: temporal resolution in the Adventist Health Study. J Clin Epidemiol 1996;49(7): 783–90.

[41] Goldberg RJ. Monitoring trends in severity of acute myocardial infarction: challenges for the next millennium. Am Heart J 2000;139(5):767–70.

[42] Hellermann JP, Reeder GS, Jacobsen SJ, et al. Longitudinal trends in the severity of acute myocardial infarction: a population study in Olmsted County, MN. Am J Epidemiol 2002; 156:246–53.

[43] Hellermann JP, Goraya TY, Jacobsen SJ, et al. Incidence of heart failure after myocardial infarction: Is it changing over time? Am J Epidemiol 2003;157:1101–7.

[44] Goldberg RJ, Samad NA, Yarzebski J, et al. Temporal trends in cardiogenic shock complicating acute myocardial infarction. N Engl J Med 1999;340(15):1162–8.

[45] Goff DC Jr, Howard G, Wang CH, et al. Trends in severity of hospitalized myocardial infarction: the atherosclerosis risk in communities (ARIC) study, 1987–1994. Am Heart J 2000; 139(5):874–80.

[46] Hellermann JP, Reeder GS, Jacobsen SJ, et al. Has the severity of acute myocardial infarction changed over time? A population-based study in Olmsted County, MN. Circulation 2001;104:II-787.

[47] Alpert JS, Thygesen K, Antman E, et al. Myocardial infarction redefined—a consensus document of The Joint European Society of Cardiology/American College of Cardiology Committee for the redefinition of myocardial infarction. J Am Coll Cardiol 2000;36(3): 959–69.

[48] Braunwald E, Antman EM, Beasley JW, et al. ACC/AHA guidelines for the management of patients with unstable angina and non-ST-segment elevation myocardial infarction. A report of the American College of Cardiology/American Heart Association Task Force on Practice Guidelines (Committee on the Management of Patients with Unstable Angina). J Am Coll Cardiol 2000;36(3):970–1062.

[49] Antman EM, Tanasijevic MJ, Thompson B, et al. Cardiac-specific troponin I levels to predict the risk of mortality in patients with acute coronary syndromes. N Engl J Med 1996; 335(18):1342–9.

[50] Ohman EM, Armstrong PW, Christenson RH, et al. Cardiac troponin T levels for risk stratification in acute myocardial ischemia. GUSTO IIA Investigators. N Engl J Med 1996; 335(18):1333–41.

[51] Norris RM. Dissent from the consensus on the redefinition of myocardial infarction. Eur Heart J 2001;22(17):1626–7.

[52] Birkhead JS, Norris RM. Redefinition of myocardial infarction. Lancet 2001;358(9283):764.

[53] Jolobe OM. Redefinition of myocardial infarction. Lancet 2001;358(9283):764.

[54] Richards AM, Lainchbury JG, Nicholls MG. Unsatisfactory redefinition of myocardial infarction. Lancet 2001;357(9269):1635–6.

[55] Tunstall-Pedoe H. Redefinition of myocardial infarction by a consensus dissenter. J Am Coll Cardiol 2001;37(5):1472–4.

[56] Tunstall-Pedoe H. Comment on the ESC/ACC redefinition of myocardial infarction by a consensus dissenter. Eur Heart J 2001;22(7):613–5.

[57] Meier MA, Al-Badr WH, Cooper JV, et al. The new definition of myocardial infarction: diagnostic and prognostic implications in patients with acute coronary syndromes. Arch Intern Med 2002;162(14):1585–9.

[58] Koukkunen H, Penttila K, Kemppainen A, et al. Differences in the diagnosis of myocardial infarction by troponin T compared with clinical and epidemiologic criteria. Am J Cardiol 2001;88(7):727–31.

[59] Kontos MC, Fritz LM, Anderson FP, et al. Impact of the troponin standard on the prevalence of acute myocardial infarction. Am Heart J 2003;146(3):446–52.

[60] Jaffe AS. Elevations of troponin—false positive, the real truth. Cardiovasc Toxicol 2001; 1(2):87–92.

[61] Apple FS, Wu AH, Jaffe AS. European Society of Cardiology and American College of Cardiology guidelines for redefinition of myocardial infarction: how to use existing assays clinically and for clinical trials. Am Heart J 2002;144(6):981–6.

[62] Jaffe AS, Katus H. Acute coronary syndrome biomarkers: the need for more adequate reporting. Circulation 2004;110(2):104–6.

[63] Jaffe A. Caveat emptor. Am J Med 2003;115(3):241–4.

[64] Apple FS, Quist HE, Doyle PJ, et al. Plasma 99th percentile reference limits for cardiac troponin and creatine kinase MB mass for use with European Society of Cardiology/American College of Cardiology consensus recommendations. Clin Chem 2003;49(8):1331–6.

[65] Salomaa V, Ketonen M, Koukkunen H, et al. The effect of correcting for troponins on trends in coronary heart disease events in Finland during 1993–2002: the FINAMI study. Eur Heart J 2006;27:2394–9.

[66] Roger VL, Killian JM, Weston SA, et al. Redefinition of myocardial infarction: prospective evaluation in the community. Circulation 2006;114(8):790–7.

[67] Ng SM, Krishnaswamy P, Morrisey R, et al. Mitigation of the clinical significance of spurious elevations of cardiac troponin I in settings of coronary ischemia using serial testing of multiple cardiac markers. Am J Cardiol 2001;87(8):994–9, A994.

[68] Tunstall-Pedoe H, Vanuzzo D, Hobbs M, et al. Estimation of contribution of changes in coronary care to improving survival, event rates, and coronary heart disease mortality across the WHO MONICA Project populations. Lancet 2000;355(9205):688–700.

[69] Laatikainen T, Critchley J, Vartiainen E, et al. Explaining the decline in coronary heart disease mortality in Finland between 1982 and 1997. Am J Epidemiol 2005;162(8):764–73.

[70] Fox KA, Birkhead J, Wilcox R, et al. British Cardiac Society Working Group on the definition of myocardial infarction. Heart 2004;90(6):603–9.

ELSEVIER
SAUNDERS

Med Clin N Am 91 (2007) 553–572

THE MEDICAL
CLINICS
OF NORTH AMERICA

Pathophysiology of Acute Myocardial Infarction

Allen P. Burke, MD*, Renu Virmani, MD

CVPath Institute, 19 Firstfield Road, Gaithersburg, MD 20878, USA

More than 80% of acute myocardial infarcts are the result of coronary atherosclerosis with superimposed luminal thrombus. Uncommon causes of myocardial infarction include coronary spasm, coronary embolism, and thrombosis in nonatherosclerotic normal vessels. Additionally, concentric subendocardial necrosis may result from global ischemia and reperfusion in cases of prolonged cardiac arrest with resuscitation. Myocardial ischemia shares features with other types of myocyte necrosis, such as that caused by inflammation, but specific changes result from myocyte hypoxia that vary based on length of occlusion of the vessel, duration between occlusion and reperfusion, and presence of collateral circulation.

Gross pathologic findings

The earliest change that can be grossly discerned in the evolution of acute myocardial infarction is pallor of the myocardium, which occurs 12 hours or later after the onset of irreversible ischemia. The gross detection of infarction can be enhanced by the use of tetrazolium salt solutions, which form a colored precipitate on gross section of fresh heart tissue in the presence of dehydrogenase-mediated activity. Myocardial necrosis can be detected as early as 2 to 3 hours in the dog and in man by this method [1,2]. In non-reperfused infarction, the area of the infarct is well defined at 2 to 3 days with a central area of yellow discoloration that is surrounded by a thin rim of highly vascularized hyperemia (Fig. 1A–C). In a reperfused infarct the infarcted region will appear red from trapping of the red cells and hemorrhage from the rupture of the necrotic capillaries (Fig. 1D). At 5 to 7 days the regions are much more distinct, with a central soft area and depressed

---

* Corresponding author.
E-mail address: aburke@cvpath.org (A.P. Burke).

0025-7125/07/$ - see front matter © 2007 Elsevier Inc. All rights reserved.
doi:10.1016/j.mcna.2007.03.005   *medical.theclinics.com*

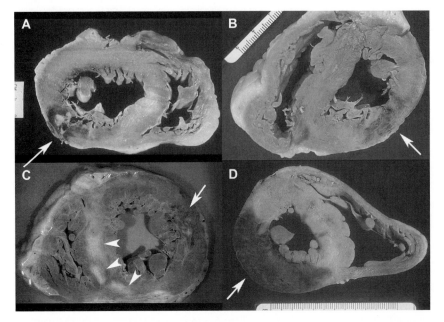

Fig. 1. Acute myocardial infarction. (*A*) Rupture of acute infarction at day 3 post symptoms (*arrow*). Note hyperemic border surrounding pale area. No reperfusion occurred. (*B*) Acute myocardial infarction, 4 days after onset of symptoms. Hemorrhagic area, with no central pallor (*arrow*). Partial reperfusion may have occurred with attempted thrombolysis up to 1 day after symptoms. (*C*) Healing myocardial infarct (*arrow*) 19 days after initial ECG changes. Note persistent pale areas in center of infarct. Older infarcts are seen (*arrowheads*) in the septum. (*D*) Acute reperfusion infarct (*arrow*). Death 2 days after thrombolysis for acute infarct. Note diffuse hemorrhage and lack of central pallor.

hyperemic border. At 1 to 2 weeks the infarct begins to be depressed (Fig. 2), especially at the margins where organization takes place, and the borders have a white hue. Healing may be complete as early as 4 to 6 weeks in small infarcts, or may take as long as 2 to 3 months when the area of infarction is large. Healed infarcts are white from the scarring and the ventricular wall may be thinned (aneurysmal), especially in transmural infarction. In general, infarcts that occupy more than 50% of the ventricular wall, from the subendocardial to the epicardial surface, are considered transmural and associated with Q-wave changes on electrocardiogram.

Light microscopic findings in nonreperfused infarction

The earliest morphologic characteristic of myocardial infarction occurs between 12 to 24 hours after onset of chest pain. Hypereosinophilia of the cytoplasm as assessed by hematoxylin–eosin staining is characteristic of myocardial ischemia (Fig. 3A). Neutrophil infiltration is present by 24 hours at the border areas. As the infarct progresses between 24 and 48 hours,

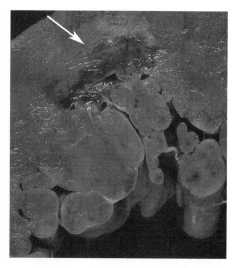

Fig. 2. Healed myocardial infarction, early. Depressed gelatinous area, with congested dark appearance, without dense scarring (*arrow*). Patient had a history of chest pain 2 months before death.

coagulation necrosis is established with various degrees of nuclear pyknosis, early karyorrhexis, and karyolysis. The myocyte striations are preserved and the sarcomeres elongate. The border areas show prominent neutrophil infiltration by 48 hours (Fig. 3B). At 3 to 5 days the central portion of the infarct shows loss of myocyte nuclei and striations; in smaller infarcts neutrophils invade within the infarct and fragment, resulting in more severe karyorrhexis (nuclear dust). Markers of ischemia include hypoxia-inducible factor-1 and cyclo-oxygenase-2, which can be shown immunohistochemically [3]. The influx of inflammatory cells, including mast cells, induces a cascade of chemokines that suppress further inflammation and result in scar tissue [4,5]. Macrophages and fibroblasts begin to appear in the border areas (Fig. 4A). By 1 week, neutrophils decline and granulation tissue is established with neocapillary invasion and lymphocytic and plasma cell infiltration. Although lymphocytes may be seen as early as 2 to 3 days, they are not prominent in any stage of infarct evolution. Eosinophils may be seen within the inflammatory infiltrate but are only present in 24% of infarcts [6]. Phagocytic removal of the necrotic myocytes by macrophages occurs, and pigment is seen within macrophages.

By the second week, fibroblasts are prominent but their appearance may be seen as early as day 4 at the periphery of the infarct (Fig. 4B). The necrotic myocytes continue to be removed as the fibroblasts are actively producing collagen, and angiogenesis occurs in the area of healing (Fig. 4C). The healing continues and, depending on the extent of necrosis, may be complete as early as 4 weeks or require 8 weeks or longer to complete.

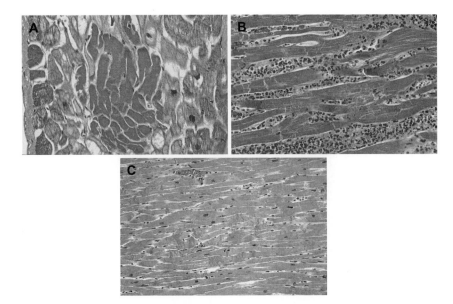

Fig. 3. Acute myocardial infarction, histologic features. (*A*) Area of hypereosinophilia (*center*) with surrounding intact myocytes. Approximately 24 hours duration. (*B*) Acute neutrophilic infiltrate at border of acute infarct, approximately 3 days duration. (*C*) Reperfusion infarct, with abundant contraction bands, and sparse diffuse inflammation.

The central area of infarction may remain unhealed, showing mummified myocytes for extended periods, despite the fact that the infarct borders are completely healed.

Light microscopic appearance of reperfused acute myocardial infarction

At 24 hours of occlusion followed by reperfusion after 6 hours in the dog model, myocytes are thin, hypereosinophilic, devoid of nuclei, or showing karyorrhexis, with ill-defined borders and interspersed areas of interstitial hemorrhage. A diffuse but mild neutrophil infiltration appears. Within 2 to 3 days, macrophage infiltration is obvious and phagocytosis of necrotic myocytes and early stages of granulation tissue are seen. The infarct healing in the dog is more rapid than in man, probably because of nondiseased adjoining coronary arteries (collaterals) and a lack of underlying myocardial disease. In humans who have acute myocardial infarction, often chronic ischemia occurs secondary to extensive atherosclerotic disease.

In man, if reperfusion occurs within 4 to 6 hours after onset of chest pain or ECG changes, myocardial salvage occurs and the infarct is likely to be subendocardial without transmural extension. A nearly confluent area of hemorrhage appears within the infarcted myocardium, with extensive contraction band necrosis (Fig. 3C). Within a few hours of reperfusion,

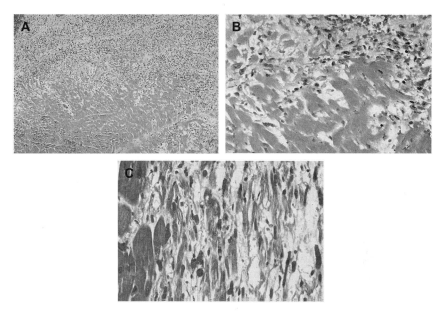

Fig. 4. Healing myocardial infarction, histologic features. (*A*) Nine-day infarct, with area of necrosis (*bottom*) and inflammation (*top*). (*B*) Higher magnification, showing inflammatory infiltrate composed primarily of lymphocytes and macrophages. (*C*) Nineteen-day infarct, with ingrowth of fibroblasts.

neutrophils are evident within the area of necrosis, but are usually sparse. Macrophages begin to appear by day 2 to 3, and by day 3 to 5 fibroblasts appear with an accelerated rate of healing compared with nonreperfused infarcts. As early as 2 to 3 weeks, subendocardial infarcts may be fully healed. Larger infarcts, and those reperfused after 6 hours, take longer to heal. Infarcts reperfused after 6 hours show larger areas of hemorrhage compared with occlusions with more immediate reperfusion.

Mechanisms of myocardial injury

Under normal aerobic conditions cardiac energy is derived from fatty acids, supplying 60% to 90% of the energy for adenosine triphosphate (ATP) synthesis. The rest of the energy (10%–40%) comes from oxidation of pyruvate formed from glycolysis and lactate oxidation. Sudden occlusion of a major branch of a coronary artery shifts aerobic or mitochondrial metabolism to anaerobic glycolysis within seconds. Reduced aerobic ATP formation stimulates glycolysis and an increase in myocardial glucose uptake and glycogen breakdown. Decreased ATP inhibits Na^+, K^+-ATPase, increasing intracellular Na^+ and Cl^-, leading to cell swelling. Derangements in transport systems in the sarcolemma and sarcoplasmic reticulum increase cytosolic Ca^{2+}, inducing activation of proteases and alterations in contractile proteins. Pyruvate is not readily oxidized in the mitochondria, leading to the production of lactate, a fall in intracellular pH, a reduction in contractile function, and a greater ATP requirement to maintain Ca^{2+} homeostasis [7].

Ultrastructurally, reversibly injured myocytes are edematous and swollen from the osmotic overload. The cell size is increased with a decrease in the glycogen content [8–10]. The myocyte fibrils are relaxed and thinned; I-bands are prominent secondary to noncontracting ischemic myocytes [11]. The nuclei show mild condensation of chromatin at the nucleoplasm. The cell membrane (sarcolemma) is intact and no breaks can be identified. The mitochondria are swollen, with loss of normal dense mitochondrial granules and incomplete clearing of the mitochondrial matrix, but without amorphous or granular flocculent densities. Irreversibly injured myocytes contain shrunken nuclei with marked chromatin margination. The two hallmarks of irreversible injury are cell membrane breaks and mitochondrial presence of small osmiophilic amorphous densities [12]. The densities are composed of lipid, denatured proteins, and calcium [13].

Irreversible ischemic injury is characterized by various processes involving the sarcolemmal membrane, eventuating in its disruption and cell death. Increased cytosolic Ca^{2+} and mitochondrial impairment cause phospholipase activation and release of lysophospholipids and free fatty acids, which are incorporated within the cell and damaged by peroxidative damage from free radicals and toxic oxygen species. Cleavage of anchoring cytoskeletal proteins and progressive increases in cell membrane permeability result in physical disruption and cell death [13].

Apoptosis, oncosis, and autophagic myocyte death

Cell death involves various pathways, with different morphologic manifestations. Myocyte oncosis, generally resulting from events exogenous to the cell, results in cell swelling and is independent of energy or caspase activity. Apoptosis, or programmed cell death, results in cell shrinkage, is ATP-dependent, and involves various pathways, including caspases. Because apoptosis is energy-dependent, it has not been classically implicated in ischemic myocyte death; however, apoptosis may be involved in the first hours of ischemic injury, especially during reperfusion. The detection of apoptosis depends on identifying the final outcome of the apoptotic pathway (double-stranded DNA fragmentation), but issues of specificity exist in detecting these fragments with the most commonly used technique, terminal deoxynucleotidyl transferase-mediated biotinylated dUTP nick end-labeling (TUNEL). Other features of apoptosis that can be assayed include activation of cytosolic aspartate–specific cysteine proteases, or caspases; cytochrome C release in mitochondria; and selective alteration of cell membranes with an increased expression of phosphatidylserine in the outer membrane, with preservation of selective membrane permeability (generally accomplished with annexin-V labeling). Various alterations have been described in ischemic myocardium, but the current consensus is that apoptosis and oncosis proceed together in ischemic myocytes, with oncosis dominating, especially in end stages [13].

Autophagic, or ubiquitin-related cell death, is characterized ultrastructurally by autophagic vacuoles, cellular degeneration, and nuclear disassembly [14]. Autophagic cell death is energy-dependent similar to apoptosis but, unlike apoptosis, is caspase-independent. The formation of autophagic vacuoles involves posttranslational modification of proteins through linkage to numerous ubiquitin molecules, making them susceptible to proteasomal digestion. Various proteins, including cathepsin D, cathepsin B, heat shock cognate protein Hsc73, beclin 1, and the processed form of microtubule-associated protein 1 light chain 3, are known to mediate autophagy. Autophagic cell death has been described in hypertrophied and failing myocardium and has been found to be increased in hibernating myocardium [15]. The initiation of autophagy does not always result in cell death, because autophagy may be responsible for the turnover of unnecessary or dysfunctional organelles and cytoplasmic proteins. In a model of repetitive ischemia in the pig, autophagic cell death has been shown to occur later than apoptosis, inversely suggesting a protective effect against ischemia-induced apoptosis [16].

Evolution of myocardial infarction, determinants of infarct size, and ventricular remodeling

Although biochemical and functional abnormalities begin almost immediately at the onset of ischemia, severe loss of myocardial contractility occurs within 60 seconds, whereas other changes take a more protracted course. For example, the loss of viability (irreversible injury) occurs at least 20 to 40 minutes after total occlusion of blood flow. The canine model showed that infarction proceeded as a "wavefront" from endocardium to epicardium [17,18]. After 15 minutes of occlusion, no infarct occurred. At 40 minutes, the infarct was subendocardial, involving only the papillary muscle, resulting in 28% of the myocardium at risk. At 3 hours after coronary artery occlusion and reperfusion, the infarct was significantly smaller compared with nonreperfused permanently occluded infarct (62% of area at risk). The infarct size was the greatest in permanent occlusion, becoming transmural and involving 75% of the area at risk [11].

Two zones of myocardial damage occur: a central zone with no flow or very low flow and a zone of collateral vessels in a surrounding marginal zone. The survival of the marginal zone depends on the level and duration of ischemia. In autopsy hearts, the size of the ischemic zone surrounding an acute myocardial infarction is associated with increased apoptosis and degree of occlusion of the infarct-related artery [3]. The extent of coronary collateral flow is among the principal determinants of infarct size. In man, approximately 40% of patients who experienced acute myocardial infarction have been shown to have well-developed collateral circulation [19]. Absence of myocardial ischemia (shown through electrocardiographic changes or angina during transient coronary balloon occlusion) is associated with the presence of well-developed collateral vessels, suggesting that patients who have well-developed collateral vessels have a low risk for developing acute myocardial infarction on abrupt closure of the culprit coronary artery [20]. Collaterals have been shown to be better-developed in patients who have angina and younger individuals compared with older patients who have acute infarcts [19].

In addition to the presence of collateral circulation, factors that influence infarct size include preconditioning, which may greatly reduce infarct size, and reperfusion.

Ischemic preconditioning

Preconditioning was initially described as a decrease in experimental infarct size after one or repeated brief episodes of occlusion before prolonged occlusion. This definition is now extended to cardiac function and arrhythmias, although arrhythmias are not as consistent [21].

The mechanisms of preconditioning are unclear, but preconditioning has been shown to reduce the energy demand of the myocardium in animals and man. Two phases of preconditioning have been described: the classical initial phase, which is operative for 1 to 2 hours before sustained coronary occlusion, and the delayed phase, which is operative 24 hours after the precondition, known as the *second window of protection* (SWOP) [13]. Classical preconditioning is associated with activation of adenosine receptors, activation of protein kinase C coupled to G proteins, and opening of ATP-dependent potassium channels. The mechanism of SWOP is less clear and is believed to involve a kinase cascade, including mitogen-activated protein kinases and nuclear factor kappa B, which increase levels of superoxide dismutase, nitric oxide synthase, cyclo-oxygenase 2 and heat shock proteins, thereby creating a protective milieu for the cardiomyocyte.

Clinically, Yellon and associates [22] have shown that intermittent aortic cross-clamping could precondition the human left ventricle during coronary artery bypass surgery, resulting in preservation of ATP levels. Other observations confirming the existence of preconditioning in patients have been observed in those undergoing percutaneous transluminal coronary angioplasty. Repeated balloon inflations of 60 to 90 seconds have been associated with decreased chest pain, reduced ST segment elevation, and decreased lactate production with subsequent inflations; these phenomena are observed irrespective of the presence or absence of collaterals [23]. In the Thrombolysis in Myocardial Infarction (TIMI)-9 trial, which studied the timing of angina in relationship to myocardial infarction, only patients who had angina within 24 hours of infarction showed smaller infract size and better clinical outcome [24].

The mediators of preconditioning are believed to involve the ATP-sensitive potassium (K_{ATP}) channel and specific isoforms of protein kinase C. The protective effect of temporary ischemia can be blocked through pretreating the myocardium with inhibitors of the K_{ATP} channel, such as glibenclamide and 5-hydrocydeconate [25,26]. Similarly, inhibitors of protein kinase C and tyrosine kinase, but not protein kinase C alone, will prevent ischemic preconditioning, and agonists of adenosine (A_1 receptor) will pharmacologically precondition the heart against ischemia [27].

The no-reflow phenomenon and reperfusion injury

A balance exists between the benefits of reperfusion to reduce infarct size and reperfusion injury, which depends on onset time. In general, if reperfusion is instituted within 2 to 3 hours of the onset of ischemia, the degree of myocardial salvage greatly exceeds damage from free radicals and calcium loading caused by reperfusion. The term *reperfusion injury* describes reperfusion-related expansion or worsening of the ischemic cardiac injury assessed through contractile performance, the arrhythmogenic threshold, conversion of reversible to irreversible myocyte injury, and microvessel dysfunction [28]. Recent studies have shown that angiographic no-reflow is a strong predictor of major cardiac events, such as congestive heart failure, malignant arrhythmias, and cardiac death after acute myocardial infarction. The major mediators of reperfusion injury are oxygen radicals, calcium loading, and neutrophils [29].

Infarct expansion and cardiac remodeling

In the late 1970s, transmural infarcts were documented to increase for weeks after the initial event, and the degree of this expansion was associated with a decrease in survival rate [30]. Transmural extent of necrosis is a major determinant of infarct expansion (remodeling) based on large infarct size and the persistence of the occlusion. Preserving islands of viable myocardium in the subepicardial regions has been associated with decreased remodeling or infarct expansion. Other factors that have been implicated in reduced ventricular remodeling include microvascular integrity [31] and initial ventricular compliance, as measured through mitral deceleration time [32]. Although the effect of reperfusion on ventricular remodeling is clear regarding early reperfusion because definite benefits exist in reducing infarct size and expansion, the benefits of late reperfusion, beyond myocardial salvage, are unclear. Studies have shown that remodeling is affected by the presence of viable zones after successful late percutaneous coronary intervention [33]. In general, the mechanisms of ventricular remodeling are poorly understood, because different techniques have been used to assess myocardial viability in human subjects, animal studies, and post-mortem specimens. The release of matrix metalloproteinases are now being linked to remodeling.

Reversible myocardial ischemia: hibernating myocardium

Reversibly dysfunctional tissue is commonly referred to as *hibernating myocardium* [34]. Sheiban and colleagues [35] have shown that 5 to 7 minutes of angioplasty balloon inflations in the coronary arteries of patients undergoing interventional procedures, followed by tracking of the resolution of the regional wall motion abnormalities over the next 5 days, showed persistence of regional wall motion abnormities for up to 36 hours. Similarly, return of left ventricular function has been studied after acute myocardial infarction. Delayed recovery of wall motion was observed in the infarct region, with a positive change in wall motion from 0.2 at 3 days to 1.0 at 6 months only in patients who underwent reperfusion, as measured through the centerline method [36].

In detecting hibernating myocardium, clinical functional techniques such as stress echocardiography and cardiac magnetic resonance are more specific but less sensitive than nuclear modalities, which assess perfusion and metabolic activity [34,37]. Several experimental studies show that ischemia is not the result of simple inadequacy of blood flow for myocardial contraction, but that a stepwise decrease in function occurs based on incremental decrease in oxygen-supplying perfusion (so-called "perfusion–contraction matching"). Evidence shows that repeated episodes of ischemia–reperfusion may result in a state of chronic hibernation, with alterations in the flow–function relationship and decreased oxygen demand. Chronically hibernating myocardium shows alterations in adrenergic control and calcium responsiveness. Substances that have been shown to be up-regulated in chronic hibernating myocardium include heat shock protein, hypoxia-inducible factor, inducible nitric oxide synthase, cyclo-oxygenase 2, and monocyte chemotactic protein. Because some of these pathways are involved in preconditioning, a relationship between cardiac hibernation and preconditioning has been postulated.

Morphologically, hibernating myocytes show loss of contractile elements, especially in the perinuclear region and occasionally throughout the cytoplasm (Fig. 5). The space left by the dissolution of the myofibrils is occupied by glycogen, as evidenced by the strong positivity for the periodic acid–Schiff reagent. The interstitium shows an increase in connective tissue. Increased numbers of apoptotic myocytes has been shown using DNA nick end-labeling [38], in addition to increased autophagic and oncotic cell death [15,39].

The composition and distribution of sarcomeric, cytoskeletal, and membrane-associated proteins has been shown to be significantly altered in chronic myocardial hibernation [40,41]. A disorderly increase in cytoskeletal desmin, tubulin, and vinculin occurs, with a decrease in contractile proteins

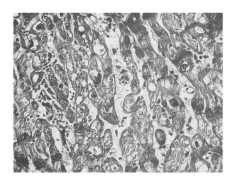

Fig. 5. Vacuolated myocytes, subendocardium, congestive heart failure, corresponding to reversible myocyte injury (hibernating myocardium).

myosin, titin, and alpha-actinin. More recently, decreased connexin43, a membrane transport protein, has been associated with reduced gap junction size and a proposed propensity for arrhythmias in the hibernating state [42].

Epicardial thrombosis and acute myocardial infarction

Incidence and type of thrombus

Most myocardial infarctions occur in patients who have coronary atherosclerosis, with more than 90% associated with superimposed luminal thrombus, most commonly plaque rupture (Fig. 6A, B) and less commonly plaque erosion (Fig. 6C). Arbustini and colleagues [43] found coronary thrombi in 98% of patients dying of clinically documented acute myocardial infarction, with 75% of these caused from plaque rupture and 25% from plaque erosion. They found gender differences in the cause of coronary thrombi that lead to acute myocardial infarcts, showing that 37% of thrombi in women were caused by erosion compared with only 18% in men. Although an individual severe stenosis is more likely to become occluded by a thrombus than a lesion with less-severe stenosis, the less severely narrowed plaques produce more occlusions because many more sites are mild to moderately narrowed [44].

The authors observed that the mean percent stenosis underlying coronary plaque erosion is 70% versus 80% at the site of plaque rupture; however, 82% of fatal plaque erosions result in total occlusions compared with only 57% of plaque ruptures [45]. The culprit coronary artery of infarction at autopsy most frequent is the left anterior descending artery (approximately one half) followed by the right coronary artery (30%–45%) and then the left circumflex (15%–20%). No thrombi are found in fewer than 5% of acute myocardial infarctions.

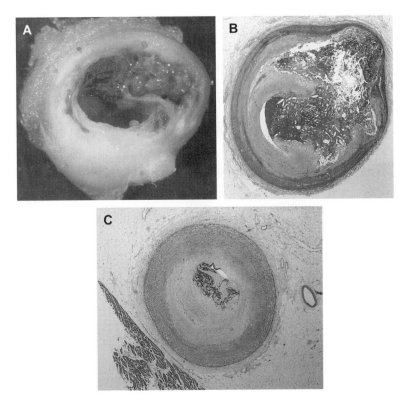

Fig. 6. Acute thrombosis, epicardial coronary arteries. (*A*) Acute plaque rupture, gross appearance. Necrotic core is at right, thrombus in lumen at left. (*B*) Acute plaque rupture, histologic appearance. Necrotic core is at top right, lumen bottom left. (*C*) Acute plaque erosion. Occlusive thrombus in the absence of necrotic core or cap disruption.

Microembolization

Acute coronary thrombosis with or without percutaneous intervention results in the embolization of microparticles, including fragments of fibrin–platelet thrombus and necrotic core. Coronary microembolization has been associated with arrhythmias, contractile dysfunction, microinfarcts, and reduced coronary reserve [46]. Autopsy studies have shown a 13% rate of microembolization in cardiac disease, often associated with focal myocyte necrosis [47]. The rate of coronary microembolization is highest in documented epicardial coronary thrombosis, reaching 30% to 54% [48,49] and even higher (79%) in acute myocardial infarcts [50]. Few data compare acute plaque rupture versus acute plaque erosion and the rate of embolization, but the authors have noted a higher rate of thrombotic microembolization with plaque erosion. In hearts with acute coronary thrombi, evidence of distal embolization was more frequent in erosions than ruptures.

Pathologic consequences of myocardial infarction

Rupture of myocardium

The incidence of rupture of the left ventricular free wall is between 10% and 20%; patients who have a first infarct have a rupture rate of about 18% [51]. In contrast, rupture of the ventricular septum is only 2% [51]. Left ventricular wall rupture is seven times more common than right ventricular rupture [52]. The ventricular apex is the most common site (Fig. 7). Although reperfusion therapy has reduced the incidence of cardiac rupture, late thrombolytic therapy may increase the risk for cardiac rupture.

Factors associated with cardiac rupture include female gender, age older than 60 years, hypertension, and first myocardial infarction. Additional risk factors include multivessel atherosclerotic disease, absence of ventricular hypertrophy, poor collateral flow, transmural infarct involving at least 20% of the wall, and location of the infarct in the mid-anterior or lateral wall of the

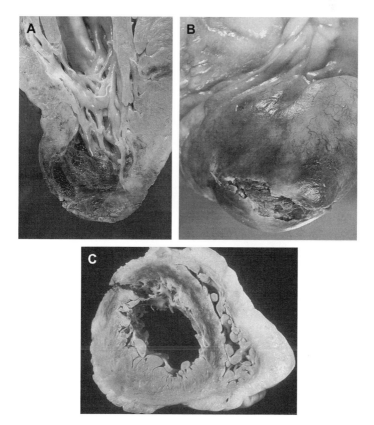

Fig. 7. Ruptured acute myocardial infarction. (*A*) Acute apical aneurysm, with transmural infarction. (*B*) Epicardial surface, showing rupture site. (*C*) Acute reperfusion infarct (hemorrhagic) with rupture of anterior left ventricular wall.

left ventricle [53]. Defective cardiac remodeling, involving matrix metalloproteinases and the extracellular matrix, may predispose the heart for rupture. In addition to surgery, management includes hemodynamic monitoring and treatment with β-blockers and angiotensin-converting enzyme inhibitors in selected cases [54].

Cardiac rupture usually occurs in the first few days (1–4 days) after the infarct, when coagulation necrosis and neutrophilic infiltration are at their peak and have weakened the left ventricular wall. However, at least 13% to 28% of rupture occurs within 24 hours of infarction onset, when inflammation and necrosis are not prominent [52]. Infarcts with rupture contain more extensive inflammation and are more likely to show eosinophils compared with nonruptured infarcts [55].

Myocardial rupture, in addition to the free wall, may involve solely the papillary muscle or the ventricular septum (Fig. 8). Simple ruptures have a discrete defect and have a direct through-and-through communication across the septum, are usually associated with anterior myocardial infarction, and are located in the apex. Complex ruptures are characterized by extensive hemorrhage with irregular serpiginous borders of the necrotic muscle, usually occur in inferior infarcts, and involve the basal inferoposterior septum [56].

Right-sided and atrial infarction

Right ventricular infarction is a common complication of inferior transmural myocardial infarction. Isolated right ventricular infarction may infrequently occur in the absence of coronary disease in patients who have

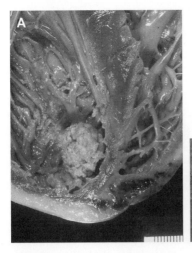
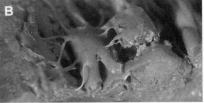

Fig. 8. Acute apical infarct with marked thinning of apical ventricular septum, mural thrombus in left ventricular apex, and hemorrhagic tract extending into right ventricular apex (acquired ventricular septal defect). Note thrombus (*white*) in left ventricular apex.

chronic lung disease and right ventricular hypertrophy [57]. Atrial infarction occurs in 10% of all left ventricular inferior wall infarcts and typically involves the right atrium [58].

Pericardial effusion and pericarditis

Pericardial effusion is reported in 25% of patients who have acute myocardial infarcts and is more common in patients who have anterior myocardial infarction, large infarcts, and congestive heart failure [59]. Pericarditis occurs less often than pericardial effusion and is seen only in transmural acute myocardial infarction. Although its incidence seems to have decreased in the era of thrombolytic therapy, the incidence of pleuropericardial chest pain has remained constant [60]. The incidence of postinfarction syndrome (Dressler syndrome), previously reported to occur in 3% to 4% of all myocardial infarction, has been greatly reduced because of the extensive use of thrombolysis and treatments that dramatically decrease the size of myocardial necrosis and modulate the immune system [61].

Chronic congestive heart failure

At autopsy, congestive heart failure is characterized by dilatation of both atria and the ventricles, which show either a large healed infarct or multiple smaller infarcts with or without a transmural scar [62]. Scarring of the inferior wall of the left ventricle often involves the posteromedial papillary muscle, which gives rise to mitral regurgitation contributing to congestive heart failure [62]. Microscopically, the subendocardial regions of ischemia show myocytes with myofibrillar loss and rich in glycogen, suggesting a state of hibernation [63]. Often areas of subendocardial replacement fibrosis are seen.

True and false aneurysm

The overall incidence of left ventricular aneurysm is currently almost 12% [64]. Single-vessel disease, absence of previous angina, totally occluded left anterior descending coronary artery, and female gender are independent determinants of left ventricular aneurysm formation after anterior infarct [65]. Patients undergoing thrombolytic therapy and showing a patent infarct-related artery have a lower incidence of aneurysm formation [64].

Four of five aneurysms involve the anteroapical wall of the left ventricle (Fig. 9) and are four times more frequent in this wall than the inferior or posterior wall. The pericardium usually adheres to the aneurysm and may calcify. True aneurysms rarely rupture, whereas rupture is more common in false aneurysms [66]. The cavity of the aneurysm usually contains an organizing thrombus and patient may present with embolic complications. Mortality is significantly higher in patients who have aneurysms than those who do not.

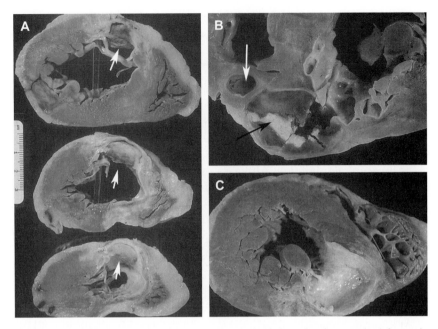

Fig. 9. Healed infarction with aneurysm. (*A*) Short axis sections showing anterior left ventricular healed infarct with aneurysm, apex to base (*arrows*). Mural thrombus appears in the aneurysm. (*B*) Apical aneurysm secondary to healed transmural infarct, with extension into right ventricle and small acquired ventricular septal defect (*white arrow*). Aneurysm is focally calcified (*black arrow*). (*C*) Healed transmural infarct with posterior left ventricular wall aneurysm, near cardiac base.

Mural thrombus and embolization

Mural thrombus forming on the endocardial surface over the area of the acute infarction occurs in 20% of all patients. However, the incidence is 40% for anterior infarcts and 60% for apical infarcts [67]. Patients who have left ventricular thrombi have poorer global left ventricular function and worse prognosis compared with those who have no thrombi [68]. The poor prognosis is secondary to complications of a large infarct and not from emboli [67]. Those that form thrombi have been reported to have endocardial inflammation during the phase of acute infarction. The thrombi tend to organize, but the superficial portions may embolize in approximately 10% of cases [68]. The usual sites of symptomatic embolization are the brain, eyes, kidney, spleen, bowel, legs, and coronary arteries. Symptomatic emboli are usually caused by larger fragments, whereas small particles of thrombus that embolize generally do not cause symptoms [69]. The risk for embolization is greatest in the first few weeks of acute myocardial infarction [70].

References

[1] Vargas SO, Sampson BA, Schoen FJ. Pathologic detection of early myocardial infarction: a critical review of the evolution and usefulness of modern techniques. Mod Pathol 1999; 12(6):635–45.

[2] Adegboyega PA, Adesokan A, Haque AK, et al. Sensitivity and specificity of triphenyl tetrazolium chloride in the gross diagnosis of acute myocardial infarcts. Arch Pathol Lab Med 1997;121(10):1063–8.

[3] Abbate A, Bussani R, Biondi-Zoccai GG, et al. Infarct-related artery occlusion, tissue markers of ischaemia, and increased apoptosis in the peri-infarct viable myocardium. Eur Heart J 2005;26(19):2039–45.

[4] Frangogiannis NG. Chemokines in the ischemic myocardium: from inflammation to fibrosis. Inflamm Res 2004;53(11):585–95.

[5] Frangogiannis NG, Entman ML. Identification of mast cells in the cellular response to myocardial infarction. Methods Mol Biol 2006;315:91–101.

[6] Cowan MJ, Reichenbach D, Turner P, et al. Cellular response of the evolving myocardial infarction after therapeutic coronary artery reperfusion. Hum Pathol 1991;22(2):154–63.

[7] Stanley WC. Cardiac energetics during ischaemia and the rationale for metabolic interventions. Coron Artery Dis 2001;12(Suppl 1):S3–7.

[8] Jennings RB, Ganote CE. Mitochondrial structure and function in acute myocardial ischemic injury. Circ Res 1976;38(5 Suppl 1):I80–91.

[9] Jennings RB, Ganote CE, Reimer KA. Ischemic tissue injury. Am J Pathol 1975;81(1): 179–98.

[10] Virmani R, Forman MB, Kolodgie FD. Myocardial reperfusion injury. Histopathological effects of perfluorochemical. Circulation 1990;81(3 Suppl):IV57–68.

[11] Jennings RB, Steenbergen C Jr, Reimer KA. Myocardial ischemia and reperfusion. Monogr Pathol 1995;37:47–80.

[12] Jennings RB, Ganote CE. Structural changes in myocardium during acute ischemia. Circ Res 1974;35(Suppl 3):156–72.

[13] Buja LM. Myocardial ischemia and reperfusion injury. Cardiovasc Pathol 2005;14(4):170–5.

[14] Knaapen MW, Davies MJ, De Bie M, et al. Apoptotic versus autophagic cell death in heart failure. Cardiovasc Res 2001;51(2):304–12.

[15] Elsasser A, Vogt AM, Nef H, et al. Human hibernating myocardium is jeopardized by apoptotic and autophagic cell death. J Am Coll Cardiol 2004;43(12):2191–9.

[16] Yan L, Vatner DE, Kim SJ, et al. Autophagy in chronically ischemic myocardium. Proc Natl Acad Sci U S A 2005;102(39):13807–12.

[17] Reimer KA, Jennings RB. The "wavefront phenomenon" of myocardial ischemic cell death. II. Transmural progression of necrosis within the framework of ischemic bed size (myocardium at risk) and collateral flow. Lab Invest 1979;40(6):633–44.

[18] Reimer KA, Jennings RB, Tatum AH. Pathobiology of acute myocardial ischemia: metabolic, functional and ultrastructural studies. Am J Cardiol 1983;52(2):72A–81A.

[19] Fujita M, Nakae I, Kihara Y, et al. Determinants of collateral development in patients with acute myocardial infarction. Clin Cardiol 1999;22(9):595–9.

[20] Miwa K, Fujita M, Kameyama T, et al. Absence of myocardial ischemia during sudden controlled occlusion of coronary arteries in patients with well-developed collateral vessels. Coron Artery Dis 1999;10(7):459–63.

[21] Hagar JM, Hale SL, Kloner RA. Effect of preconditioning ischemia on reperfusion arrhythmias after coronary artery occlusion and reperfusion in the rat. Circ Res 1991; 68(1):61–8.

[22] Yellon DM, Alkhulaifi AM, Pugsley WB. Preconditioning the human myocardium. Lancet 1993;342(8866):276–7.

[23] Kloner RA, Yellon D. Does ischemic preconditioning occur in patients? J Am Coll Cardiol 1994;24(4):1133–42.

[24] Kloner RA, Shook T, Antman EM, et al. Prospective temporal analysis of the onset of pre-infarction angina versus outcome: an ancillary study in TIMI-9B. Circulation 1998;97(11): 1042–5.

[25] Critz SD, Liu GS, Chujo M, et al. Pinacidil but not nicorandil opens ATP-sensitive K+ chan-nels and protects against simulated ischemia in rabbit myocytes. J Mol Cell Cardiol 1997; 29(4):1123–30.

[26] Kloner RA, Jennings RB. Consequences of brief ischemia: stunning, preconditioning, and their clinical implications: part 2. Circulation 2001;104(25):3158–67.

[27] Takano H, Bolli R, Black RG Jr, et al. A(1) or A(3) adenosine receptors induce late precon-ditioning against infarction in conscious rabbits by different mechanisms. Circ Res 2001; 88(5):520–8.

[28] Kloner RA, Ganote CE, Jennings RB. The "no-reflow" phenomenon after temporary cor-onary occlusion in the dog. J Clin Invest 1974;54(6):1496–508.

[29] Moens AL, Claeys MJ, Timmermans JP, et al. Myocardial ischemia/reperfusion-injury, a clinical view on a complex pathophysiological process. Int J Cardiol 2005;100(2): 179–90.

[30] Eaton LW, Weiss JL, Bulkley BH, et al. Regional cardiac dilatation after acute myocardial infarction: recognition by two-dimensional echocardiography. N Engl J Med 1979;300(2): 57–62.

[31] Bolognese L, Carrabba N, Parodi G, et al. Impact of microvascular dysfunction on left ven-tricular remodeling and long-term clinical outcome after primary coronary angioplasty for acute myocardial infarction. Circulation 2004;109(9):1121–6.

[32] Cerisano G, Bolognese L, Carrabba N, et al. Doppler-derived mitral deceleration time: an early strong predictor of left ventricular remodeling after reperfused anterior acute myocar-dial infarction. Circulation 1999;99(2):230–6.

[33] Bellenger NG, Yousef Z, Rajappan K, et al. Infarct zone viability influences ventricular re-modelling after late recanalisation of an occluded infarct related artery. Heart 2005;91(4): 478–83.

[34] Bhatia G, Sosin M, Leahy JF, et al. Hibernating myocardium in heart failure. Expert Rev Cardiovasc Ther 2005;3(1):111–22.

[35] Sheiban I, Tonni S, Marini A, et al. Clinical and therapeutic implications of chronic left ven-tricular dysfunction in coronary artery disease. Am J Cardiol 1995;75(13):23E–30E.

[36] Schmidt WG, Sheehan FH, von Essen R, et al. Evolution of left ventricular function after intracoronary thrombolysis for acute myocardial infarction. Am J Cardiol 1989;63(9): 497–502.

[37] Gerber BL, Belge B, Legros GJ, et al. Characterization of acute and chronic myocardial in-farcts by multidetector computed tomography: comparison with contrast-enhanced mag-netic resonance. Circulation 2006;113(6):823–33 [Epub 2006 Feb 2006].

[38] Lim H, Fallavollita JA, Hard R, et al. Profound apoptosis-mediated regional myocyte loss and compensatory hypertrophy in pigs with hibernating myocardium. Circulation 1999; 100(23):2380–6.

[39] Schwarz ER, Schaper J, vom Dahl J, et al. Myocyte degeneration and cell death in hibernat-ing human myocardium. J Am Coll Cardiol 1996;27(7):1577–85.

[40] Elsasser A, Schaper J. Hibernating myocardium: adaptation or degeneration? Basic Res Cardiol 1995;90(1):47–8.

[41] Elsasser A, Schlepper M, Klovekorn WP, et al. Hibernating myocardium: an incomplete ad-aptation to ischemia. Circulation 1997;96(9):2920–31.

[42] Kaprielian RR, Gunning M, Dupont E, et al. Downregulation of immunodetectable connex-in43 and decreased gap junction size in the pathogenesis of chronic hibernation in the human left ventricle. Circulation 1998;97(7):651–60.

[43] Arbustini E, Dal Bello B, Morbini P, et al. Plaque erosion is a major substrate for coronary thrombosis in acute myocardial infarction. Heart 1999;82(3):269–72.

[44] Falk E, Shah PK, Fuster V. Coronary plaque disruption. Circulation 1995;92(3):657–71.

[45] Farb A, Burke AP, Tang AL, et al. Coronary plaque erosion without rupture into a lipid core. A frequent cause of coronary thrombosis in sudden coronary death. Circulation 1996;93(7):1354–63.

[46] Heusch G, Schulz R, Haude M, et al. Coronary microembolization. J Mol Cell Cardiol 2004; 37(1):23–31.

[47] El-Maraghi N, Genton E. The relevance of platelet and fibrin thromboembolism of the coronary microcirculation, with special reference to sudden cardiac death. Circulation 1980; 62(5):936–44.

[48] Davies MJ, Thomas AC, Knapman PA, et al. Intramyocardial platelet aggregation in patients with unstable angina suffering sudden ischemic cardiac death. Circulation 1986; 73(3):418–27.

[49] Falk E. Unstable angina with fatal outcome: dynamic coronary thrombosis leading to infarction and/or sudden death. Autopsy evidence of recurrent mural thrombosis with peripheral embolization culminating in total vascular occlusion. Circulation 1985;71(4):699–708.

[50] Frink RJ, Rooney PA Jr, Trowbridge JO, et al. Coronary thrombosis and platelet/fibrin microemboli in death associated with acute myocardial infarction. Br Heart J 1988;59(2): 196–200.

[51] Figueras J, Cortadellas J, Soler-Soler J. Left ventricular free wall rupture: clinical presentation and management. Heart 2000;83(5):499–504.

[52] Batts KP, Ackermann DM, Edwards WD. Postinfarction rupture of the left ventricular free wall: clinicopathologic correlates in 100 consecutive autopsy cases. Hum Pathol 1990;21(5): 530–5.

[53] Pohjola-Sintonen S, Muller JE, Stone PH, et al. Ventricular septal and free wall rupture complicating acute myocardial infarction: experience in the Multicenter Investigation of Limitation of Infarct Size. Am Heart J 1989;117(4):809–18.

[54] Wehrens XH, Doevendans PA. Cardiac rupture complicating myocardial infarction. Int J Cardiol 2004;95(2–3):285–92.

[55] Atkinson JB, Robinowitz M, McAllister HA, et al. Association of eosinophils with cardiac rupture. Hum Pathol 1985;16(6):562–8.

[56] Birnbaum Y, Fishbein MC, Blanche C, et al. Ventricular septal rupture after acute myocardial infarction. N Engl J Med 2002;347(18):1426–32.

[57] Kopelman HA, Forman MB, Wilson BH, et al. Right ventricular myocardial infarction in patients with chronic lung disease: possible role of right ventricular hypertrophy. J Am Coll Cardiol 1985;5(6):1302–7.

[58] Lazar EJ, Goldberger J, Peled H, et al. Atrial infarction: diagnosis and management. Am Heart J 1988;116(4):1058–63.

[59] Sugiura T, Iwasaka T, Takayama Y, et al. Factors associated with pericardial effusion in acute Q wave myocardial infarction. Circulation 1990;81(2):477–81.

[60] Aydinalp A, Wishniak A, van den Akker-Berman L, et al. Pericarditis and pericardial effusion in acute ST-elevation myocardial infarction in the thrombolytic era. Isr Med Assoc J 2002;4(3):181–3.

[61] Bendjelid K, Pugin J. Is Dressler syndrome dead? Chest 2004;126(5):1680–2.

[62] Virmani R, Roberts WC. Quantification of coronary arterial narrowing and of left ventricular myocardial scarring in healed myocardial infarction with chronic, eventually fatal, congestive cardiac failure. Am J Med 1980;68(6):831–8.

[63] Kloner RA, Bolli R, Marban E, et al. Medical and cellular implications of stunning, hibernation, and preconditioning: an NHLBI workshop. Circulation 1998;97(18):1848–67.

[64] Tikiz H, Balbay Y, Atak R, et al. The effect of thrombolytic therapy on left ventricular aneurysm formation in acute myocardial infarction: relationship to successful reperfusion and vessel patency. Clin Cardiol 2001;24(10):656–62.

[65] Tikiz H, Atak R, Balbay Y, et al. Left ventricular aneurysm formation after anterior myocardial infarction: clinical and angiographic determinants in 809 patients. Int J Cardiol 2002;82(1):7–14 [discussion: 14–6].

[66] MacDonald ST, Mitchell AR, Timperley J, et al. Left ventricular pseudoaneurysm and rupture after limited myocardial infarction. J Am Soc Echocardiogr 2005;18(9):980.

[67] Fuster V, Halperin JL. Left ventricular thrombi and cerebral embolism. N Engl J Med 1989; 320(6):392–4.

[68] Keeley EC, Hillis LD. Left ventricular mural thrombus after acute myocardial infarction. Clin Cardiol 1996;19(2):83–6.

[69] Meltzer RS, Visser CA, Fuster V. Intracardiac thrombi and systemic embolization. Ann Intern Med 1986;104(5):689–98.

[70] Kupper AJ, Verheugt FW, Peels CH, et al. Left ventricular thrombus incidence and behavior studied by serial two-dimensional echocardiography in acute anterior myocardial infarction: left ventricular wall motion, systemic embolism and oral anticoagulation. J Am Coll Cardiol 1989;13(7):1514–20.

ELSEVIER
SAUNDERS

THE MEDICAL
CLINICS
OF NORTH AMERICA

Med Clin N Am 91 (2007) 573–601

Vulnerable Plaque: Detection and Management

Mario Gössl, MD[a], Daniele Versari, MD[a],
Heike Hildebrandt[a], Dallit Mannheim, MD[a],
Monica L. Olson, BS[a], Lilach O. Lerman, MD, PhD[b],
Amir Lerman, MD[a],*

[a]Division of Cardiovascular Diseases, Mayo Clinic, Mary Brigh 4-523,
200 First Street SW, Rochester, MN 55905, USA
[b]Division of Nephrology and Hypertension, Mayo Clinic, Mary Brigh 4-523,
200 First Street SW, Rochester, MN 55905, USA

Characteristics of the vulnerable plaque

Because most myocardial infarctions result from the rupture of a plaque that did not significantly compromise the coronary lumen before the event [1], experts widely accept that the morphology, composition, and degree of inflammation of a coronary atherosclerotic plaque is more important than the degree of luminal stenosis. Two depicting examples are the concentric, calcified lesion that shows significant luminal stenosis but is stable because of the stabilizing clasp of calcification. In contrast, a smaller but inflamed thin fibrous cap atheroma with a big lipid/necrotic core may rupture and cause an immediate fatal coronary occlusion.

Although the precise definition of the term *vulnerable plaque* is still debated, most basic researchers, clinical scientists, and clinicians would probably agree on the major features of a plaque that is prone to rupture and is thus vulnerable. According to recent literature, including most recent histopathologic findings, four important characteristics seem to make an atherosclerotic plaque vulnerable [2,3]. Besides a large lipid/necrotic core and a thin fibrous cap, macrophage infiltration (ie, inflammation) and vasa vasorum neovascularization seem to play a significant role in its genesis.

Because the term *vulnerable* has been extended to plaques that are not only prone to rupture but also at risk for rapid progression to become

---

* Corresponding author.
E-mail address: lerman.amir@mayo.edu (A. Lerman).

0025-7125/07/$ - see front matter © 2007 Elsevier Inc. All rights reserved.
doi:10.1016/j.mcna.2007.03.004

culprit lesions, researchers are trying to establish a unifying terminology and major and minor criteria to define the vulnerable plaque. However, this process may have somewhat diluted the original implications of the term. Box 1 summarizes major and minor criteria recommended by the Center of Vulnerable Plaque Research [3].

This article focuses on the dilemma interventional cardiologists face in daily practice in deciding whether to treat vulnerable, nonstenotic coronary lesions invasively or conservatively and, most importantly, whether the imaging technology and evidence-based guidelines are available to help identify the vulnerable plaque and make the treatment decision. In contrast to this scenario is the high-grade stenosis (>90%), which is also one of the recommended major criteria, for which interventional cardiologists to only need angiography to decide on immediate invasive treatment in symptomatic patients. However, in daily practice cardiologists worry more about the thin fibrous cap atheroma with a big lipid core that reached neither the status of a culprit lesion nor a significant degree of stenosis (40%–60% lumen area stenosis). Currently, no guidelines are available recommending a defined treatment, because results from appropriate prospective, randomized studies are not available. Moreover, which and how many imaging tools clinicians need to reliably differentiate vulnerable from stable plaques are unclear.

Therefore, this review evaluates the currently available invasive and noninvasive imaging tools with regard to their ability and potential to image as many of the vulnerable plaque criteria as possible. It also briefly evaluates treatment options for the nonculprit, vulnerable plaque from a preventive perspective.

Although several older and newer invasive and noninvasive imaging techniques are available, none is capable of identifying all major features of a vulnerable plaque. No documentation exists of a plaque rupture; a vulnerable

---

Box 1. Criteria for defining vulnerable plaque

Major criteria
Active inflammation (monocyte/macrophage/T-cell infiltration)
Thin cap with large lipid core
Endothelial denudation with superficial platelet aggregation
Fissured plaque
Stenosis greater than 90%

Minor criteria
Superficial calcified nodule
Glistening yellow
Intraplaque hemorrhage
Endothelial dysfunction
Outward (positive) remodeling

plaque can only be seen before it ruptures or becomes the culprit lesion, or the end result of a plaque rupture is seen.

Imaging tools

Invasive

Coronary angiography

Coronary angiography provides only a luminal view of a lesion. Based on the radiographic silhouette produced by the intracoronary contrast, plaques have been classified into stable (smooth borders, no intraluminal lucencies, more concentric) or unstable (irregular borders, with intraluminal lucencies, eccentric) lesions with good histopathologic correlations (Fig. 1) [4,5].

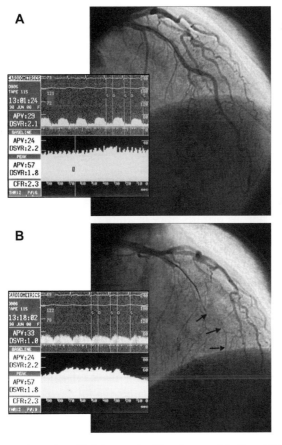

Fig. 1. Coronary angiography with intravascular Doppler coregistration. (*A*) Baseline angiogram of a patient's left anterior descending coronary artery (LAD) before acetylcholine challenge (the intracoronary catheter is already in place). (*B*) Significant LAD vasospasm after intracoronary injection of acetylcholine 10^{-4} M (*black arrows*).

However, because angiography cannot assess vessel wall morphology or plaque composition, it is not the optimal modality to correctly identify a vulnerable plaque [6] and therefore has not been able to predict the site of a future cardiac event in multiple serial angiographic studies [7,8]. Nevertheless, coronary angiography is still the most widely used imaging tool for in vivo imaging of luminal, obstructive disease in coronary arteries.

The vascular endothelium is strategically located between the vascular wall and the circulation and plays a major role in the regulation of vascular tone and response to injury [9]. Endothelial dysfunction is considered the early stage of atherosclerosis and is independently associated with cardiovascular events [10]. Thus, it is conceivable that coronary segments with endothelial dysfunction represent the potential sites and initiation of vulnerable plaques. Endothelial dysfunction is characterized by attenuated vasodilatation or vasoconstriction response to the endothelium-dependent vasodilator acetylcholine. Thus, the intracoronary administration of acetylcholine in high-risk patients who do not have significant obstructive coronary artery disease may detect the future site of vulnerable plaques and rupture (Fig. 1) [9,10].

Hence, coronary angiography may be a tool to diagnose the degree of coronary atherosclerosis and to assess changes in coronary artery diameter in response to provocative tests. Angiography could thus be used to reliably identify one major criterion (stenosis $> 90\%$) and one minor criterion (endothelial dysfunction).

Coronary angioscopy

Coronary angioscopy allows a direct view of the plaque and therefore provides indirect information about plaque composition and stability of the cap. Lipid-rich plaques often have an irregular surface and appear yellow, whereas more fibrous plaques appear white (Fig. 2). In the early 1990s, angioscopy was used to show that patients who had acute coronary syndromes typically had irregular, lipid-rich xanthomatous plaques with overlying thrombus [11]. In another 12-month follow-up study in 157 patients who had stable angina pectoris with yellow plaque showed significantly higher progression to plaque rupture than those who had white plaques. Among the yellow plaques, glistening yellow plaques showed an even higher incidence of plaque rupture [12]. Hence, although coronary angioscopy cannot provide an inside or cross-sectional view of the plaque, it can still identify at least two major (endothelial denudation with superficial platelet aggregation and plaque fissure) and two minor criteria (glistening yellow and superficial calcified nodule) of a vulnerable plaque [3]. However, angioscopy has major disadvantages that prevent it from becoming the ideal tool for identifying vulnerable plaque, including the need to occlude the coronary artery distal to the lesion of interest to perform saline flushing for image quality, which may not be tolerated by an unstable patient. Other limitations include the inability to pass a high-grade stenosis or that the first 2 cm of the coronaries, which often contain the culprit lesion, cannot be visualized [13].

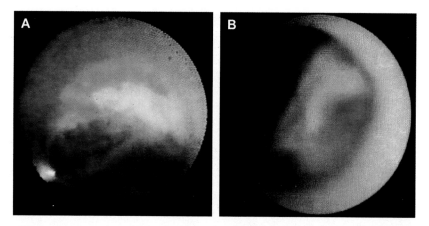

Fig. 2. Coronary angioscopy. Representative angioscopic images of culprit lesions with (*A*) and without (*B*) ruptured plaque. (*A*) Large protruding thrombus and yellow plaque content occupying more than 50% of luminal area is observed. (*B*) Mural thrombus with yellow plaque is observed. (From Mizote I, Ueda Y, Ohtani T, et al. Distal protection improved reperfusion and reduced left ventricular dysfunction in patients with acute myocardial infarction who had angioscopically defined ruptured plaque. Circulation 2005;112(7):1001–7; with permission.)

Intravascular ultrasound

Intravascular ultrasound provides in vivo histology of lesions and is therefore the gold standard for evaluating coronary plaque, lumen, and vessel wall dimensions. Current Intravascular ultrasound (IVUS) systems can image as deep as 8 to 10 mm inside the plaque with axial resolutions of 150 μm and lateral resolutions of 250 μm. In contrast to coronary angiography and angioscopy, IVUS provides a series of tomographic images of the vessel wall, including the lesion of interest, enabling cardiologists to evaluate plaque size, composition, and morphology. Newer systems even allow thee-dimensional visualization of the plaque morphology (Fig. 3) [14]. Plaque morphology is characterized by different echo signal intensities and gray scales. The signal intensity of the adventitia can be used as a reference: fibrous tissue has a comparable signal intensity, soft tissue has a lower signal intensity, and calcified tissue, including microcalcifications [15], has a higher signal intensity with distal shadowing [16]. Thrombi may have a glittery appearance in IVUS images [17] but, depending on their size, are generally more difficult to distinguish.

Although the current IVUS resolutions do not allow visualization of the thin fibrous cap (typically <65 μm), a plaque rupture or fissure and the washed-out necrotic core can be feasibly visualized, especially if intracoronary contrast injections are also used [14].

Several studies show a high correlation between IVUS and histology and that angiography fails to identify the true extent of atherosclerotic disease [18,19]. Because of positive remodeling, as introduced by Glagov and

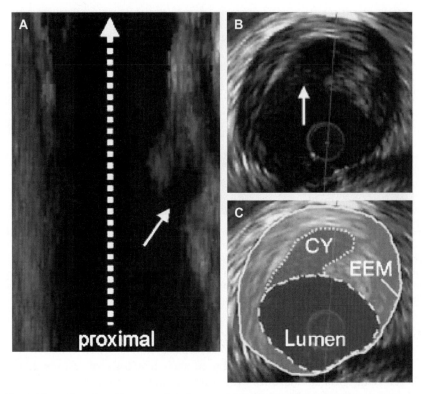

Fig. 3. Three-dimensional intravascular ultrasound (IVUS). Longitudinal IVUS reconstruction of ruptured plaque in the mid right coronary artery. Small arrowheads in the longitudinal (*A*) and transversal (*B*) IVUS images indicate the site of the plaque rupture, which was located in the proximal (upstream) shoulder of the plaque. Large dotted arrowhead indicates direction of blood flow. External elastic membrane (EEM), lumen and plaque cavity (CY) area were measured on each image slice of the lesion segment (*C*). Thin lines in (*B*) and (*C*) indicate the plane of the longitudinal reconstruction (*A*). (*From* Gossl M, von Birgelen C, Mintz GS, et al. Volumetric assessment of ulcerated ruptured coronary plaques with three-dimensional intravascular ultrasound in vivo. Am J Cardiol 2003;91(8):992–6, A997; with permission.)

colleagues [20] in 1987, the angiographic luminal silhouette may still seem unchanged although considerable plaque burden exists in the coronary artery wall. Studies comparing IVUS with angioscopy and histopathology clearly show a high sensitivity and specificity of IVUS in identifying characteristics of a vulnerable plaque [21,22].

Based on the aforementioned facts, IVUS can identify four major criteria (lipid core, endothelial denudation with superficial platelet aggregation, fissured plaque, and stenosis > 90%) and three minor criteria (superficial calcified nodule, endothelial dysfunction, and outward [positive] remodeling) of a vulnerable plaque and thus may be considered the current gold standard for vulnerable plaque imaging.

Intravascular ultrasound–based virtual histology

Because IVUS alone provides only gray scale images of the lesion of interest, differentiating between fibrous and lipid-rich lesions is difficult. With the introduction of spectral analysis of IVUS radiofrequency data (IVUS virtual histology) (Fig. 4), a more exact analysis of plaque composition became available, with first data showing a high accuracy in discerning calcified necrotic and fibrolipidic regions [23]. In a more recent study, correlation of virtual histology with histopathology showed high accuracy in stable and unstable patients who had coronary artery disease [24]. In another study, the detailed analysis of plaque composition with virtual histology showed that the percentage of lipid core in the nonculprit coronary was significantly larger in patients who had acute coronary syndromes [25]. Further ongoing studies will show whether the more detailed definition of plaque morphology and composition with virtual histology in culprit and nonculprit vessels can predict future outcome.

Moreover, despite the scientific merit of further development of the ultrasound technique, neither imaging modality has proven to prospectively identify the vulnerable plaque in the vulnerable patient, meaning that an acute cardiovascular event like plaque rupture currently cannot be predicted.

In summary, IVUS-based virtual histology improves the quality of IVUS alone but does not identify additional criteria of a vulnerable plaque.

Optical coherence tomography

Optical coherence tomography (OCT) generally uses near-infrared light with a wavelength of 130 nm and achieves a spatial resolution of 4 to 16 μm with a penetration depth of 2 to 3 mm. The light pulses are split by a beam splitter, which directs 50% of the light at the sample and 50% at a moving mirror. OCT measures the interference of light from both arms and uses it to represent backreflection intensity [26]. In patients who had mild to moderate coronary artery lesions, OCT image time was 10 minutes longer (imposing no harm to the patients) than IVUS [27,28], but detected the same vessel wall structures without the problem of acoustic shadowing in calcified plaques (Fig. 5). Moreover, OCT characterized intimal hyperplasia and lipid/necrotic cores not evident with IVUS. The approximately nine-times-higher resolution of OCT provides clear advantages in assessing stent–strut deployment and describing the detailed anatomy of the intima–media area. Correlations with immunohistochemistry have shown that OCT provides reliable information about macrophage accumulation within the neointima, an important feature to better characterize the vulnerable plaque [29]. Although one can argue that, with the current penetration depth, most cardinal features of a vulnerable plaque are readily assessed, OCT has additional limitations that prevent its routine clinical use.

The limitation in penetration depth probably does not allow plaque neovascularization (vasa vasorum) to be assessed. Because recent pathohistologic data indicate that plaque neovascularization may be a main feature

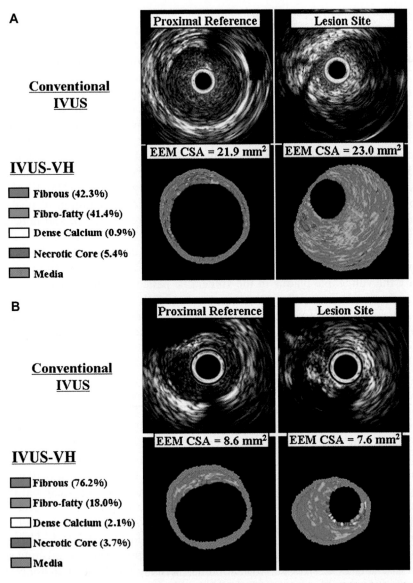

Fig. 4. Virtual histology. Examples of conventional IVUS image and virtual histology color-coded map side by side. (*A*) Lesion with acute coronary syndrome indicates positive remodeling, with a remodeling index of 1.05, external elastic membrane (EEM) CSA of 23.0 mm², plaque burden of 87%, and lumen CSA of 3.0 mm²; in this segment, fibrous and fibrofatty plaques distribute evenly (*lower right*). (*B*) Lesion with stable angina indicates negative remodeling, with a remodeling index of 0.88, an external elastic membrane CSA of 7.6 mm², plaque burden of 79%, and lumen CSA of 1.6 mm²; this segment is predominantly fibrous (*lower right*). (*From* Fujii K, Carlier SG, Mintz GS, et al. Association of plaque characterization by intravascular ultrasound virtual histology and arterial remodeling. Am J Cardiol 2005;96:1480; with permission.)

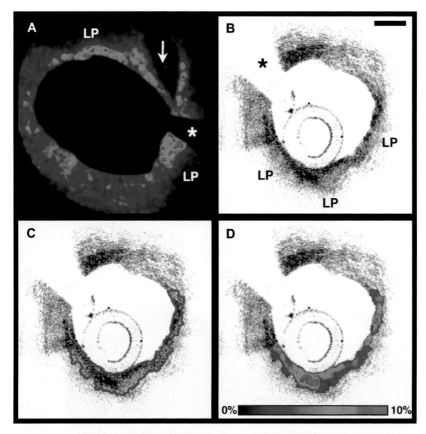

Fig. 5. Optical coherence tomography (OCT). Fibrous cap segmentation and macrophage density images for lipid-rich plaques. (*A*) A normalized standard deviation (NSD) image demonstrating high macrophage density (*blue → red*) at a site of disruption (*arrow*) within a lipid-rich plaque (LP). The * represents guide wire shadow artifact. (*B*) OCT image of an LP. The * represents guide wire shadow artifact. A 500-μm scale bar is shown in the top right corner. (*C*) Outline (*red*) of the segmented fibrous cap of the OCT image depicted in panel b. (*D*) Normalized standard deviation image superimposed over a standard intensity image shows locations (*blue → red*) corresponding to increased macrophage density. The color scale bar represents the color mapping of the NSD parameter. (*From* MacNeill BD, Jang I-K, Bouma BE, et al. Focal and multi-focal plaque macrophage distributions in patients with acute and stable presentations of coronary artery disease. J Am Coll Cardiol 2004;44(5):972–9. Copyright © 2004, with permission from the American College of Cardiology Foundation.)

of a vulnerable plaque [2], the inability of OCT to evaluate this may preclude it from becoming a major future imaging modality. In addition, reliable delineation of morphoantomic structures is limited to a radius of approximately 2 to 3 mm, meaning that it cannot image a complete plaque, and it requires the catheter to be placed adjacent to the coronary vessel wall. Moreover, OCT, like angioscopy, needs a saline-flushed, blood-free vessel segment for best image quality. Therefore, cardiologists either have only a 2-second scan-time window for analysis or must used a static saline column, which may not be tolerated by the patient. In addition, because of cardiac motion and imprecise catheter localization, repeat sampling of the same side is difficult if not impossible. Potential improvements of this technique are being developed, but OCT is still far from becoming part of routine clinical practice.

Therefore, OCT would be able to identify four major criteria (active inflammation, thin cap with lipid core, endothelial denudation, and fissure) and one minor criterion (superficial calcified nodule).

Intravascular ultrasound–based palpography and gray scale echogenicity

The concept of palpography is to provide an imaging tool that assesses not only plaque morphology and composition but also the response of the tissue to the pulsating force applied by the blood pressure. Because the lipid/necrotic core cannot oppose the mechanical forces of blood pressure, the fibrous cap undergoes major radial and circumferential mechanical stresses that under certain circumstances cause rupture of the fibrous cap with the well-known sequelae (Fig. 6). The factors that seem to most

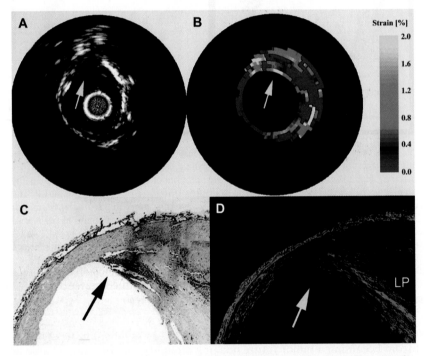

Fig. 6. Palpography. Vulnerable plaque marked in IVUS (*A*), elastogram (*B*), macrophage staining (*C*), and collagen staining (*D*). In the elastogram, a vulnerable plaque is indicated by a high strain on the surface. In the corresponding histology, a high amount of macrophages (*C*) is visible with a thin cap (*D*) and a lipid pool (LP). (*From* Schaar JA, De Korte CL, Mastik F, et al. Characterizing vulnerable plaque features with intravascular elastography. Circulation 2003;108(21):2636–41; with permission.)

influence the stability of the fibrous cap are its thickness and degree of inflammation.

Palpography has the potential to inform cardiologists as to which region of a plaque is exposed to the highest strain. In addition, palpography can identify different plaque components because of their different mechanical properties. In vitro validation has shown that a high-strain region demonstrated with IVUS-based palpography has a high sensitivity and specificity (88% and 89%, respectively) in identifying vulnerable plaques, defined histologically by a large atheroma, a thin fibrous cap, and a moderate to heavy infiltration of macrophages [30]. In addition, the recently published results of the Integrated Biomarker and Imaging Study (IBIS) trial [31] showed that, in contrast to conventional IVUS measurements and angiography, palpography measurements of strain were the only plaque characteristic that correlated well with clinical presentation and could show the success of medical treatment. However, because no in vivo data are currently available, the question remains if and when plaques that are palpographically classified as vulnerable will eventually rupture, whether the concepts of treating these plaques appropriately are available, and whether a plaque that shows reduction in strain measurement but no change in plaque morphology and composition still bears the risk for rupture. Otherwise, one may question whether additional information (on top of pure IVUS measurements) is helpful at all.

The question remains whether a plaque exists that is more vulnerable or more prone to rupture. In other words, can a plaque with a thin fibrous cap and a considerable lipid/necrotic core only be classified as vulnerable if the amount of strain within the fibrous cap is known.

These questions cannot yet be answered. Palpography, however, requires acquisition of additional data, and would therefore be used in addition to angiography and IVUS. Thus, the value of this additional piece of information in identifying the vulnerable plaque must be proven in future prospective studies.

Intravascular MRI

To overcome the difficulty of imaging coronary lesions with MRI caused by motion artifacts and the impracticability of MRI magnets in the catheterization laboratory, intravascular MRI has been introduced recently. In vitro intravascular MRI showed a high sensitivity and specificity in identifying thin- and thick-cap fibroatheromas in human aortas and coronaries through a simplified representation of the plaques lipid content and its extension into the superficial and deeper vessel wall layers [32]. Another in vivo study used intravascular MRI to image 25 human iliac arteries and results were compared with those of IVUS. Intravascular MRI showed the heterogeneity of atherosclerotic plaque content (calcification, lipid, and fibrous tissue), with sensitivity and specificity values ranging from 73% to 100% and 81% to 97%, respectively (Fig. 7). In addition, the level of inter- and

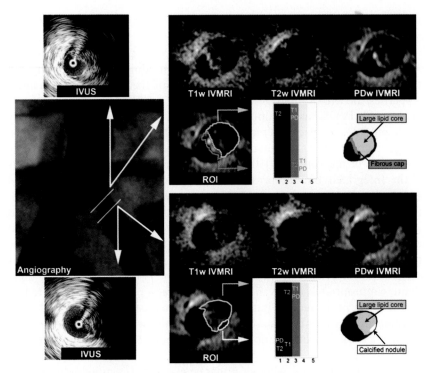

Fig. 7. Intravascular MRI (IVMRI) of common iliac artery in vivo. Angiogram (*left*) of a common iliac artery and corresponding IVUS and IVMRI images of the iliac artery at its origin (*top half*) and 6 mm distal to the bifurcation (*bottom half*). In both segments, the artery is characterized by angiographic narrowing and IVUS that images the outside edges of the artery and plaque incompletely, whereas the corresponding IVMRI depicts the entire plaque morphology. The validated approach to tissue characterization ex vivo applied to this in vivo study shows a predominantly lipid core with overlying fibrous cap at the origin of the iliac artery (*top half*) and a large lipid core with a calcium nodule in the more distal segment (*bottom half*). (*From* Larose E, Yeghiazarians Y, Libby P, et al. Characterization of human atherosclerotic plaques by intravascular magnetic resonance imaging. Circulation 2005;112(15):2324–31; with permission.)

intraobserver variability was higher for intravascular MRI [33]. However, before this exciting technique can be applied in coronary arteries in vivo, several technical limitations must be overcome, including limited resolution and bulky detector coils. Hence, intravascular MRI currently cannot be considered an imaging tool to identify coronary vulnerable plaques, but it certainly has the potential to determine three major criteria (thin cap and lipid core, fissure, and >90% stenosis) and three minor criteria (calcified nodules, intraplaque hemorrhage, and positive remodeling).

Near-infrared spectroscopy and intracoronary thermography

Near-infrared (NIR) spectroscopy, which is still in the experimental stage, is based on the principle that emitted NIR light interacts with the different tissue entities and the differential absorbance spectrum defines the plaque composition (Fig. 8). Early experimental data in aortic and coronary plaques showed high sensitivities and specificities for identifying a thin fibrous cap and the presence of inflammatory cells [34]. However, it has not been translated into the in vivo setting yet because of technical limitations [35].

Intracoronary thermography uses the fact that an active (potentially vulnerable) plaque shows a high metabolic rate caused by the processes involved in inflammation and neoangiogenesis and hence show higher surface temperatures. Human in vivo studies in patients with acute coronary syndromes showed that plaque surface temperature correlated well with the severity of symptoms and was associated with adverse cardiac events in follow up [36]. Ongoing clinical trials will determine whether thermography may become a widely used imaging method. Because it only gives indirect information on tissue inflammation and thus may identify one major criteria (active inflammation) the advantage over IVUS based platforms as discussed above is, however, doubtful.

Imaging tools

Noninvasive

MRI

In immediate comparison with coronary angiography, MRI shows high sensitivity and accuracy but low specificity in detecting atherosclerotic disease in all three major coronary arteries [37,38]. The next step, of course, is to not only identify plaque but also characterize the plaque so that its

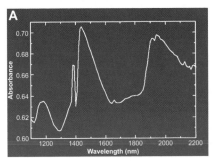 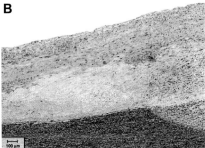

Fig. 8. Near-infrared (NIR) spectroscopy. NIR spectra collected from atheromatous, lipid-rich aortic plaque. (*A*) NIR absorbance tracing from spectra collected with an InfraAlyzer 500 spectrophotometer. Absorbance values were collected from 1100- to 2200-nm wavelength window at 10-nm intervals (see text for details). (*B*) Lipid-rich aortic plaque (elastic trichrome staining). (*From* Moreno PR, Lodder RA, Purushothaman KR, et al. Detection of lipid pool, thin fibrous cap, and inflammatory cells in human aortic atherosclerotic plaques by near-infrared spectroscopy. Circulation 2002;105(8):923–7; with permission.)

vulnerability can be defined. In a recent case report [39] the use of a 3.0T MRI combined with multicontrast black blood transverse images and three-dimensional time in flight transverse images provided visualization of a vulnerable plaque in an internal carotid artery (Fig. 9). Subsequent correlation with histology showed that MRI was capable of discerning the lipid core, the fibrous cap, and calcification. In retrospect, 3.0T MRI was found to be able to identify macrophage-rich regions in the shoulder of the plaque because of the improved signal-to-noise-ratio, excellent fat suppression, and enhanced tissue contrast. In contrast, 1.5T imaging did not identify the macrophage-rich region and had worse signal-to-noise and contrast-to-noise ratios. Considering that 3.0T MRI is not readily available for most patients and that motion artifacts will make imaging of coronary arteries more difficult than fixed carotids, MRI does not readily qualify as the tool for imaging coronary vulnerable plaque. The addition of a gadolinium-based agent has been shown to enhance plaque areas of neovascularization in carotid arteries [40]. Using superparamagnetic iron oxides that are phagocytosed by macrophages in atherosclerotic plaques [41,42] or agents that target metalloproteinases and thus enhance plaque areas with high proteolytic activity [43,44] may be other means of visualizing the vulnerable plaque (see the section on molecular imaging).

Respiratory and cardiac motion, coronary artery location, size, and tortuosity are probably the main limitations in using MRI for reliably evaluating vulnerable coronary plaques. Free breathing navigator gating, which assesses cardiac and diaphragmatic positions and compensates for motion artifacts in combination with slice tracking, has been shown to reduce residual motion of the coronaries [45]. Further improvements like an obliquely oriented reinversion slab with adiabatic pulses [46] may eventually lead to reliable, noninvasive imaging of vulnerable plaques with MRI.

If MRI technique is assembled in an intravascular, self-contained MRI probe, it has the capability to visualize histologically verified thin fibrous cap fibroatheromas in vitro [32]; in vivo feasibility, however, has not been proven.

Therefore, MRI alone without combined molecular imaging may be able to reliably detect coronary artery stenosis of more than 90% with a thin cap with lipid core as two major criteria and outward remodeling plus intraplaque hemorrhage (Fig. 10) as two minor criteria [47,48], but it currently fails to assess the other criteria. Future technical and contrast agent developments and various combinations with molecular imaging, however, are promising and may make MRI a strong diagnostic tool for detecting vulnerable plaques in future.

Multislice CT/electron beam CT
    Many improvements in CT technology (eg, higher gantry speed, up to 64 detector rows, the decrease in slice thickness to submillimetric levels) have increased the diagnostic accuracy of multislice computed tomography

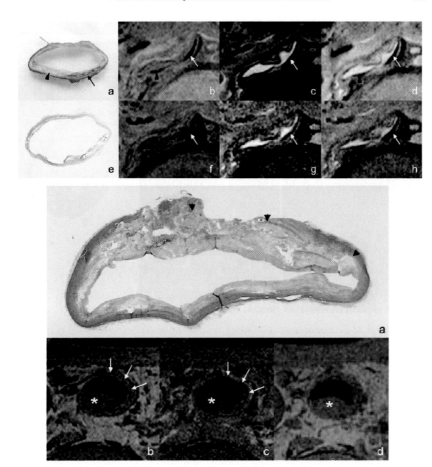

Fig. 9. MRI. (*Top*) Cross-sectional macroscopic (*A*) and histologic (h & e) (e) image of the aorta at the branching of the inferior mesenteric artery, corresponding multicontrast MR images at 3.0 Tesla (*B–D* are T1-weighted, T2-weighted, and proton density [PD]–weighted) and at 1.5 Tesla (*F–H* are T1-weighted, T2-weighted, and PD-weighted). Superior depiction of the vessel wall components at 3.0 Tesla, showing a large calcified plaque opposite the branching artery (*arrow*) and smaller calculus at the right-sided circumference (*arrowhead*). (*Bottom*) (*A*) Cross-sectional histological slide (Masson-Goldner-Elastica); (*B*) T1-weighted and (*C*) T2-weighted MRI images at 3.0 Tesla; (*D*) T1-weighted at 1.5 Tesla. Bands of hyperintensity in T1-weighted and hypointensity in T2-weighted image at 3.0 Tesla (*arrows*) in correlation with light zones in the enlarged intimal layer of the histological image (*arrowheads*) representing lipid cores. These T1-weighted hyperintense areas/lipid cores could not be sufficiently discriminated at 1.5 Tesla and were here falsely categorized as a fibrotic plaque. In the lumen of the MRI images, postmortal blood clotting can be seen (*asterisk*), which was eliminated in the histologic slide because of preparation. (*From* Koops A, Ittrich H, Petri S, et al. Multicontrast-weighted magnetic resonance imaging of atherosclerotic plaques at 3.0 and 1.5 Tesla: ex-vivo comparison with histopathologic correlation. Eur Radiol 2006:1–8; with kind permission of Springer Science and Business Media.)

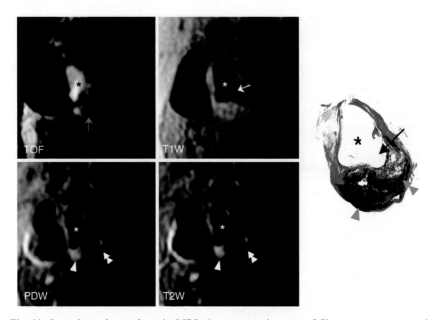

Fig. 10. Intraplaque hemorrhage in MRI. A representative case of fibrous cap rupture and hemorrhage into a carotid atherosclerotic plaque on baseline MRI. The subject experienced an ipsilateral stroke 24 months later and subsequently underwent carotid endarterectomy. Signal intensity patterns of hemorrhage (*red arrow in time-of-flight* [*TOF*]) are hyperintensity on the TOF and T1 W images and hypointensity (*double arrowhead*) and hyperintensity (*arrowhead*) on the PDW/T2 W images, suggesting a mixed of type I and type II intraplaque hemorrhage. A Mallory trichrome-stained matching histology section shows the presence of the hemorrhage (*arrowhead* and *double arrowhead*) and surface disruption (*arrow*). The hemorrhage near to the disrupted surface (*double arrowhead*) is more recent than the hemorrhage deep in the plaque (*arrowhead*). Asterisks indicate the lumen. (*From* Takaya N, Yuan C, Chu B, et al. Association between carotid plaque characteristics and subsequent ischemic cerebrovascular events: a prospective assessment with MRI—initial results. Stroke 2006;37(3):818–23; with permission.)

(MSCT) in noninvasive assessment of coronary atherosclerosis (Figs. 11 and 12) [49,50]. In a recent report directly comparing IVUS and contrast-enhanced 16-slice CT of 252 plaques in patients undergoing coronary angiography for clinical reasons, a significant difference was seen in the mean CT attenuation within atherosclerotic lesions of hypo- and hyperechogenic appearance in IVUS but, because of significant overlap of attenuation values, differentiation between lipid-rich and fibrous was not reliable [51]. Another study comparing a 64-slice CT scanner against IVUS in detecting coronary stenoses of less than 50%, showed that 64-sclice CT correctly identified noncalcified, mixed, and calcified plaques in 83%, 94%, and 95% of cases (overall sensitivity and specificity 84% and 91%, respectively, in detecting nonsignificant plaques). Moreover, 64-slice CT identified a lipid pool in 70% of cases [49].

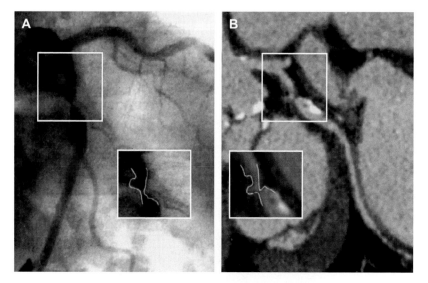

Fig. 11. CT. Correlation of quantitative coronary angiography (QCA) and 64-slice CT angiography: visualization and quantification of a high-grade stenosis in the left circumflex artery. (Diameter in the reference section 3.1 mm on QCA, 3.0 mm on 64-slice CT; minimal diameter within the stenotic section 0.6 mm on QCA, 0.5 mm on 64-slice CT). (*A*) Invasive coronary angiogram of the left coronary artery (right anterior oblique projection). (*B*) Multiplanar reformatted projection of the left circumflex artery using 64-slice CT. (*From* Leber AW, Knez A, von Ziegler F, et al. Quantification of obstructive and nonobstructive coronary lesions by 64-slice computed tomography: a comparative study with quantitative coronary angiography and intravascular ultrasound. J Am Coll Cardiol 2005;46(1):147–54. Copyright © 2005, with permission from the American College of Cardiology Foundation.)

Despite systematic overestimation of cross-sectional areas, the assessment of positive remodeling also seems feasible and accurate, at least in selected coronary artery data sets with good image quality [52].

Obviously, depending on the CT technology used (eg, from 4- to 64-slice CT, dimension of slice thickness) and intergroup variances in applied reconstruction algorithms, the accuracy, sensitivity, and specificity in detecting coronary lesions vary. However, technical improvements will probably increase the accuracy of MSCT and make it a powerful imaging modality for imaging and follow-up of vulnerable plaques in future clinical studies.

Recent expert statements list the electron-bean CT (EBCT)–derived quantity of coronary artery calcification (CAC) as a modality to measure the extent of coronary atherosclerosis [53], and several clinical studies have used CAC scoring to evaluate the risk for future cardiovascular events or as a surrogate for plaque burden before and after treatment [54,55]. However, because the resolution of EBCT is not high enough to visualize plaque composition and structure, and the absence of calcium does not exclude atherosclerotic lesions, EBCT is unlikely to be a future diagnostic tool for detecting vulnerable plaques.

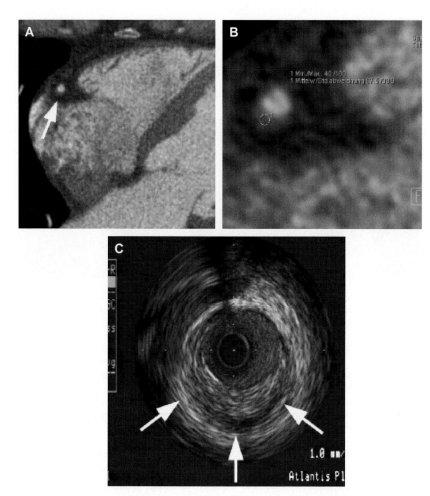

Fig. 12. CT II. Visualization of a noncalcified atherosclerotic plaque (*arrows*) in the mid right coronary artery using multidetector CT (MDCT) (*A, B*) and IVUS (*C*). In MDCT, the mean CT attenuation in a standard region of interest (1.5 mm^2) is 88 HU (*B*). In IVUS, the echogenicity of the lesion is lower than the surrounding tissue (*C*). (*From* Pohle K, Achenbach S, Macneill B, et al. Characterization of non-calcified coronary atherosclerotic plaque by multidetector row CT: comparison to IVUS. Atherosclerosis 2006;190:176; with permission.)

Although CT technique is finding its place as a noninvasive tool for detecting and quantifying coronary lesions, high-quality and accuracy of image analysis, especially regarding plaque composition, seems currently reserved for specialized centers. In addition, current resolutions do not allow visualization of minimal changes at the plaque surface; for example, the identification of plaque fissures or thrombus aggregation and the diagnosis of in-stent restenosis are not accurate enough because of stent artifacts (except for stents in the left main coronary artery imaged under perfect conditions [56]).

In summary, both CT techniques provide the advantage of noninvasiveness but currently have technical limitations preventing them from reliably identifying a vulnerable plaque. In addition, high-resolution scanning, which holds the highest promises for the reliable detection of vulnerable plaques, can currently only be provided for a few patients who have coronary artery disease.

MSCT and EBCT are currently able to reliably identify stenosis of more than 90% as a major criterion for detecting vulnerable plaque, and MSCT can reliably detect positive remodeling and possibly superficial calcified nodules as two minor criteria.

Molecular imaging

In contrast to the more morphoanatomically-oriented methods, molecular imaging aims to image biological properties of atherosclerotic plaques in vivo [57]. Potential targets for molecular imaging are macrophages, [18]fluorodeoxyglucose ([18]FDG) metabolism, and protease and myeloperoxidase activity. As one of the major players in vessel wall inflammation, macrophages can be visualized using MRI with or without concomitant near-infrared fluorescence (NIRF) using magnetic nanoparticles (MNP) with carbohydrate coatings that undergo endocytosis by the macrophages [42,58]. Possible future technical developments, such as intravascular NIRF catheters and better MNP, may lead to applications in coronary arteries. Currently, however, this technique must be considered experimental.

In combination with CT or MRI, [18]FDG positron emission tomography (PET) is another option to visualize inflammatory processes within the plaque because it competes with glucose for uptake in metabolically active cells (eg, macrophages). In a recent study, FDG-PET combined with high-resolution MRI was able to assess the degree of inflammation in stenotic and nonstenotic plaques in carotid arteries of patients who had a recent transient ischemic attack [59]. However, PET cannot detect FDG-labeled coronary plaques because of respiratory and heart motion artifacts and the small size and low activity of these plaques [60].

Increased protease activity (eg, cathepsin B) as a marker for atherosclerosis and potential cause of plaque rupture from extracellular matrix degradation has been visualized with noninvasive fluorescence-mediated tomography coregistered with MRI in western-type diet-fed apoE and apoE/endothelial nitric oxide synthase double knockout mice (Fig. 13) [61,62]. Likewise, matrix metalloproteinase activity has been visualized with single-photon emission CT (SPECT) in carotid plaques of Apo E−/− mice [63]. Because future improvements in these imaging devices (and combinations with CT) and the agents are expected, these techniques have the potential to identify inflamed coronary plaque in vivo.

Similar methods are currently under investigation to visualize myeloperoxidase, lipoproteins, apoptosis, and angiogenesis. They all have in common the ability to identify one major criteria (active inflammation) and, combined

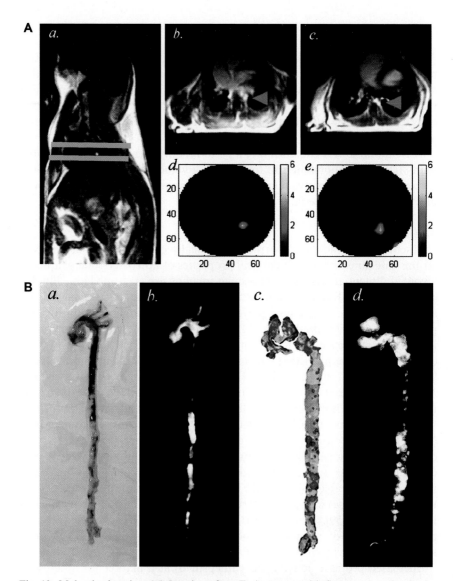

Fig. 13. Molecular imaging. (*A*) Imaging of apoE−/− mouse with fluorescent molecular tomography (FMT). (*A*) Sagittal MR image showing highlighted axial sections (*B*, *C*) for anatomic reference. (*D*, *E*) FMT images corresponding to the MR sections shown in *B* and *C*. Note that signal is emanating from descending aorta in a distribution similar to that shown in *B* (color map, 0–6 × 10-7 mol/L concentration of Cy 5.5; numbers on *x* and *y* axes represent millimeter bars). (*B*) Aortas from two apoE−/− mice fed western-type diet. *A* and *B* represent intact vessel, and *C* and *D* represent vessel opened longitudinally. (*A*) Photograph of unstained intact vessel, with normal areas filled with blood (*red*) and atherosclerotic lesions appearing white. (*B*) Corresponding near-infrared fluorescent (NIRF) image, showing cathepsin B–activated fluorescent areas in the arch and abdominal aorta. (*C*) Sudan IV staining of the longitudinally opened aorta, where red areas represent lipid-rich areas stained with Sudan IV. (*D*) Corresponding NIRF image showing prominent cathepsin B signal from atherosclerotic lesions that matches Sudan staining. (*From* Chen J, Tung CH, Mahmood U, et al. In vivo imaging of proteolytic activity in atherosclerosis. Circulation 2002;105(23):2766–71; with permission.)

with MRI or CT, possibly additional criteria. However, because these methods and in vivo human coronary artery imaging are still at the experimental stage, future studies must show their usefulness.

Besides inflammatory processes, high-resolution MRI combined with a fibrin-specific MR contrast agent has been shown to be capable of visualizing microthrombi on an atherosclerotic plaque (Fig. 14) [64].

In summary, noninvasive imaging methods (excluding the more experimental molecular imaging for now) can certainly be used as initial screening tools in symptomatic patients, but currently massive screening of the general population for coronary calcification and vulnerable plaques cannot be recommended.

Management

Even if the perfect imaging modality was available to identify the truly unstable plaque, how would this information be used? Would this lesion be stented although it did not produce a significant stenosis yet? Or, is the patient treated vigorously with high doses of statins and anti-inflammatory drugs?

REVERSAL, ASTEROID trials

Using serial IVUS measurements, the Reversal of Atherosclerosis with Aggressive Lipid Lowering (REVERSAL) trial [65] showed that intensive

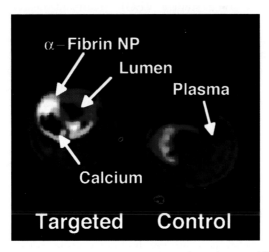

Fig. 14. Fibrin-specific imaging with MRI. Color-enhanced MR images of fibrin-targeted and control carotid endarterectomy specimens revealing contrast enhancement (*white*) of small fibrin deposit on symptomatic ruptured plaque. Calcium deposit (*black*). Three-dimensional, fat-suppressed, T1-weighted, fast gradient echo signal. NP indicates nanoparticle. (*From* Flacke S, Fischer S, Scott MJ, et al. Novel MRI contrast agent for molecular imaging of fibrin: implications for detecting vulnerable plaques. Circulation 2001;104(11):1280–5; with permission.)

lipid-lowering therapy with 80 mg of atorvastatin led to preservation of the pretreatment coronary plaque burden. Earlier this year, using very high–intensity statin therapy (rosuvastatin 40 mg/d) and serial IVUS measurements, the A Study to Evaluate the Effect of Rosuvastatin on Intravascular Ultrasound-Derived Coronary Atheroma Burden (ASTEROID) trial [66] showed that a further reduction of low-density lipoprotein levels even leads to a regression of atherosclerosis (at least by means of three prespecified IVUS measures of disease burden). Another interesting therapeutic option is the enzyme acyl-coenzyme A:cholesterol acyltransferase (ACAT), which was recently tested in The ACAT Intravascular Atherosclerosis Treatment Evaluation (ACTIVATE) trial in addition to standard statin therapy [67]. Unfortunately, patients treated with ACAT showed no effect on atheroma volume but actually an adverse effect on two major secondary efficacy measures assessed by IVUS.

Based on these results, future guidelines will probably recommend high-dose treatment with statins for every patient who has coronary artery disease. A future study design may specifically examine the potentially beneficial effect of high-dose statin treatment on the reversal of a plaque from vulnerable to stable. A possible future extension of that design may be another arm in which patients who have a vulnerable plaque are treated with coronary artery stenting (ie, drug-eluting stent).

Another potential treatment of coronary artery disease and specifically the vulnerable plaque is the vascular endothelial growth factor (VEGF). However, the literature shows conflicting results in animal and human studies. Although in some studies VEGF treatment decreased neointimal thickening or had no effect [68,69], it induced progression of neointima formation in others [70]. Antiangiogenic treatment with various factors mainly decreases neointima formation, although VEGF-trap in a mouse model increased neointima formation [71]. Possible explanations for these discrepancies are the choice of species, choice of vascular bed, route of drug delivery, and possibly the stage of atherosclerotic disease when VEGF is delivered. Because plaque neovascularization may play a significant role in the progression and complication of atherosclerosis, species that do not have vasa vasorum might react differently from humans who have vasa vasorum in almost every vascular bed. In addition, recent human and animal studies show that different vascular beds have a different spatial density and distribution of vasa vasorum. Thus, before possible therapeutic interventions can be included or excluded, future animal experiments and human studies must show whether specific treatments must be designed for the different stages of the atherosclerotic process and the different vascular beds.

Another concept might be the intracoronary infusion of endothelial progenitor cells. This approach, however, is certainly in its earliest stages and future experimental studies must show first whether endothelial progenitor cells actually stabilize or even destabilize coronary plaques through influencing various intraplaque processes such as neovascularization and inflammation.

The introduction of drug-eluting stents has been shown to reduce the rate of significant restenosis to less than 5% of cases. Hence, experts have proposed that these stents also be used for vulnerable, nonstenotic plaques. However, a considerable number of acute and subacute stent thromboses (0.5%–1%) still exist that are potentially fatal which, in a prophylactic treatment, might be unacceptable. In addition, the impact of a metal stent deployment on vessel wall and vasa vasorum compression is significant, which has been shown to lead to vessel wall inflammation and vasa vasorum neovascularization, both potential sources for neointima proliferation and restenosis. A recent study reported that the sirolimus-eluting stent implantation may also be associated with endothelial dysfunction [72]. Based on these data, prophylactic drug-eluting stent deployment cannot be recommended.

The recent introduction of bioresolvable stents [73,74] may offer a new approach for treating coronary artery disease, especially vulnerable plaques. These stents literally disappear after several weeks, and therefore do not cause permanent irritation to the coronary vessel wall, especially the vasa vasorum. Deployment of bioresolvable stents at vulnerable plaques compared with medical treatment alone may be a future study design if upcoming research warrants no ethical problems.

Currently, no prospective data are available defining the vulnerable plaque that will eventually become a culprit lesion (ie, a lesion that is responsible for an acute coronary event). One earlier IVUS-based serial study, however, showed that the pre-examined lesions (<50% diameter stenosis) at which an acute occlusion occurred within the 22-month follow-up (12 of 114) were characteristically large and eccentric, and contained a lipid core in most cases (>80%) [75]. In addition, extensive histopathologic studies have shown that of the 60% of sudden deaths caused by acute coronary artery thrombosis, an eroded lesion and not a ruptured plaque is the culprit in 30% to 35% [76]; in acute myocardial infarction, culprit erosions account for 20% to 25% of deaths [77]. These data also imply that in approximately 40% of sudden deaths, no acute coronary artery thrombosis occurred. Thus, interventional cardiologists practicing evidenced-based medicine currently have no data that reliably recommend interventional treatment of a vulnerable plaque. Nevertheless, the quest for imaging modalities that allow prospective follow-up of vulnerable plaques might lead to studies that may change treatment of the vulnerable plaque or patient.

The ideal (perfect) imaging tool

From a patient's viewpoint, the ideal imaging modality for assessing a vulnerable plaque should be noninvasive but capable of reliably visualizing the cardinal features of the plaque, such as a thin fibrous cap, the lipid/necrotic core, markers of inflammation like macrophage accumulation, and

Table 1
Characteristics of a vulnerable plaque and available imaging modalities

Lesion characteristic	Available imaging modalities	Exemplary figures
Inflammation/macrophage invasion	Inv: OCT [79], Mol-Imaging [57,62], thermography [36], IVMRI [80] Non-inv: MRI [42]	5, 7, 9, and 13
Thin cap/lipid core	Inv: IVUS-VH [14,81], OCT [79], palpography [82], IVMRI [80], NIR-spectroscopy [34] Non-inv: MRI [39], CT	4–9
Erosion ± thrombus	Inv: IVUS-VH [14,81], OCT [79], angioscopy [12] Non-inv: MRI [64]	2, 4, 5, and 14
Fissure ± thrombus	Inv: IVUS-VH [14,81], OCT [79], angioscopy [12] Non-inv: MRI [64]	2, 4, 5, 9, and 14
>90% Luminal stenosis	Inv: Angio [4], IVUS-VH [14,81] Non-inv: CT [49,51], MRI [83]	1, 4, 9, 11, and 12
Microcalcification	Inv: IVUS-VH [14,81,84], OCT [79], IVMRI [33] Non-inv: MRI [85], CT	4, 5, 7, and 9
Yellow appearance	Inv: Angioscopy [86]	2
Hemorrhage	Inv: IVUS-VH [14,81], NIR-spectroscopy [34], IVMRI [80] Non-inv: MRI [80,87]	4, 7, 8, and 10
Endothelial dysfunction	Inv: Angio [9] (with intravascular Doppler)	1
Positive remodeling	Inv: IVUS-VH [88] Non-inv: CT [49,51], MRI [89]	4, 9, 11, and 12

Abbreviations: Angio, coronary angiography; Angioscopy, coronary angioscopy; Inv, invasive; IVMRI, intravascular magnetic resonance imaging; IVUS-VH, intravascular ultrasound ± virtual histology; Mol-Imaging, molecular imaging; NIR-spectroscopy, near-infrared spectroscopy; Non-inv, noninvasive; OCT, optical coherence tomography.

vasa vasorum neovascularization/intraplaque hemorrhage. Potentially, it should also offer the capability of imaging stented lesions for the same features in follow-ups. Based on the facts presented in this article, however, only catheter-based, invasive methods based on an IVUS platform with or without expansions such as virtual histology or palpography currently allow a satisfying number of vulnerable plaque criteria to be visualized. Hence, among the invasive methods, a high-resolution IVUS-based platform combined with virtual histology and features like OCT and palpography to assess inflammation and local tissue strain might be the perfect tool. With the recent promising development of high-resolution IVUS combined with echo-contrast injections, even vasa vasorum neovascularization may be readily assessed in future [78]. Ideally, this invasive imaging tool should have all the necessary features integrated within one single catheter.

Among the noninvasive methods, a technical combination of molecular imaging to assess vessel wall inflammation with MRI or MSCT for morphologic assessments would be necessary to cover most criteria of a vulnerable plaque. Based on this article, MRI would need to be the major feature of that combined tool to be able to visualize the lipid core with a thin fibrous cap and intraplaque hemorrhage in addition to other dimensional measurements.

In conclusion, although the ideal imaging tool currently does not exist, many are available to choose from (Table 1) [49,79–89]. In the presence of increasing health care costs, future studies will have to determine which imaging modalities must be concentrated on, at least for widespread use in daily cardiovascular medicine.

Future prospective studies must show whether visualizing additional plaque characteristics such as inflammation, tissue strain, and vascularization helps identify the vulnerable plaque earlier, but also which characteristics eventually justify an early, preventive, specifically designed, local or systemic treatment of a vulnerable plaque that did not yet produce a significant luminal stenosis. Based on those results, the ideal tool or tool combination to image the vulnerable plaque may be determined.

Acknowledgments

This work was supported in part by NIH grant K24 HL69840 and the Mayo Clinic.

References

[1] Falk E, Shah PK, Fuster V. Coronary plaque disruption. Circulation 1995;92(3):657–71.
[2] Kolodgie FD, Gold HK, Burke AP, et al. Intraplaque hemorrhage and progression of coronary atheroma. N Engl J Med 2003;349(24):2316–25.
[3] Naghavi M, Libby P, Falk E, et al. From vulnerable plaque to vulnerable patient: a call for new definitions and risk assessment strategies: part I. Circulation 2003;108(14): 1664–72.
[4] Ambrose JA, Israel DH. Angiography in unstable angina. Am J Cardiol 1991;68(7): 78B–84B.
[5] Levin DC, Fallon JT. Significance of the angiographic morphology of localized coronary stenoses: histopathologic correlations. Circulation 1982;66(2):316–20.
[6] Romagnoli E, Burzotta F, Giannico F, et al. Images in cardiovascular medicine. Culprit lesion seen 1 hour before occlusion: limits of coronary angiography in detecting vulnerable plaques. Circulation 2006;113(5):e61–2.
[7] Little WC, Constantinescu M, Applegate RJ, et al. Can coronary angiography predict the site of a subsequent myocardial infarction in patients with mild-to-moderate coronary artery disease? Circulation 1988;78(5 Pt 1):1157–66.
[8] Ambrose JA, Tannenbaum MA, Alexopoulos D, et al. Angiographic progression of coronary artery disease and the development of myocardial infarction. J Am Coll Cardiol 1988;12(1):56–62.
[9] Bonetti PO, Lerman LO, Lerman A. Endothelial dysfunction: a marker of atherosclerotic risk. Arterioscler Thromb Vasc Biol 2003;23(2):168–75.
[10] Lerman A, Zeiher AM. Endothelial function: cardiac events. Circulation 2005;111(3):363–8.
[11] Mizuno K, Miyamoto A, Satomura K, et al. Angioscopic coronary macromorphology in patients with acute coronary disorders. Lancet 1991;337(8745):809–12.

[12] Uchida Y, Nakamura F, Tomaru T, et al. Prediction of acute coronary syndromes by percutaneous coronary angioscopy in patients with stable angina. Am Heart J 1995;130(2): 195–203.

[13] Wang JC, Normand SL, Mauri L, et al. Coronary artery spatial distribution of acute myocardial infarction occlusions. Circulation 2004;110(3):278–84.

[14] Gossl M, von Birgelen C, Mintz GS, et al. Volumetric assessment of ulcerated ruptured coronary plaques with three-dimensional intravascular ultrasound in vivo. Am J Cardiol 2003; 91(8):992–6, A997.

[15] Friedrich GJ, Moes NY, Muhlberger VA, et al. Detection of intralesional calcium by intracoronary ultrasound depends on the histologic pattern. Am Heart J 1994;128(3):435–41.

[16] Nissen SE, Gurley JC, Booth DC, et al. Intravascular ultrasound of the coronary arteries: current applications and future directions. Am J Cardiol 1992;69(20):18H–29H.

[17] Pandian NG, Kreis A, Brockway B. Detection of intraarterial thrombus by intravascular high frequency two-dimensional ultrasound imaging in vitro and in vivo studies. Am J Cardiol 1990;65(18):1280–3.

[18] Mintz GS, Popma JJ, Pichard AD, et al. Limitations of angiography in the assessment of plaque distribution in coronary artery disease: a systematic study of target lesion eccentricity in 1446 lesions. Circulation 1996;93(5):924–31.

[19] Gussenhoven EJ, Essed CE, Lancee CT, et al. Arterial wall characteristics determined by intravascular ultrasound imaging: an in vitro study. J Am Coll Cardiol 1989;14(4):947–52.

[20] Glagov S, Weisenberg E, Zarins CK, et al. Compensatory enlargement of human atherosclerotic coronary arteries. N Engl J Med 1987;316(22):1371–5.

[21] Siegel RJ, Ariani M, Fishbein MC, et al. Histopathologic validation of angioscopy and intravascular ultrasound. Circulation 1991;84(1):109–17.

[22] Palmer ND, Northridge D, Lessells A, et al. In vitro analysis of coronary atheromatous lesions by intravascular ultrasound; reproducibility and histological correlation of lesion morphology. Eur Heart J 1999;20(23):1701–6.

[23] Nair A, Kuban BD, Tuzcu EM, et al. Coronary plaque classification with intravascular ultrasound radiofrequency data analysis. Circulation 2002;106(17):2200–6.

[24] Nasu K, Tsuchikane E, Katoh O, et al. Accuracy of in vivo coronary plaque morphology assessment: a validation study of in vivo virtual histology compared with in vitro histopathology. J Am Coll Cardiol 2006;47(12):2405–12.

[25] Rodriguez-Granillo GA, McFadden EP, Valgimigli M, et al. Coronary plaque composition of nonculprit lesions, assessed by in vivo intracoronary ultrasound radio frequency data analysis, is related to clinical presentation. Am Heart J 2006;151(5):1020–4.

[26] Brezinski ME, Tearney GJ, Bouma BE, et al. Optical coherence tomography for optical biopsy. Properties and demonstration of vascular pathology. Circulation 1996;93(6):1206–13.

[27] Jang IK, Tearney GJ, MacNeill B, et al. In vivo characterization of coronary atherosclerotic plaque by use of optical coherence tomography. Circulation 2005;111(12):1551–5.

[28] Jang IK, Bouma BE, Kang DH, et al. Visualization of coronary atherosclerotic plaques in patients using optical coherence tomography: comparison with intravascular ultrasound. J Am Coll Cardiol 2002;39(4):604–9.

[29] Tearney GJ, Yabushita H, Houser SL, et al. Quantification of macrophage content in atherosclerotic plaques by optical coherence tomography. Circulation 2003;107(1):113–9.

[30] Schaar JA, De Korte CL, Mastik F, et al. Characterizing vulnerable plaque features with intravascular elastography. Circulation 2003;108(21):2636–41.

[31] Van Mieghem CA, McFadden EP, de Feyter PJ, et al. Noninvasive detection of subclinical coronary atherosclerosis coupled with assessment of changes in plaque characteristics using novel invasive imaging modalities: the Integrated Biomarker and Imaging Study (IBIS). J Am Coll Cardiol 2006;47(6):1134–42.

[32] Schneiderman J, Wilensky RL, Weiss A, et al. Diagnosis of thin-cap fibroatheromas by a self-contained intravascular magnetic resonance imaging probe in ex vivo human aortas and in situ coronary arteries. J Am Coll Cardiol 2005;45(12):1961–9.

[33] Larose E, Yeghiazarians Y, Libby P, et al. Characterization of human atherosclerotic plaques by intravascular magnetic resonance imaging. Circulation 2005;112(15):2324–31.

[34] Moreno PR, Lodder RA, Purushothaman KR, et al. Detection of lipid pool, thin fibrous cap, and inflammatory cells in human aortic atherosclerotic plaques by near-infrared spectroscopy. Circulation 2002;105(8):923–7.

[35] Caplan JD, Waxman S, Nesto RW, et al. Near-infrared spectroscopy for the detection of vulnerable coronary artery plaques. J Am Coll Cardiol 2006;47(8 Suppl):C92–6.

[36] Stefanadis C, Toutouzas K, Tsiamis E, et al. Increased local temperature in human coronary atherosclerotic plaques: an independent predictor of clinical outcome in patients undergoing a percutaneous coronary intervention. J Am Coll Cardiol 2001;37(5):1277–83.

[37] Krittayaphong R, Mahanonda N, Kangkagate C, et al. Accuracy of magnetic resonance imaging in the diagnosis of coronary artery disease. J Med Assoc Thai 2003;86(Suppl 1): S59–66.

[38] Kim WY, Danias PG, Stuber M, et al. Coronary magnetic resonance angiography for the detection of coronary stenoses. N Engl J Med 2001;345(26):1863–9.

[39] Cury RC, Houser SL, Furie KL, et al. Vulnerable plaque detection by 3.0 Tesla magnetic resonance imaging. Invest Radiol 2006;41(2):112–5.

[40] Yuan C, Kerwin WS, Ferguson MS, et al. Contrast-enhanced high resolution MRI for atherosclerotic carotid artery tissue characterization. J Magn Reson Imaging 2002;15(1): 62–7.

[41] Ruehm SG, Corot C, Vogt P, et al. Magnetic resonance imaging of atherosclerotic plaque with ultrasmall superparamagnetic particles of iron oxide in hyperlipidemic rabbits. Circulation 2001;103(3):415–22.

[42] Kooi ME, Cappendijk VC, Cleutjens KB, et al. Accumulation of ultrasmall superparamagnetic particles of iron oxide in human atherosclerotic plaques can be detected by in vivo magnetic resonance imaging. Circulation 2003;107(19):2453–8.

[43] Choudhury RP, Fuster V, Badimon JJ, et al. MRI and characterization of atherosclerotic plaque: emerging applications and molecular imaging. Arterioscler Thromb Vasc Biol 2002;22(7):1065–74.

[44] Choudhury RP, Fuster V, Fayad ZA. Molecular, cellular and functional imaging of atherothrombosis. Nat Rev Drug Discov 2004;3(11):913–25.

[45] Fischer RW, Botnar RM, Nehrke K, et al. Analysis of residual coronary artery motion for breath hold and navigator approaches using real-time coronary MRI. Magn Reson Med 2006;55(3):612–8.

[46] Priest AN, Bansmann PM, Kaul MG, et al. Magnetic resonance imaging of the coronary vessel wall at 3 T using an obliquely oriented reinversion slab with adiabatic pulses. Magn Reson Med 2005;54(5):1115–22.

[47] Worthley SG, Helft G, Fuster V, et al. Serial in vivo MRI documents arterial remodeling in experimental atherosclerosis. Circulation 2000;101(6):586–9.

[48] Wilensky RL, Song HK, Ferrari VA. Role of magnetic resonance and intravascular magnetic resonance in the detection of vulnerable plaques. J Am Coll Cardiol 2006;47 (8 Suppl):C48–56.

[49] Leber AW, Knez A, von Ziegler F, et al. Quantification of obstructive and nonobstructive coronary lesions by 64-slice computed tomography: a comparative study with quantitative coronary angiography and intravascular ultrasound. J Am Coll Cardiol 2005;46(1): 147–54.

[50] Cordeiro MA, Miller JM, Schmidt A, et al. Non-invasive half millimetre 32 detector row computed tomography angiography accurately excludes significant stenoses in patients with advanced coronary artery disease and high calcium scores. Heart 2006; 92(5):589–97.

[51] Pohle K, Achenbach S, Macneill B, et al. Characterization of non-calcified coronary atherosclerotic plaque by multi-detector row CT: comparison to IVUS. Atherosclerosis 2006; 190(1):174–80.

[52] Achenbach S, Ropers D, Hoffmann U, et al. Assessment of coronary remodeling in stenotic and nonstenotic coronary atherosclerotic lesions by multidetector spiral computed tomography. J Am Coll Cardiol 2004;43(5):842–7.

[53] Third Report of the National Cholesterol Education Program (NCEP) expert panel on detection, evaluation, and treatment of high blood cholesterol in adults (Adult Treatment Panel III) final report. Circulation 2002;106(25):3143–421.

[54] Keelan PC, Bielak LF, Ashai K, et al. Long-term prognostic value of coronary calcification detected by electron-beam computed tomography in patients undergoing coronary angiography. Circulation 2001;104(4):412–7.

[55] Schmermund A, Achenbach S, Budde T, et al. Effect of intensive versus standard lipid-lowering treatment with atorvastatin on the progression of calcified coronary atherosclerosis over 12 months: a multicenter, randomized, double-blind trial. Circulation 2006;113(3): 427–37.

[56] Van Mieghem CA, Cademartiri F, Mollet NR, et al. Multislice spiral computed tomography for the evaluation of stent patency after left main coronary artery stenting. A comparison with conventional coronary angiography and intravascular ultrasound. Circulation 2006; 114(7):645–53.

[57] Jaffer FA, Libby P, Weissleder R. Molecular and cellular imaging of atherosclerosis: emerging applications. J Am Coll Cardiol 2006;47(7):1328–38.

[58] Jaffer FA, Nahrendorf M, Sosnovic DE, et al. Cellular imaging of inflammation an atherosclerosis using magnetofluorescent nanomaterials. Mol Imaging 2006;5(2):85–92.

[59] Davies JR, Rudd JH, Fryer TD, et al. Identification of culprit lesions after transient ischemic attack by combined 18F fluorodeoxyglucose positron-emission tomography and high-resolution magnetic resonance imaging. Stroke 2005;36(12):2642–7.

[60] Shikhaliev PM, Xu T, Ducote JL, et al. Positron autoradiography for intravascular imaging: feasibility evaluation. Phys Med Biol 2006;51(4):963–79.

[61] Chen J, Tung CH, Mahmood U, et al. In vivo imaging of proteolytic activity in atherosclerosis. Circulation 2002;105(23):2766–71.

[62] Ntziachristos V, Tung CH, Bremer C, et al. Fluorescence molecular tomography resolves protease activity in vivo. Nat Med 2002;8(7):757–60.

[63] Schafers M, Riemann B, Kopka K, et al. Scintigraphic imaging of matrix metalloproteinase activity in the arterial wall in vivo. Circulation 2004;109(21):2554–9.

[64] Flacke S, Fischer S, Scott MJ, et al. Novel MRI contrast agent for molecular imaging of fibrin: implications for detecting vulnerable plaques. Circulation 2001;104(11):1280–5.

[65] Nissen SE. Effect of intensive lipid lowering on progression of coronary atherosclerosis: evidence for an early benefit from the Reversal of Atherosclerosis with Aggressive Lipid Lowering (REVERSAL) trial. Am J Cardiol 2005;96(5A):61F–8F.

[66] Nissen SE, Nicholls SJ, Sipahi I, et al. Effect of very high-intensity statin therapy on regression of coronary atherosclerosis: the ASTEROID trial. JAMA 2006;295(13):1556–65.

[67] Nissen SE, Tuzcu EM, Brewer HB, et al. Effect of ACAT inhibition on the progression of coronary atherosclerosis. N Engl J Med 2006;354(12):1253–63.

[68] Leppanen P, Koota S, Kholova I, et al. Gene transfers of vascular endothelial growth factor-A, vascular endothelial growth factor-B, vascular endothelial growth factor-C, and vascular endothelial growth factor-D have no effects on atherosclerosis in hypercholesterolemic low-density lipoprotein-receptor/apolipoprotein B48-deficient mice. Circulation 2005;112(9): 1347–52.

[69] Khurana R, Moons L, Shafi S, et al. Placental growth factor promotes atherosclerotic intimal thickening and macrophage accumulation. Circulation 2005;111(21):2828–36.

[70] Celletti FL, Waugh JM, Amabile PG, et al. Vascular endothelial growth factor enhances atherosclerotic plaque progression. Nat Med 2001;7(4):425–9.

[71] Hutter R, Carrick FE, Valdiviezo C, et al. Vascular endothelial growth factor regulates re-endothelialization and neointima formation in a mouse model of arterial injury. Circulation 2004;110(16):2430–5.

[72] Hofma SH, van der Giessen WJ, van Dalen BM, et al. Indication of long-term endothelial dysfunction after sirolimus-eluting stent implantation. Eur Heart J 2005;27(2):166–70.

[73] Heublein B, Rohde R, Kaese V, et al. Biocorrosion of magnesium alloys: a new principle in cardiovascular implant technology? Heart 2003;89(6):651–6.

[74] Eggebrecht H, Rodermann J, Hunold P, et al. Images in cardiovascular medicine. Novel magnetic resonance-compatible coronary stent: the absorbable magnesium-alloy stent. Circulation 2005;112(18):e303–4.

[75] Yamagishi M, Terashima M, Awano K, et al. Morphology of vulnerable coronary plaque: insights from follow-up of patients examined by intravascular ultrasound before an acute coronary syndrome. J Am Coll Cardiol 2000;35(1):106–11.

[76] Virmani R, Burke AP, Farb A, et al. Pathology of the vulnerable plaque. J Am Coll Cardiol 2006;47(8):C13–8.

[77] Arbustini E, Dal Bello B, Morbini P, et al. Plaque erosion is a major substrate for coronary thrombosis in acute myocardial infarction. Heart 1999;82(3):269–72.

[78] Carlier S, Kakadiaris IA, Dib N, et al. Vasa vasorum imaging: a new window to the clinical detection of vulnerable atherosclerotic plaques. Curr Atheroscler Rep 2005;7(2):164–9.

[79] MacNeill BD, Jang I-K, Bouma BE, et al. Focal and multi-focal plaque macrophage distributions in patients with acute and stable presentations of coronary artery disease. J Am Coll Cardiol 2004;44(5):972–9.

[80] Koops A, Ittrich H, Petri S, et al. Multicontrast-weighted magnetic resonance imaging of atherosclerotic plaques at 3.0 and 1.5 Tesla: ex-vivo comparison with histopathologic correlation. Eur Radiol 2007;17(1):276–86.

[81] Fujii K, Carlier SG, Mintz GS, et al. Association of plaque characterization by intravascular ultrasound virtual histology and arterial remodeling. J Am Coll Cardiol 2005;96(11): 1476–83.

[82] Schaar J, Korte C, Mastik F, et al. Intravascular palpography for high-risk vulnerable plaque assessment. Herz 2003;28(6):488–95.

[83] Kefer J, Coche E, Legros G, et al. Head-to-head comparison of three-dimensional navigator-gated magnetic resonance imaging and 16-slice computed tomography to detect coronary artery stenosis in patients. J Am Coll Cardiol 2005;46(1):92–100.

[84] Ehara S, Kobayashi Y, Yoshiyama M, et al. Spotty calcification typifies the culprit plaque in patients with acute myocardial infarction: an intravascular ultrasound study. Circulation 2004;110(22):3424–9.

[85] Clarke SE, Hammond RR, Mitchell JR, et al. Quantitative assessment of carotid plaque composition using multicontrast MRI and registered histology. Magn Reson Med 2003; 50(6):1199–208.

[86] Mizote I, Ueda Y, Ohtani T, et al. Distal protection improved reperfusion and reduced left ventricular dysfunction in patients with acute myocardial infarction who had angioscopically defined ruptured plaque. Circulation 2005;112(7):1001–7.

[87] Takaya N, Yuan C, Chu B, et al. Association between carotid plaque characteristics and subsequent ischemic cerebrovascular events: a prospective assessment with MRI—initial results. Stroke 2006;37(3):818–23.

[88] von Birgelen C, Hartmann M, Mintz GS, et al. Remodeling index compared to actual vascular remodeling in atherosclerotic left main coronary arteries as assessed with long-term (> or = 12 months) serial intravascular ultrasound. J Am Coll Cardiol 2006;47(7):1363–8.

[89] Kim WY, Stuber M, Bornert P, et al. Three-dimensional black-blood cardiac magnetic resonance coronary vessel wall imaging detects positive arterial remodeling in patients with nonsignificant coronary artery disease. Circulation 2002;106(3):296–9.

THE MEDICAL
CLINICS
OF NORTH AMERICA

ELSEVIER
SAUNDERS

Med Clin N Am 91 (2007) 603–616

Risk Stratification Following Acute Myocardial Infarction

Mandeep Singh, MD, MPH[a,b,*]

[a]Division of Cardiovascular Diseases and Internal Medicine, Mayo Clinic College of Medicine,
200 1st Street South West, Rochester, MN 55905, USA
[b]Division of Biostatistics, Mayo Clinic College of Medicine, 200 1st Street South West,
Rochester, MN 55905, USA

Risk stratification is an integral part of managing patients presenting with acute myocardial infarction (MI). Early risk assessment guides triage to clinical pathways of patient care and optimizes use of hospital resources, with pharmacologic and technologic high-intensity care directed to patients who have a higher risk for early and late adverse outcomes after MI. Despite well-characterized predictors of outcomes, reliable risk estimation remains a challenge, because patients present with a spectrum of risk profiles requiring assimilation of numerous data. The available models for risk stratification in MI range from simple bedside risk assessment tools that are both effective and convenient to use at patient presentation to more robust although complicated models that incorporate data during hospitalization.

This article reviews the current risk assessment models available for patients presenting with MI. These practical tools enhance the health care provider's ability to rapidly and accurately assess patient risk from the event or revascularization therapy, and are of paramount importance in managing patients presenting with MI. This article highlights the models used for ST-elevation MI (STEMI) and non-ST elevation MI (NSTEMI) and provides an additional description of models used to assess risks after primary angioplasty (ie, angioplasty performed for STEMI).

Several models have been developed to assess risks for adverse outcome after MI. Most models limit to either STEMI or NSTEMI, but few models encompass the whole spectrum of acute coronary syndrome. The available models also vary in outcomes studied. Most models predict mortality, but several others provide information on other major adverse cardiovascular events (MACE), such as recurrent MI and severe recurrent ischemia

* Mayo Clinic, 200 First Street SW, Rochester, MN 55905.
E-mail address: singh.mandeep@mayo.edu

requiring urgent revascularization. The risk prediction tools also vary in simplicity, validity in internal or external datasets, covariates used, and derivation from population- or trial-based dataset.

Development of a model: statistical considerations

A good predictive model should be both accurate and discriminatory. An accurate model, on average, is not biased toward over- or underprediction. If the true average risk of an event in a population is 5%, accuracy could be achieved through predicting 5% risk for every patient. These estimates would lack precision, however, because the same prognosis is given for both low- and high-risk patients. Discriminatory ability is related to precision (distinguishing high- from low-risk patients). Prediction is the probability that an event will occur; a high-risk patient may have a predicted risk of 0.50, but they will not experience a half-event. Therefore, assessments of these models tend to focus more on discriminatory ability than accuracy. Logistic regression is the standard statistical model used for binary outcomes. Typically, logistic regression is used to express the log–odds of an event as a linear function of the explanatory variables (ie, risk factors). This model produces odds–ratios as measures of the associations between risk factors and the event.

Once a final model is chosen, the Hosmer-Lemeshow goodness-of-fit test may be used to determine if the model adequately reflects the observed data. The test is constructed through dividing the overall sample into groups, often by deciles, with similar predicted values of risk. Observed and expected event rates are then compared within these groups. If the observed and expected totals generally agree throughout, then the test returns a nonsignificant result. The discriminatory ability of a model may be quantified by the C-statistic (C for concordance). The C-statistic, or area under the receiver operating characteristic (ROC) curve, is the proportion of times that the model correctly ranks the risks for a pair of subjects. If two patients have MI, and if one experiences an event (eg, death), it is the rate at which the model assigns a higher level of risk to that patient. Thus, a C-statistic of 0.50 indicates that the model performs as well as risk assigned through tossing a coin. Perfect discrimination results in a C-statistic of 1.00.

The simplification of the statistical model to an additive integer-scoring tool is commonly used for patient counseling. The goal is to assign integer coefficients to risk factors significantly associated with an event so that the physician may quickly sum the coefficients for a numerical ranking of the patient's risk. Once the logistic regression model is finalized, the simplified scoring tool may be defined by selecting integer coefficients roughly proportional to the log-odds ratio coefficients (ie, parameter estimates) of the logistic regression model variables. Various risk models to predict outcomes after MI are listed in Box 1.

Box 1. Risk models predicting outcomes after myocardial infarction

Risk Models for STEMI
Thrombolysis in Myocardial Infarction (TIMI) risk score [1,2]
Global Utilization of Streptokinase and t-PA for Occluded
  Coronary Arteries (GUSTO) [3]
Thrombolytic Predictive Instrument (TPI) [4]

Risk Models for NSTEMI
TIMI [5]
Platelet glycoprotein IIb/IIIa in unstable angina: receptor
  suppression using Integrilin therapy (PURSUIT) [6]

Risk Models for both STEMI and NSTEMI
Predicting Risk of Death in Cardiac Disease Tool (PREDICT) [7]
Global Registry of Acute Coronary Events (GRACE) [8,9]

Risk Models for Primary Angioplasty for STEMI
Controlled Abciximab and Device Investigation to Lower Late
  Angioplasty Complications (CADILLAC) [9]
Primary Angioplasty in Myocardial Infarction (PAMI) [10]

Risk models for NSTEMI

The heterogeneity of presentation of patients who have acute coronary syndrome (ACS) and the early hazard of adverse outcomes after presentation makes the strategy of early evaluation and management paramount. Patients who do not have coronary heart disease can be triaged over the phone. However, a physician should refer patients who have symptoms suggesting possible ACS to a facility that allows evaluation, including recording of a 12-lead EKG. Patients who have suspected ACS with chest discomfort at rest for greater than 20 minutes, hemodynamic instability, or recent syncope or presyncope should be considered for immediate referral to an emergency department or a chest pain facility [11].

The current American College of Cardiology/American Heart Association (ACC/AHA) Class I recommendations for the early risk stratification are as follows:

1. Determination of patients who have chest discomfort of the likelihood of acute ischemia caused by coronary heart disease as high, intermediate, or low (level of evidence: C).
2. Patients who have chest discomfort should undergo early risk stratification that focuses on symptoms, physical and EKG findings, and biomarkers of cardiac injury (level of evidence: B).

3. A 12-lead EKG should be obtained immediately (within 10 minutes) in patients who have ongoing chest discomfort and as soon as possible in patients who have chest discomfort consistent with ACS but whose chest discomfort has resolved by the evaluation (level of evidence: C).

4. Biomarkers of cardiac injury should be measured in all patients who present with chest discomfort consistent with ACS. A cardiac-specific troponin is the preferred marker. In patients who have negative markers within 6 hours of the onset of chest pain, another sample should be drawn in the 6- to 12-hour timeframe.

Whether the symptoms are a manifestation of ACS and, if so, what is the patient's prognosis are the two key questions that can help physicians select the site of care (coronary care unit or step-down facility), management (glycoprotein IIb/IIIa receptor inhibitor), and whether the patient should be transferred to a facility with coronary angiographic/coronary artery bypass surgery capability (Tables 1 and 2) [11–13]. These tables show characteristics that are associated with high likelihood of ACS, and patients who have high likelihood of short-term risk for death/nonfatal MI. The early hazard after presenting with ACS is well characterized, and this risk declines to a level observed by patients who have chronic stable angina within 2 months, highlighting the need to rapidly triage patients into different risk categories [14].

The clinical features associated with increased risk for death were age (>65 years), presence of positive cardiac markers for myonecrosis, lighter weight, more severe (Canadian Cardiovascular Society class III or IV) chronic angina before the index admission, rales on physical examination, and ST-segment depression on the admission EKG [15]. In another trial, tachycardia, bradycardia, and lower blood pressure were associated with higher risk for death or MI [6]. These characteristics help physicians stratify patients into different risks and are the basis for the available models. In patients who have possible ACS, presence of hypertension, hyperlipidemia, or smoking is only weakly predictive of the likelihood of ischemia, and therefore the presence or absence of these risk factors should not be used to determine admission or management of these patients. Presence of diabetes mellitus and extracardiac peripheral vascular disease are major risk factors for adverse outcome (see Table 1).

Estimation of early risk at presentation

Several studies have used the clinical, EKG, and abnormal cardiac biomarkers to develop risk models that can predict outcomes, including, death, reinfarction, or need for urgent revascularization. Three major determinants of prognosis in ACS include (1) the extent of myocardial injury; (2) the extent of coronary artery disease; and (3) the instability of the disease and its refractoriness to management [16]. The GRACE and PURSUIT scores

Table 1
Likelihood that signs and symptoms represent an acute coronary syndrome secondary to coronary artery disease

Feature	High likelihood (any of the below features)	Intermediate likelihood (absence of high-likelihood features and presence of any of the below features)	Low likelihood (absence of high- or intermediate-likelihood features, but may have any of the below features)
History	Chest or left arm pain or discomfort as chief symptom reproducing prior documented angina Known history of coronary artery disease, including myocardial infarction	Chest or left arm pain or discomfort as chief symptom Age > 70 years Male sex Diabetes mellitus	Probable ischemic symptoms in absence of any of the intermediate likelihood characteristics Recent cocaine use
Examination	Transient mitral regurgitation, hypotension, diaphoresis, pulmonary edema, or rales	Extracardiac vascular disease	Chest discomfort reproduced by palpation
ECG	New, or presumably new, transient ST-segment deviation (≥ 0.05 mV) or T- wave inversion (≥ 0.2 mV) with symptoms	Fixed Q-waves Abnormal ST-segments or T-waves not documented to be new	T-wave flattening or inversion in leads with dominant R-waves Normal ECG
Cardiac markers	Elevated cardiac troponin I, troponin T, or creatine kinase MB	Normal	Normal

From Braunwald E, Mark DB, Jones RH, et al. Unstable angina: diagnosis and management. Rockville, MD: Agency for Health Care policy and Research and the National Heart, Lung, and Blood Institute, US Public Health Service, US Department of Health and Human Services; 1994; AHCPR Publication No. 94-0602; with permission.

provided excellent prediction of in-hospital and short-term mortality [8,9]. The TIMI risk score developed a seven-point risk score (Table 3) [5]. The risk for development of an adverse outcome, death, (re)infarction, or recurrent severe ischemia ranged from 5% to 41%. The TIMI risk score was defined as the sum of individual risk factors, and higher scores were associated with higher short-term risk and also greater benefit with glycoprotein IIb/IIIa inhibitors and more invasive revascularization therapy in patients who had higher risk scores. Higher PURSUIT risk score was associated with lower ejection fraction, higher prevalence of severe coronary artery

Table 2
Short-term risk for death or nonfatal myocardial infarction in patients who have unstable angina[a]

Feature	High-risk (at least one of the below features must be present)	Intermediate-risk (no high-risk feature, but must have one of the below features)	Low-risk (no high- or intermediate-risk feature, but may have any of the below features)
History	Accelerating tempo of ischemic symptoms in preceding 48 hours	Prior myocardial infarction, peripheral or cerebrovascular disease, or coronary artery bypass graft; prior aspirin use	
Character of pain	Prolonged ongoing (>20 min) rest pain	Prolonged (>20 min) rest angina, now resolved, with moderate or high likelihood of coronary artery disease Rest angina (<20 min) or relieved with rest or sublingual nitroglycerin	New-onset or progressive Canadian Cardiovascular Society class III or IV angina in the past 2 weeks without prolonged (>20 min) rest pain but with moderate or high likelihood of coronary artery disease
Clinical findings	Pulmonary edema, most likely caused by ischemia New or worsening mitral regurgitation murmur S_3 or new/worsening rales Hypotension, bradycardia, tachycardia Age >75 years	Age >70 years	

	High	Intermediate	Low
ECG	Angina at rest with transient ST-segment changes >0.05 mV Bundle branch block, new or presumed new Sustained ventricular tachycardia	T-wave inversions >0.2 mV Pathologic Q-waves	Normal or unchanged ECG during an episode of chest discomfort
Cardiac markers	Elevated (eg, troponin T or I >0.1 ng/mL)	Slightly elevated (eg, troponin T >0.01 but <0.1 ng/mL)	Normal

[a] An estimation of the short-term risks of death and nonfatal cardiac ischemic events in unstable angina is a complex multivariable problem that cannot be fully specified in a table such as this; therefore, this table is meant to offer general guidance and illustration rather than rigid algorithms.

Adapted from Braunwald E, Mark DB, Jones RH, et al. Unstable angina: diagnosis and management. Rockville, MD: Agency for Health Care Policy and Research and the National Heart, Lung, and Blood Institute, US Public Health Service, US Department of Health and Human Services; 1994; AHCPR Publication No. 94-0602; with permission.

Table 3
Various risk models for prediction of outcome in unstable angina/non-ST and ST-segment elevation myocardial infarction

TIMI score (0–7) (each variable has a score of 1)	GRACE model 6 months post-discharge death (1–263)		GRACE model (in-hospital death)		PURSUIT model	mortality	mortality/MI
Age ≥65 y	Age, y		Age, y		Age, y		
	<40	0	≤30	0	50	0	8 (11)
	40–49	18	30–39	25	60	2 (3)	9 (12)
	50–59	36	40–49	41	70	4 (6)	11 (13)
	60–69	55	50–59	58	80	6 (9)	12 (14)
	70–79	73	60–69	75			
	80–89	91	70–79	91			
	≥90	100	80–89	100			
			≥90				
At least 3 risk factors or CAD (DM, hypertension, hypercholesterolemia, diabetes, current smoker)	H/O myocardial infarction 24		Cardiac arrest at admission 39		Gender		
					Female	0	0
					Male	1	1
ST Deviation	ST-segment depression 11		28		ST depression on presenting ECG		
					No	0	0
					Yes	3	1

Severe angina

Resting heart rate (beats/min)	
≤49.9	0
50–69.9	3
70–89.9	9
90–109.9	14
110–149	23
150–199.9	35
≥200	43

Systolic BP mm Hg	
≤79.9	24
80–99.9	22
100–119.9	18
120–139.9	14
140–159.9	10
160–199.9	4
≥200	0
	15

Elevation of serum cardiac markers

Significant coronary stenosis

Initial serum creatinine, mg/dL	
0–0.39	1
0.4–0.79	3
0.8–1.19	5
1.2–1.59	7
1.6–1.99	9
2–3.99	15
≥4	24

H/O CHF

No in-hospital PCI   14

Resting heart rate (beats/min)	
≤50	0
50–69	3
70–89	9
90–109	15
110–149	24
150–199	38
≥200	46

Systolic BP mm Hg	
≤80	58
80–99	53
100–119	43
120–139	34
140–159	24
160–199	10
≥200	0
	14

Serum creatinine, mg/dL	
0–0.39	1
0.4–0.79	4
0.8–1.19	7
1.2–1.59	10
1.6–1.99	13
2–3.99	21
≥4	28

Heart rate		
80	0	0
100	1 (2)	0
120	2 (5)	0

Systolic BP mm Hg		
120	0	0
100	1	0
80	2	0

Worse Canadian Cardiovascular Society class in previous 6 weeks		
No angina;	0	0
I or II	2	2
III or IV		

Signs of heart failure (rales)		
No	0	0
Yes	3	2

disease, and higher short- and long-term mortality in a nonselected, community-based population presenting with NSTEMI [17].

Risk models for ST-elevation myocardial infarction

Global risk assessment tools integrate various demographic, presentation, and EKG variables into a single score that not only conveys overall
estimate for patient prognosis from STEMI but also helps plan clinical strategies, with high-risk interventions geared toward higher-risk patients. The
use of these tools should not delay time-sensitive coronary revascularization
of these patients. In addition to the GRACE model described earlier, several
other risk-assessment tools have been proposed for patients presenting with
STEMI [1,2,4,7]. Several predictors of high risk for complications have been
identified for patients who have STEMI. The TIMI risk group has proposed
two models [1,2] that are both derived from the In TIME trial. The first uses
a simple algorithm using only age, heart rate, and systolic blood pressure
(heart rate $\times$ [age/10]^2/systolic blood pressure). Ten baseline variables
(age ≥ 75 years, Killip II–IV, heart rate > 100 bpm, anterior MI or left bundle branch block, systolic blood pressure < 100 mm Hg, time to reperfusion
> 4 hours, weight < 67 kg, prior angina, diabetes, and hypertension) consti-
tuted the other TIMI risk score that showed a greater than 40-fold graded
increase in mortality, with scores ranging from 0 to more than 8. Other
models with similar discriminatory ability are available. In the setting of
STEMI, it is paramount have a risk model that is simple, accurate, and
can be easily applied by prehospital care providers, emergency department
physicians, or other health care professionals involved in the management
of these patients. Several available models are listed in Fig. 1 [18].

Several key points must be underscored: (1) The C-statistic of most of
these models are above 0.75, indicating good discriminatory ability; (2)

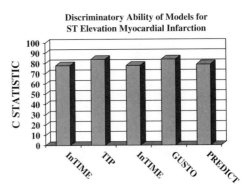

Fig. 1. Various models available for STEMI. All models contain simple and easily obtainable
variables and maintain high discriminatory ability as shown with high C-statistic.

most models are derived from trial settings and derived from patients eligible for thrombolysis, limiting generalizability of these models to general population; (3) variables included in most models are the same and easily obtainable; (4) most prognostic information is contained in only a few presentation variables (eg, age, lower systolic blood pressure, higher heart rate, Killip class, anterior infarction); and (5) the discriminatory ability of these models can be further improved with inclusion of comorbid conditions and evaluation of ejection fraction [18]. Many of these models have been externally validated in Registries and Cohort studies with modest to excellent success [19]. The strategy of risk stratification was also tested to identify patients benefiting most from higher-risk primary angioplasty procedures. In the Danish Multicenter Randomized Study on Fibrinolytic Therapy Versus Acute Coronary Angioplasty in Acute Myocardial Infarction (DANAMI-2) trial, 1527 patients were classified into low-risk (TIMI risk score 0–4), or high-risk (TIMI risk score ≥5) [20]. In the low-risk group, no difference was seen in mortality (primary angioplasty, 8%; fibrinolysis, 5.6%;

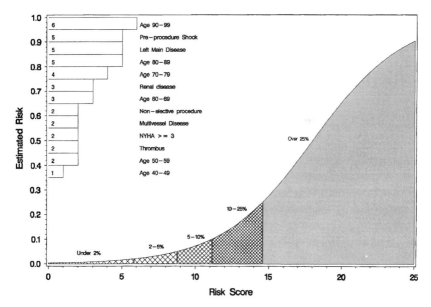

Fig. 2. Mayo Clinic Risk Score. Major adverse cardiovascular complications on the y axis (in-hospital death, Q-myocardial infarction, stroke, and emergent coronary artery bypass grafting) go up with increase in the risk score (*horizontal axis*). Estimated rates of procedural complications for the integer scoring system. The integers are proportional to the estimated continuous coefficient from the logistic model. Percentages at risk are shown for each of the five risk categories: ≤2% is very low risk for complications with coronary angioplasty; >2% to 5%, low risk; >5% to 10%, moderate risk; >10% to 25%, high risk; and >25%, very high risk. NYHA, New York Heart Association classification. (*From* Singh M, Lennon RJ, Holmes Jr DR, et al. Correlates of procedural complications and a simple integer risk score for percutaneous coronary intervention. J Am Coll Cardiol 2002;40(3):391; with permission.)

Table 4
Risk models for primary angioplasty

Variable	PAMI	Risk score	CADILLAC	Risk score
Age	>75 y	7	>65	2
	65–75	3		
Killip class	>1	2	2 or 3	3
Heart rate (bpm)	>100	2		
Diabetes mellitus	Yes	2		
Anterior myocardial infarction or left bundle branch block	Yes	2		
Baseline ejection fraction <40%				4
Renal insufficiency				3
Anemia				2
Final TIMI flow 0–2				2
Three-vessel disease				2
Outcome measured	6-month mortality		30-day, and 1-year mortality	

$P = .11$). In the high-risk group, however, significant reduction in mortality was noted with primary angioplasty compared with fibrinolysis (25.3% versus 36.2%; $P = .02$), highlighting identification of high-risk patients benefiting from primary angioplasty. The discriminant accuracy of the TIMI models was significantly improved with the addition of measures of comorbidity (PREDICT model) [7], or measure of ejection fraction [18]. However, adding these variables adds complexity to the models, limiting their applicability where time-dependent reperfusion is paramount.

Risk models for primary angioplasty

Several models are available for health care professionals to risk-stratify patients undergoing percutaneous coronary interventions (PCI) (Fig. 2). Most models also include patients undergoing primary PCI for STEMI. Older age, presence of cardiogenic shock, presentation with MI within 24 hours of symptoms, nonelective nature of the procedure, low ejection fraction, and chronic kidney disease are important baseline and noninvasive variables associated with poor outcome [21–27]. Few angiographic features (left main or three-vessel disease) not used in the other models for MI appear in some models predicting risk during PCI. Two risk models from the CADILLAC trial [28] and pooled analyses of the PAMI trial [10] were developed and validated in a population of MI undergoing primary PCI (Table 4). These models were developed from trials that excluded patients who had cardiogenic shock.

Summary

Risk stratification is an integral part of patients presenting with MI. It helps identify patients who have a high probability of this diagnosis and also recognizes patients likely to have high early hazard for major adverse cardiovascular events. Higher-risk patients benefit from glycoprotein IIb/ IIIa inhibitor and invasive revascularization procedures. These stratification models, therefore, not only help identify high-risk patients but also guide therapy. The availability of risk models encompassing the whole spectrum of ACS (GRACE) makes their use easier despite presenting diagnosis with or without ST-segment elevation. Additionally, including easily obtainable variables at presentation, determining longer-term prognosis, and validating these models in other datasets make them hugely attractive. Specific models are available for STEMI, NSTEMI, or patients undergoing PCI for NSTEMI or primary PCI for STEMI. Future challenges lie in applying these models to the management of patients who have MI. Early identification of higher-risk status should help health care providers triage these patients to undergo therapies guided by their risk status.

References

[1] Morrow DA, Antman EM, Giugliano RP, et al. A simple risk index for rapid initial triage of patients with ST-elevation myocardial infarction: an InTIME II substudy. Lancet 2001; 358(9293):1571–5.

[2] Morrow DA, Antman EM, Charlesworth A, et al. TIMI risk score for ST-elevation myocardial infarction: A convenient, bedside, clinical score for risk assessment at presentation: an intravenous nPA for treatment of infarcting myocardium early II trial substudy. Circulation 2000;102(17):2031–7.

[3] Lee KL, Woodlief LH, Topol EJ, et al. Predictors of 30-day mortality in the era of reperfusion for acute myocardial infarction. Results from an international trial of 41,021 patients. GUSTO-I Investigators. Circulation 1995;91(6):1659–68.

[4] Selker HP, Griffith JL, Beshansky JR, et al. Patient-specific predictions of outcomes in myocardial infarction for real-time emergency use: a thrombolytic predictive instrument. Ann Intern Med 1997;127(7):538–56.

[5] Antman EM, Cohen M, Bernink PJ, et al. The TIMI risk score for unstable angina/non-ST elevation MI: a method for prognostication and therapeutic decision making. JAMA 2000; 284(7):835–42.

[6] Boersma E, Pieper KS, Steyerberg EW, et al. Predictors of outcome in patients with acute coronary syndromes without persistent ST-segment elevation. Results from an international trial of 9461 patients. The PURSUIT Investigators. Circulation 2000;101(22):2557–67.

[7] Jacobs DR Jr, Kroenke C, Crow R, et al. PREDICT: a simple risk score for clinical severity and long-term prognosis after hospitalization for acute myocardial infarction or unstable angina: the Minnesota heart survey. Circulation 1999;100(6):599–607.

[8] Granger CB, Goldberg RJ, Dabbous O, et al. Predictors of hospital mortality in the global registry of acute coronary events. Arch Intern Med 2003;163(19):2345–53.

[9] Eagle KA, Lim MJ, Dabbous OH, et al. A validated prediction model for all forms of acute coronary syndrome: estimating the risk of 6-month postdischarge death in an international registry. JAMA 2004;291(22):2727–33.

[10] Addala S, Grines CL, Dixon SR, et al. Predicting mortality in patients with ST-elevation myocardial infarction treated with primary percutaneous coronary intervention (PAMI risk score). Am J Cardiol 2004;93(5):629–32.

[11] Braunwald E, Antman EM, Beasley JW, et al. ACC/AHA guideline update for the management of patients with unstable angina and non-ST-segment elevation myocardial infarction–2002: summary article: a report of the American College of Cardiology/American Heart

Association Task Force on Practice Guidelines (Committee on the Management of Patients With Unstable Angina). Circulation 2002;106(14):1893–900.

[12] Anderson HV, Cannon CP, Stone PH, et al. One-year results of the Thrombolysis in Myocardial Infarction (TIMI) IIIB clinical trial. A randomized comparison of tissue-type plasminogen activator versus placebo and early invasive versus early conservative strategies in unstable angina and non-Q wave myocardial infarction. J Am Coll Cardiol 1995;26(7): 1643–50.

[13] Inhibition of platelet glycoprotein IIb/IIIa with eptifibatide in patients with acute coronary syndromes. The PURSUIT Trial Investigators. Platelet glycoprotein IIb/IIIa in unstable angina: receptor suppression using integrilin therapy. N Engl J Med 1998;339(7):436–43.

[14] Braunwald E, Jones RH, Mark DB, et al. Diagnosing and managing unstable angina. Agency for Health Care Policy and Research. Circulation 1994;90(1):613–22.

[15] Cohen M, Stinnett SS, Weatherley BD, et al. Predictors of recurrent ischemic events and death in unstable coronary artery disease after treatment with combination antithrombotic therapy. Am Heart J 2000;139(6):962–70.

[16] Bugiardini R. Risk stratification in acute coronary syndrome: focus on unstable angina/non-ST segment elevation myocardial infarction. Heart 2004;90(7):729–31.

[17] Brilakis ES, Wright RS, Kopecky SL, et al. Association of the PURSUIT risk score with predischarge ejection fraction, angiographic severity of coronary artery disease, and mortality in a nonselected, community-based population with non-ST-elevation acute myocardial infarction. Am Heart J 2003;146(5):811–8.

[18] Singh M, Reeder GS, Jacobsen SJ, et al. Scores for post-myocardial infarction risk stratification in the community. Circulation 2002;106(18):2309–14.

[19] Morrow DA, Antman EM, Parsons L, et al. Application of the TIMI risk score for ST-elevation MI in the National Registry of Myocardial Infarction 3. JAMA 2001;286(11):1356–9.

[20] Thune JJ, Hoefsten DE, Lindholm MG, et al. Simple risk stratification at admission to identify patients with reduced mortality from primary angioplasty. Circulation 2005;112(13): 2017–21.

[21] Holmes DR Jr, Berger PB, Garratt KN, et al. Application of the New York State PTCA mortality model in patients undergoing stent implantation. Circulation 2000;102(5):517–22.

[22] Kimmel SE, Berlin JA, Strom BL, et al. Development and validation of simplified predictive index for major complications in contemporary percutaneous transluminal coronary angioplasty practice. The Registry Committee of the Society for Cardiac Angiography and Interventions. J Am Coll Cardiol 1995;26(4):931–8.

[23] Moscucci M, Kline-Rogers E, Share D, et al. Simple bedside additive tool for prediction of in-hospital mortality after percutaneous coronary interventions. Circulation 2001;104(3): 263–8.

[24] Qureshi MA, Safian RD, Grines CL, et al. Simplified scoring system for predicting mortality after percutaneous coronary intervention. J Am Coll Cardiol 2003;41(11):1890–5.

[25] Singh M, Lennon RJ, Holmes DR Jr, et al. Correlates of procedural complications and a simple integer risk score for percutaneous coronary intervention. J Am Coll Cardiol 2002;40(3): 387–93.

[26] Singh M, Rihal CS, Selzer F, et al. Validation of Mayo Clinic risk adjustment model for in-hospital complications after percutaneous coronary interventions, using the National Heart, Lung, and Blood Institute dynamic registry. J Am Coll Cardiol 2003;42(10):1722–8.

[27] Singh M, Rihal CS, Lennon RJ, et al. A critical appraisal of current models of risk stratification for percutaneous coronary interventions. Am Heart J 2005;149(5):753–60.

[28] Halkin A, Singh M, Nikolsky E, et al. Prediction of mortality after primary percutaneous coronary intervention for acute myocardial infarction: the CADILLAC risk score. J Am Coll Cardiol 2005;45(9):1397–405.

ELSEVIER
SAUNDERS

THE MEDICAL
CLINICS
OF NORTH AMERICA

Med Clin N Am 91 (2007) 617–637

Thrombolysis in Acute Myocardial Infarction: Current Status

Thomas J. Kiernan, MD, MRCPI,
Bernard J. Gersh, MB, ChB, DPhil*

*Division of Cardiovascular Diseases, Mayo Clinic, 200 First Street SW,
Rochester, MN 55905, USA*

Despite improvements in therapy, acute ST-segment elevation myocardial infarction (STEMI) remains an enormous public health problem in industrialized countries, and recent trends emphasize the growing effects of this disease in the developing world [1]. An estimated 700,000 persons in the United States will have a first myocardial infarction (MI) in 2006, and about 500,000 will have recurrent attacks [2]. Estimates of the percentage of patients with acute coronary syndrome who have STEMI range from 30% to 45% [3]. During the last decade, a progressive increase has occurred in the proportion of patients who present with non-STEMI compared with STEMI [4]. Nonetheless, the risk of mortality associated with STEMI increases for every 30 minutes that elapse before the patient's condition is recognized and treated [5]. In addition, most sudden cardiac deaths are believed to have an ischemic basis [6].

The most generally accepted pathophysiologic mechanism underlying acute MI involves erosion or sudden rupture of an atherosclerotic cap that has been weakened by internal metalloproteinase activity [7]. Exposure of blood to collagen and other matrix elements stimulates platelet adhesion, activation, and aggregation; thrombin generation; and fibrin formation. Coronary vasospasm has a variable contributory role. When these processes lead to reduction or interruption of coronary blood flow, MI is the usual consequence. Postmortem studies of MI have shown thromboemboli and distal atheroemboli in small intramyocardial arteries in a high proportion of cases [8]. Animal models have shown that myocardial cell death begins within 15 minutes of coronary occlusion and proceeds rapidly in a wave

* Corresponding author.
E-mail address: gersh.bernard@mayo.edu (B.J. Gersh).

doi:10.1016/j.mcna.2007.02.005
medical.theclinics.com

front from endocardium to epicardium [9]. Timely reperfusion (within about 3 hours) achieves partial myocardial salvage, with the extent of necrosis being modified by metabolic demands and collateral blood supply.

Currently, the general consensus is that primary percutaneous coronary intervention (PPCI) is the preferred approach to reperfusion therapy when delivered in expert centers [10]. Rapid administration of fibrinolytic therapy is associated with excellent outcomes and may be the preferred therapy in patients presenting very early (within 2 hours) after symptom onset [11]. Providing PPCI to all patients can be difficult, especially with geographic constraints from one region to another. It is important to understand the dynamic relationship among reperfusion, myocardial salvage, and mortality reduction (Fig. 1) to select the correct reperfusion strategy, especially if no facilities for PPCI are available [12].

Coronary fibrinolysis: historical perspective

In 1933, Tillet and Garner [13] isolated a fibrinolytic substance from beta-hemolytic *Streptococcus* species; it was later named streptokinase. Rentrop and associates [14] used coronary angiography to show that the intracoronary administration of streptokinase caused lysis of coronary thrombi in patients with acute MI. In 1971, a European Working Party [15] led by Marc Verstraete showed in a multicenter trial that use of streptokinase with MI decreased the rate of hospital mortality from 26.3% to 18.5%. Markis and colleagues [16] showed in 1981 that intracoronary streptokinase administration indeed salvaged ischemic myocardium in patients with evolving MI.

During the early 1980s, Rijken and Collen [17] were able to purify from melanoma cell lines a substance called human extrinsic plasminogen activator that was later renamed tissue plasminogen activator (tPA). In 1984, melanoma-derived tPA was tested in seven patients with acute MI; prompt thrombolysis occurred in six patients [18].

Fibrinolytic agents

Fibrinolysis is mediated by plasmin, a nonspecific serine protease that degrades clot-associated fibrin and fibrinogen, disrupting evolving thrombus. Thrombolytic agents are all plasminogen activators, directly or indirectly converting the proenzyme plasminogen to plasmin. Plasmin degrades several proteins including fibrin, fibrinogen, prothrombin, and factors V and VII. The most frequently used thrombolytics worldwide are streptokinase (Streptase), tenecteplase (TNKase), and reteplase (Retavase) (Table 1).

Streptokinase is a 415–amino acid bacterial protein. Streptokinase, the least expensive fibrinolytic and still widely used globally, is administered by short-term infusions. This enzyme, however, is antigenic, has little fibrin

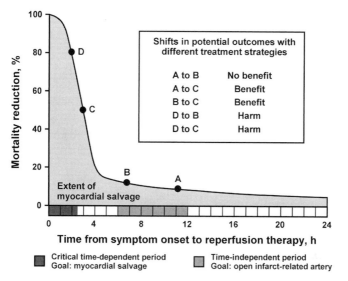

Fig. 1. Hypothetical construct of the relationship among the duration of symptoms of acute MI before reperfusion therapy, mortality reduction, and extent of myocardial salvage. Mortality reduction as a benefit of reperfusion therapy is greatest in the first 2 to 3 hours after symptom onset, which is mainly a result of myocardial salvage. The exact duration of this critical early period may be modified by several factors, including the presence of functioning collateral coronary arteries, ischemic preconditioning, myocardial oxygen demands, and duration of sustained ischemia. After this early period, the magnitude of the mortality benefit is much reduced, and as the mortality reduction curve flattens, time to reperfusion therapy is less critical. If a treatment strategy is able to move patients back up the curve, a benefit would be expected. The benefit of a shift from points A or B to point C would be substantial, but the benefit of a shift from point A to point B would be small. A treatment strategy that delays therapy during the early critical period, such as patient transfer for percutaneous coronary intervention, would be harmful (shift from point D to point C or B). Between 6 and 12 hours after the onset of symptoms, opening the infarct-related artery is the primary goal of reperfusion therapy, and primary percutaneous coronary intervention is preferred over fibrinolytic therapy. The possible contribution to mortality reduction of opening the infarct-related artery, independent of myocardial salvage, is not shown. (*From* Gersh BJ, Stone GW, White HD, et al. Pharmacological facilitation of primary percutaneous coronary intervention for acute myocardial infarction: is the slope of the curve the shape of the future? JAMA 2005;293(8):979–86; with permission. Copyright © 2004, American Medical Association. All rights reserved.)

specificity, and causes substantial systemic lytic effects in clinical doses. Because streptokinase is produced by hemolytic streptococci, antistreptococcal antibodies invariably develop in patients who receive streptokinase, which precludes readministration of the enzyme.

Tenecteplase is a genetically modified version of tPA (alteplase) with a triple-site substitution that increases the plasma half-life, fibrin binding, and resistance to plasminogen activator inhibitor-1. Its slower plasma clearance allows convenient single-bolus administration, and tenecteplase has higher fibrin specificity than all other thrombolytic agents. It is currently the most widely used agent in the United States. Reteplase, a second-generation

Table 1
Comparison of fibrinolytic agents

	Characteristic						
Agent	Immunogenicity	Plasminogen activator	Relative fibrin specificity	Plasma half-life (min)	Dosage	PAI-1 resistance	Genetic alteration to native tPA
Streptokinase	Yes	Direct	−	23	1.5 MU in 30–60 min	No	Not related to native tPA; produced by β-hemolytic streptococci
Alteplase	No	Direct	++	4–6	15-mg bolus + 90-min infusion up to 85 mg	No	No; recombinant version
Reteplase	No	Direct	+	18	10-MU + 10-MU double bolus, 30 min apart	NK	Yes; finger, EGF, and kringle-1 regions deleted
Tenecteplase	No	Direct	+++	20	≈ 0.5 mg/kg single bolus	Yes	Yes; 2 single-AA substitutions in kringle-1 and substitution of 4 AAs in catalytic domain
Lanoteplase	NK	Direct	+	37	120 kU/kg single bolus	NK	Yes; finger and EGF regions deleted, glycosylation sites in kringle-1 domain modified

Abbreviations: AA, amino acid; EGF, epidermal growth factor; kU, thousand units; MU, million units; NK, not known; PAI-1, plasminogen activator inhibitor-1.

thrombolytic agent, is also a mutant version of tPA, but unlike tenecteplase it has a single-chain deletion mutation. The deletion results in decreased plasma clearance, allowing double-bolus administration. Fibrin specificity is lower than that of tenecteplase owing to the removal of the finger domain.

Selected investigational fibrinolytics

Saruplase (Rescupase) is a recombinant nonglycosylated form of human prourokinase that has less fibrin specificity and stability than glycosylated prourokinase [19]. Comparative clinical studies of saruplase versus strepto-kinase and tPA have shown early coronary patency rates greater than for streptokinase and similar to that for 3-hour tPA infusions, but the intracranial hemorrhage (ICH) rates for saruplase were greater than for streptokinase [20]. Lanoteplase (nPA) is another tPA mutant, but further development of this drug has been terminated because of increased rates of ICH in early clinical studies. Staphylokinase is a single-chain, 136–amino acid protein secreted by strains of *Staphylococcus aureus* and manufactured by recombinant DNA technology for clinical use [21]. Staphylokinase is antigenic, inducing neutralizing antibodies within 1 week. Of note, a staphylokinase variant has been produced with 4 domains: a plasminogen activator domain derived from staphylokinase, a fibrin affinity domain containing a K2 motif derived from tPA, an antiplatelet domain with Arg-Gly-Asp sequences, and an anticoagulant domain derived from hirudin [22]. This variant has been tested in vitro and remains a theoretically attractive lytic agent, but it has not been tested clinically.

Effects on mortality

The main trials of thrombolysis from the 1980s, which examined mortal-ity, are summarized in Table 2 [23]. The GISSI-1 (Gruppo Italiano per lo Studio della Streptochinasi nell'Infarto Miocardico-1) study [24] was the first prospective megatrial that showed convincingly that thrombolytic ther-apy decreased mortality rates in acute MI. This trial showed a statistically significant 18% relative reduction in overall in-hospital mortality rates in patients treated with streptokinase within 12 hours of the onset of symptoms [24]. The ISIS-2 (Second International Study of Infarct Survival) trial showed that the 35-day cardiac mortality rate was decreased 23% by aspirin alone, 25% by streptokinase alone, and 42% by combined aspirin and streptokinase [25].

The AIMS (effect of intravenous APSAC on mortality after acute myo-cardial infarction: preliminary report of a placebo-controlled trial) trial of the anisoylated plasminogen streptokinase activator complex (APSAC) showed decreases in 30-day mortality rates from 12.2% to 6.4% and in 1-year mortality rates from 17.8% to 11.1% with the use of APSAC [26]. The FTT (Fibrinolytic Therapy Trialists') Collaborative Group [27] pooled

Table 2
Early mortality trials of streptokinase, tPA, and APSAC

| Trial | Characteristic | | | | | | |
	No. of sites	Agent	Dose/duration	Enrollment dates	Placebo/ blinding	Age criteria (y)	Symptom duration (h)
GISSI-1 [24] (N = 11,806)	176	SK	1.5 MU/1 h	2/84–6/85	No	All	<12
ISIS-2 [25] (N = 17,187)	417	SK	1.5 MU/1 h	3/85–12/87	Yes	All	<24
AIMS [26] (N = 1,258)	39	APSAC	30 U/5 min	9/85–10/87	Yes	<75	<6
ASSET [23] (N = 5,011)	52	tPA	100 mg/3 h	11/86–2/88	Yes	<75	<5

Abbreviations: APSAC, anisoylated plasminogen streptokinase activator complex; MU, million units; SK, streptokinase.

data from nine controlled trials of patients with suspected acute MI. The 45,000 patients who presented with ST-segment elevation or complete left bundle branch block had an absolute mortality reduction of 30 per 1,000 for treatment within the first 6 hours, 20 per 1,000 for treatment in 7 to 12 hours, and a statistically uncertain reduction of 13 per 1,000 for treatment beyond 12 hours (Fig. 2). These large trials provided clinical evidence that thrombolytic-induced reperfusion, when administered in a timely manner, produced an improvement in mortality beyond that achieved with placebo.

Prehospital fibrinolysis

The benefit of fibrinolysis is greatest when administered early after the onset of symptoms and decreases rapidly after the first several hours [28]. A meta-analysis of six trials with 6434 patients showed a decrease in all-cause hospital mortality with prehospital fibrinolysis versus in-hospital thrombolysis [29]. Pooled data were insufficient to show a statistically significant difference in longer-term mortality at 1 or 2 years. Nonetheless, the GREAT (Grampian Region Early Anistreplase Trial) [30] study's follow-up results showed that the benefit of prehospital thrombolysis is maintained

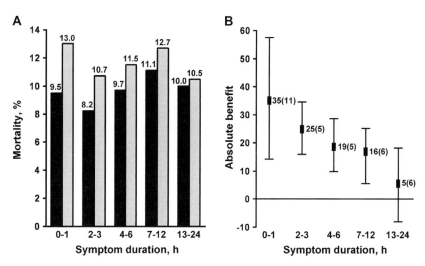

Fig. 2. Outcomes of fibrinolytic therapy according to duration of symptoms before treatment. (*A*) Graph shows the effect of fibrinolytic therapy (*black bars*) versus placebo (*white bars*) on mortality in patients classified according to duration of symptoms before treatment. (*B*) Graph shows absolute benefit of fibrinolytic therapy (lives saved per 1,000 treated, standard deviation in parentheses) with confidence intervals. (*From* Fibrinolytic Therapy Trialists' (FTT) Collaborative Group. Indications for fibrinolytic therapy in suspected acute myocardial infarction: collaborative overview of early mortality and major morbidity results from all randomised trials of more than 1000 patients. Lancet 1994;343(8893):311–22. Erratum in: Lancet 1994;343(8899):742A; with permission.

at 5 years in patients treated out of hospital among whom transport times to a hospital were prolonged.

Kalla and colleagues [31] recently showed that in the first 2 hours of symptom onset, thrombolytic therapy was associated with a lower mortality rate (5.1%) than was PPCI (7.8%), although the difference was not statistically significant ($P = .37$). Of the 1,053 consecutive patients evaluated in this registry, 34 received prehospital thrombolytic therapy at a median of 76 minutes after symptom onset [31]. This result corresponds with those of the randomized PRAGUE-2 (Primary Angioplasty in Patients Transferred From General Community Hospitals to Specialized PTCA Units With or Without Emergency Thrombolysis) [32] and CAPTIM (Comparison of Angioplasty and Prehospital Thrombolysis in Acute Myocardial Infarction) trials [33]. The results to date of prehospital thrombolysis for acute MI are indeed encouraging, but the implementation of corresponding clinical policies is subject to the logistic constraints of different health care systems and geographic regions throughout the world.

Early comparative fibrinolytic trials

After establishing the general utility of fibrinolysis in STEMI, clinical trials focused on comparisons of new drug regimens. The salient features of major early comparative outcomes trials are presented in Table 3. The GISSI-2 [34] and ISIS-3 [35] studies did not show any difference in mortality between streptokinase and tPA. The GUSTO-1 (Global Use of Streptokinase and tPA for Occluded Coronary Arteries-1) study [36] showed a marginal benefit of tPA over streptokinase in terms of mortality, with a 14% risk reduction.

Comparative trials with bolus fibrinolytics

The ASSENT-2 (Assessment of the Safety and Efficacy of a New Thrombolytic-2) trial [37] showed that 30-day mortality and ICH rates were identical when comparing weight-adjusted tenecteplase and accelerated tPA

Table 3
Early comparative fibrinolytic trials

| Trial | Characteristic | | |
	Agents tested	30-d mortality (%)	ICH rate (%)
GISSI-2 [34] ($N = 20,891$)	SK	8.5	0.3
	tPA	8.9	0.4
ISIS-3 [35] ($N = 40,775$)	SK	10.6	0.2
	tPA	10.3	0.7
	APSAC	10.5	0.6
GUSTO-1 [36] ($N = 41,021$)	SK	7.3	0.5
	tPA	6.3	0.7
	SK+tPA	7.0	0.9

Abbreviations: APSAC, anisoylated plasminogen streptokinase activator complex; SK, streptokinase.

(Table 4). The GUSTO-III trial [38] did not show any survival advantage for double-bolus reteplase over accelerated tPA. The In-TIME II (Intravenous nPA for Treating Infarcting Myocardium Early-2) trial [39] showed that 30-day mortality rates were similar with use of either lanoteplase or tPA, but a significantly higher ICH rate occurred in patients receiving lanoteplase, which has now been withdrawn from the market.

Thus, in terms of efficacy, the bolus fibrinolytic agents have not surpassed accelerated tPA, but tenecteplase and reteplase proved equivalent in efficacy to tPA. The ease of administration of these agents, especially tenecteplase, and their reduced transfusion requirements paved the way for these bolus agents to become the standard of care for thrombolytic therapy.

Combinations of fibrinolytic therapy and platelet inhibitors or low-molecular-weight heparins

Fibrinolytics and glycoprotein IIb/IIIa inhibitors

Various clinical trials have evaluated the addition of glycoprotein IIb/IIIa inhibitors or low-molecular-weight heparins (LMWH) to thrombolytic therapy. The hypothesis was that combined fibrinolysis and major platelet inhibition would lead to improved 30-day mortality. Studies such as TIMI-14 [40] and SPEED (strategies for patency enhancement in the emergency department) [41] used tPA and reteplase, respectively, in conjunction with abciximab (ReoPro). In these trials, combination therapy was associated with higher Thrombolysis in Myocardial Infarction (TIMI) 3 flow rates in the infarct-related artery, but the trials were not powered to address mortality. This improvement in TIMI 3 flow, however, came at the expense of a higher rate of major bleeding complications and transfusions. Two of the largest trials published regarding the combination of fibrinolysis and glycoprotein IIb/IIIa inhibition are the GUSTO-V acute MI trial [42] and the ASSENT-3 trial (Table 5) [43]. These trials showed that patients receiving reduced-dose fibrinolytics in combination with abciximab had fewer ischemic complications after acute MI, albeit without any incremental benefit in mortality. However, the incidence of bleeding complications was increased, especially with the use

Table 4
Comparative trials with bolus fibrinolytics

	Characteristic		
Trial	Agents used	30-d mortality (%)	ICH rate (%)
ASSENT-2 [37] ($N = 16,949$)	tPA	6.15	0.94
	Tenecteplase	6.18	0.93
GUSTO-III [38] ($N = 15,059$)	tPA	7.24	0.87
	Reteplase	7.47	0.91
InTIME-II [39] ($N = 15,060$)	tPA	6.61	0.64
	Lanoteplase	6.75	1.12

Table 5
Comparative outcomes trials with combined fibrinolytic and glycoprotein IIb/IIIa inhibitor therapy

Trial	Agents used	30-d mortality (%)	ICH rate (%)	Major bleeding rate (%)
GUSTO V [42] (N = 16,588)	Reteplase	6.2	0.6	2.3
	Half-dose reteplase + abciximab	5.9	0.6	4.6
ASSENT-3 [43] (N = 6,095)	Tenecteplase + heparin	6.0	0.93	2.2
	Tenecteplase + enoxaparin	5.4	0.88	3.0
	Half-dose tenecteplase + abciximab	6.6	0.94	4.3

of abciximab as a combination agent. In ASSENT-3 [43] an increased rate of bleeding was also seen with tenecteplase plus enoxaparin (Lovenox) in comparison with the tenecteplase/heparin control.

Fibrinolytics and aspirin

At a dose of 162 mg or more, aspirin produces a rapid clinical antithrombotic effect caused by immediate and near-total inhibition of thromboxane A_2 production. The ISIS-2 trial [25] conclusively showed the efficacy of aspirin alone for treatment of evolving acute MI, with an absolute risk difference in 35-day mortality of 2.4% (relative risk reduction, 23%). When aspirin was combined with streptokinase, the absolute risk difference in mortality was 5.2% (relative risk reduction, 42%). The use of aspirin is contraindicated in those with hypersensitivity to salicylate. In patients with true aspirin allergy (hives, nasal polyps, bronchospasm, or anaphylaxis), clopidogrel (Plavix) or ticlopidine (Ticlid) may be substituted.

Fibrinolytics and clopidogrel

In the CLARITY-TIMI 28 Trial [44], patients who received clopidogrel and LMWH within 12 hours of STEMI had particularly low rates of cardiovascular death (3.2%) and recurrent MI (3.0%) without a significant increase in major or minor bleeding. The COMMIT (clopidogrel and metoprolol in myocardial infarction trial) Trial [45], which enrolled 45,852 patients admitted within 24 hours of suspected acute MI, also showed a highly significant 9% proportional decrease in the primary composite end points of death, reinfarction, or stroke with clopidogrel. Clopidogrel, therefore, is important as an adjunctive agent in the treatment of STEMI.

Fibrinolytics and LMWH

The recently published ExTRACT-TIMI 25 trial [46] showed a significant 33% decrease in the relative risk of myocardial reinfarction at 30 days with enoxaparin versus unfractionated heparin, which suggests that the antithrombotic effect of this agent is superior to that achieved with the currently recommended regimen of unfractionated heparin. Despite adjusting the dosage of enoxaparin for age and renal function, however, a significant increase in major bleeding episodes was associated with its use. In a substudy analysis of the CLARITY-TIMI 28 Trial [47], treatment with LMWH, compared with unfractionated heparin, was associated with improved late patency and a lower rate of cardiovascular death or recurrent MI, without a significant increase in major or minor bleeding. LMWH has proven its worth in terms of efficacy with regard to major cardiovascular end points, but caution is still warranted concerning the association with major bleeding, especially in the elderly and patients with established renal impairment.

Fibrinolytic therapy and direct antithrombins

The TIMI 9A [48] and HIT-III (Hirudin for Improvement of Thrombolysis-III) [49] trials focused on patients with STEMI, testing the direct antithrombin desirudin (Iprivask) versus heparin. These trials were terminated prematurely because of unacceptable rates of serious bleeding, particularly ICH. The HERO-2 trial [50] randomly assigned 17,073 patients with acute MI to receive unfractionated heparin or bivalirudin (Angiomax); 30-day mortality, the primary end point, did not differ between the bivalirudin and heparin groups (10.8% versus 10.9%). However, adjudicated 30-day reinfarction was decreased with bivalirudin (2.8% versus 3.6%, $P = .004$) at the expense of increased moderate to severe bleeding and increased ICH. In the PRIME (Promotion of Reperfusion in Myocardial Infarction Evolution) trial [51], efegatran appeared to offer no clear advantage over heparin as an adjunct to thrombolysis for STEMI. The direct thrombin inhibitors are associated with an increased rate of adverse bleeding.

Risks and adverse effects of thrombolysis

Bleeding

Bleeding is the predominant risk of thrombolytic therapy. ICH is the most feared bleeding risk, occurring in about 0.5% to 1.0% of those who receive thrombolytic therapy, with substantial risk of fatality or disability [52]. Noncerebral bleeding risk has benefited from increased fibrin selectivity, but cerebral bleeding has not. The four independent predictors of increased ICH risk are age older than 65 years, weight of less than 70 kg, hypertension on admission, and female sex (Fig. 3) [53].

Allergy, hypotension, and fever

Streptokinase is antigenic and may be allergenic, but serious anaphylaxis or bronchoconstriction are rarely associated with its use (<0.2% to 0.5%

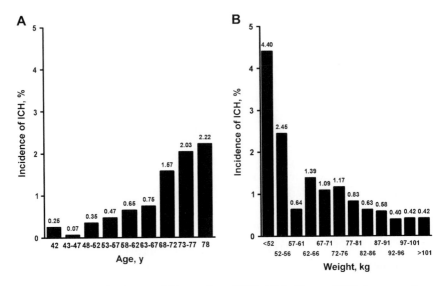

Fig. 3. Risk factors for intracranial hemorrhage (ICH). (*A*) Incidence of ICH shown as a function of age group. (*B*) Incidence of ICH shown as a function of body weight. (*From* Van de Werf F, Barron HV, Armstrong PW, et al, ASSENT-2 Investigators. Assessment of Safety and Efficacy of a New Thrombolytic. Incidence and predictors of bleeding events after fibrinolytic therapy with fibrin-specific agents: a comparison of TNK-tPA and rt-PA. Eur Heart J 2001; 22(24):2253–61; with permission.)

incidence) [25]. In the ISIS-3 trial [35], any allergic-type reaction was reported in 3.6% of those given streptokinase and in 0.8% of those taking tPA. Angioneurotic and periorbital edema, hypersensitivity vasculitis, and purpuric rashes have been reported rarely, especially after repeat administration, and prior exposure (more than 5 days earlier) or prior allergic reaction are relative contraindications to using streptokinase [26]. If an antigenic-based adverse effect occurs, an alteplase-based or nonstreptokinase-based agent should be used if thrombolysis is required in the future.

Contraindications and cautions for the use of fibrinolysis in STEMI are shown in Box 1 [54]. The American College of Cardiology/American Heart Association guidelines for the use of fibrinolytics in acute MI (as of 2004) are detailed in Box 2 [54].

Fibrinolysis in the elderly

Recent data from a meta-analysis of 11 published randomized, clinical trials of fibrinolysis in STEMI concluded that, despite established mortality reductions with fibrinolysis, elderly compared with younger patients still have a three to fourfold increased risk of mortality and adverse events when treated with fibrinolysis and antithrombin therapy [55]. The trials have found variable and conflicting results over time concerning fibrinolytic

Box 1. Contraindications and cautions for fibrinolysis in STEMI

Absolute contraindications to thrombolysis:
Any prior ICH
Known structural cerebrovascular lesion (eg, arteriovenous malformation)
Known malignant intracranial neoplasm (primary or metastatic)
Ischemic stroke within 3 months *except* acute ischemic stroke within 3 hours
Suspected aortic dissection
Active bleeding or bleeding diathesis (except menses)

Relative contraindications to thrombolysis:
History of chronic, severe, poorly controlled hypertension
Severe uncontrolled hypertension on presentation (systolic blood pressure >180 mm Hg or diastolic blood pressure >110 mm Hg)
Traumatic or prolonged (>10 min) cardiopulmonary resuscitation or major surgery (within <3 weeks)
Recent (within 2 to 4 weeks) internal bleeding
Noncompressible vascular punctures
For streptokinase/anistreplase: prior exposure (>5 days) or prior allergic reaction to these agents
Pregnancy
Active peptic ulcer
History of prior ischemic stroke (>3 months), dementia, or known intracranial pathology not covered in absolute contraindications
Current use of anticoagulants: the higher the INR, the higher the risk of bleeding

---

From Antman EM, Anbe DT, Armstrong PW, et al, American College of Cardiology, American Heart Association, Canadian Cardiovascular Society. ACC/AHA guidelines for the management of patients with ST-elevation myocardial infarction: executive summary. A report of the American College of Cardiology/American Heart Association Task Force on Practice Guidelines. J Am Coll Cardiol 2004;44(3):671–719. Erratum in J Am Coll Cardiol 2005;45(8):1376; with permission. Copyright © 2004, American Heart Association, Inc.

therapy in elderly patients. A Medicare analysis suggested that fibrinolytic therapy may even be harmful in those older than 75 years [56]. In contrast, a large Swedish registry found a 12% risk reduction in the composite end point of cerebral bleeding and 1-year mortality in elderly patients receiving

Box 2. Current guidelines for use of fibrinolytics in acute MI, American College of Cardiology/American Heart Association 2004

Class I

1. In the absence of contraindications, fibrinolytic therapy should be administered to STEMI patients with symptom onset within the prior 12 hours and ST-segment elevation > 0.1 mV in at least two contiguous precordial leads or at least two adjacent limb leads (level of evidence: A).

2. In the absence of contraindications, fibrinolytic therapy should be administered to STEMI patients with symptom onset within the prior 12 hours and new or presumably new left bundle branch block (level of evidence: A).

Class IIa

1. In the absence of contraindications, it is reasonable to administer fibrinolytic therapy to STEMI patients with symptom onset within the prior 12 hours and 12-lead electrocardiography findings consistent with a true posterior MI (level of evidence: C).

2. In the absence of contraindications, it is reasonable to administer fibrinolytic therapy to patients with symptoms of STEMI beginning within the prior 12 to 24 hours who have continuing ischemic symptoms and ST elevation greater than 0.1 mV in at least two contiguous precordial leads or at least two adjacent limb leads (level of evidence: B).

Class III

1. Fibrinolytic therapy should not be administered to asymptomatic patients whose initial symptoms of STEMI began more than 24 hours earlier (level of evidence: C).

2. Fibrinolytic therapy should not be administered to patients whose 12-lead ECG shows only ST-segment depression except if a true posterior MI is suspected (level of evidence: A).

From Antman EM, Anbe DT, Armstrong PW, et al, American College of Cardiology, American Heart Association, Canadian Cardiovascular Society. ACC/AHA guidelines for the management of patients with ST-elevation myocardial infarction: executive summary. A report of the American College of Cardiology/American Heart Association Task Force on Practice Guidelines. J Am Coll Cardiol 2004;44(3):671–719. Erratum in J Am Coll Cardiol 2005;45(8):1376; with permission. Copyright © 2004, American Heart Association, Inc.

thrombolytic therapy [57]. Similarly, the FTT overview of randomized trial data in patients older than 75 years reported 35-day mortality rate to be decreased with fibrinolytic therapy [27]. The consensus is that older patients should never be denied reperfusion therapy on the basis of age alone, but the risks of bleeding are significantly increased, particularly in some subsets of patients.

Adjunctive therapies

Nitrates

The physiologic effects of nitrates include decreased preload and afterload through peripheral arterial and venous dilation, relaxation of epicardial coronary arteries to improve coronary flow, and dilation of collateral vessels, potentially creating a more favorable subendocardial-to-epicardial flow ratio. Nitrate-induced vasodilatation may also have particular utility in those rare patients with coronary spasm presenting as STEMI. However, the large GISSI-3 [58] and ISIS-4 [59] trials did not show any mortality benefit for patients receiving nitrate therapy.

Beta-blockers

The ISIS-1 investigators showed that the use of atenolol (Tenormin) was associated with a 15% decrease in vascular mortality during the acute treatment period [60]. In the TIMI-II trial, in which all patients received intravenous alteplase, those randomly assigned to receive intravenous metoprolol followed by oral metoprolol daily had a decreased incidence of subsequent nonfatal reinfarction and recurrent ischemia compared with those started on oral metoprolol 6 days after the acute event [61]. The COMMIT Trial [45] randomly assigned 45,852 patients admitted within 24 hours of acute MI to initial intravenous then daily oral metoprolol versus placebo. Metoprolol in acute MI patients did not significantly decrease in-hospital mortality. However, it decreased the absolute risks both of reinfarction and of ventricular fibrillation by 5 per 1,000. Overall, metoprolol increased the risk of cardiogenic shock by 11 per 1,000. In acute MI, it is essential to start beta-blocker therapy when the patient is hemodynamically stable and then continue long-term therapy. Intravenous beta-blocker therapy should not be implemented routinely in acute MI, but each patient should be considered and assessed individually from a hemodynamic standpoint.

Magnesium

The MAGIC (Magnesium in Coronaries) trial [62] enrolled 6,213 high-risk MI patients, defined as aged 65 years or older or unsuitable for acute reperfusion therapy. Magnesium or placebo was administered within 6 hours of symptom onset, but no beneficial effect of magnesium was seen on heart failure, ventricular arrhythmias, or mortality. The report concluded that routine administration of intravenous magnesium had no role in the treatment of high-risk patients with acute MI.

Angiotensin-converting enzyme inhibitors

The CONSENSUS II study [63], in which intravenous enalapril was administered within 24 hours or less of an acute MI, showed no improvement in survival during the 180 days after infarction. Other studies have shown that high-risk post-MI patients definitely benefit from oral angiotensin-converting enzyme inhibitor therapy [64]. The data indicate that intravenous angiotensin-converting enzyme inhibition within the first 24 hours of STEMI is not beneficial, but oral therapy started early and continued is of great benefit, especially in high-risk patients.

Potential postlytic strategies

Patients with persistent ST-segment elevation who do not respond to thrombolytic therapy should be identified early and transferred promptly for rescue angioplasty to a center with the appropriate facilities (Fig. 4). Stable patients can undergo angiography at any time during their hospital course depending on symptoms or results of functional assessment such as exercise electrocardiography. This strategy is essentially different from using

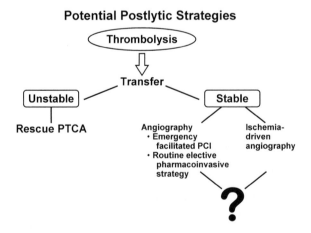

Fig. 4. Potential postlytic strategies. Potential strategies after thrombolysis include prompt transfer of patients with persistent ST-segment elevation or ongoing chest pain to a center for rescue percutaneous transluminal coronary angioplasty (PTCA). Patients who are stable and have already received thrombolysis can be transferred for immediate angiography and, if coronary anatomy permits, facilitated percutaneous coronary intervention (PCI). Other stable patients can be sent for angiography at a later stage, dictated by results of stress testing or by ongoing anginal symptoms.

"facilitated PCI," in which patients are transferred immediately after thrombolysis for angiography and PCI if anatomically suitable; indeed, recent studies [65] have shown that lytic-associated facilitated PCI may be ineffective and unsafe.

Summary

In the current era, thrombolytic therapy still has much to offer, especially when administered early in the "golden window" of the first 3 hours after symptom onset. Further development of prehospital fibrinolytic regimens may be beneficial in the future management of STEMI. PPCI may still be the preferred treatment option for STEMI in the modern world, but globally not all STEMI patients have access to such a facility. Therefore, thrombolytic therapy likely will continue to be part of everyday clinical practice for the foreseeable future and beyond.

Acknowledgment

Editing, proofreading, and reference verification were provided by the Section of Scientific Publications, Mayo Clinic.

References

[1] Thom T, Haase N, Rosamond W, et al. American Heart Association Statistics Committee and Stroke Statistics Subcommittee. Heart disease and stroke statistics—2006 update: a report from the American Heart Association Statistics Committee and Stroke Statistics Subcommittee. Circulation 2006;113(6):e85–151 [Epub 2006 Jan 11]. Erratum in: Circulation 2006;113(14):e696.

[2] Atherosclerosis risk in communities (ARIC, 1987–2000): NHLBI.

[3] Wiviott SD, Morrow DA, Frederick PD, et al. Performance of the thrombolysis in myocardial infarction risk index in the National Registry of Myocardial Infarction-3 and -4: a simple index that predicts mortality in ST-segment elevation myocardial infarction. J Am Coll Cardiol 2004;44(4):783–9.

[4] Rogers WJ, Canto JG, Lambrew CT, et al. Temporal trends in the treatment of over 1.5 million patients with myocardial infarction in the US from 1990 through 1999: the National Registry of Myocardial Infarction 1, 2 and 3. J Am Coll Cardiol 2000;36(7):2056–63.

[5] French WJ. Trends in acute myocardial infarction management: use of the National Registry of Myocardial Infarction in quality improvement. Am J Cardiol 2000;85(5A):5B–9B.

[6] Priori SG, Aliot E, Blomstrom-Lundqvist C, et al. Task force on sudden cardiac death of the European Society of Cardiology. Eur Heart J 2001;22(16):1374–450. Erratum in: Eur Heart J 2002;23(3):257.

[7] Shah PK, Falk E, Badimon JJ, et al. Human monocyte-derived macrophages induce collagen breakdown in fibrous caps of atherosclerotic plaques: potential role of matrix-degrading metalloproteinases and implications for plaque rupture. Circulation 1995;92(6):1565–9.

[8] Falk E. Unstable angina with fatal outcome: dynamic coronary thrombosis leading to infarction and/or sudden death: autopsy evidence of recurrent mural thrombosis with peripheral embolization culminating in total vascular occlusion. Circulation 1985;71(4):699–708.

[9] Reimer KA, Jennings RB. The "wavefront phenomenon" of myocardial ischemic cell death. II. Transmural progression of necrosis within the framework of ischemic bed size (myocardium at risk) and collateral flow. Lab Invest 1979;40(6):633–44.

[10] Keeley EC, Boura JA, Grines CL. Primary angioplasty versus intravenous thrombolytic therapy for acute myocardial infarction: a quantitative review of 23 randomised trials. Lancet 2003;361(9351):13–20.

[11] Nallamothu BK, Bates ER. Percutaneous coronary intervention versus fibrinolytic therapy in acute myocardial infarction: is timing (almost) everything? Am J Cardiol 2003;92(7): 824–6.

[12] Gersh BJ, Anderson JL. Thrombolysis and myocardial salvage: results of clinical trials and the animal paradigm—paradoxic or predictable? Circulation 1993;88(1):296–306.

[13] Tillett WS, Garner RL. Fibrinolytic activity of hemolytic streptococci. J Exp Med 1933;58: 485–502.

[14] Rentrop P, Blanke H, Karsch KR, et al. Selective intracoronary thrombolysis in acute myocardial infarction and unstable angina pectoris. Circulation 1981;63(2):307–17.

[15] European Working Party. Streptokinase in recent myocardial infarction: a controlled multicentre trial. Br Med J 1971;3(770):325–31.

[16] Markis JE, Malagold M, Parker JA, et al. Myocardial salvage after intracoronary thrombolysis with streptokinase in acute myocardial infarction. N Engl J Med 1981;305(14): 777–82.

[17] Rijken DC, Collen D. Purification and characterization of the plasminogen activator secreted by human melanoma cells in culture. J Biol Chem 1981;256(13):7035–41.

[18] Van de Werf F, Ludbrook PA, Bergmann SR, et al. Coronary thrombolysis with tissue-type plasminogen activator in patients with evolving myocardial infarction. N Engl J Med 1984; 310(10):609–13.

[19] Armstrong PW, Collen D. Fibrinolysis for acute myocardial infarction: current status and new horizons for pharmacological reperfusion, part 2. Circulation 2001;103(24):2987–92.

[20] Tebbe U, Michels R, Adgey J, et al. Comparison Trial of Saruplase and Streptokinase (COMPASS) Investigators. Randomized, double-blind study comparing saruplase with streptokinase therapy in acute myocardial infarction: the COMPASS Equivalence Trial. J Am Coll Cardiol 1998;31(3):487–93.

[21] Collen D, Lijnen HR. Staphylokinase, a fibrin-specific plasminogen activator with therapeutic potential? Blood 1994;84(3):680–6.

[22] Matsuo O. An ideal thrombolytic and antithrombotic agent? J Thromb Haemost 2005;3(10): 2154–5.

[23] Wilcox RG, von der Lippe G, Olsson CG, et al. Trial of tissue plasminogen activator for mortality reduction in acute myocardial infarction: Anglo-Scandinavian Study of Early Thrombolysis (ASSET). Lancet 1988;2(8610):525–30.

[24] Gruppo Italiano per lo Studio della Streptochinasi nell'Infarto Miocardico (GISSI). Effectiveness of intravenous thrombolytic treatment in acute myocardial infarction. Lancet 1986;1(8478):397–402.

[25] ISIS-2 (Second International Study of Infarct Survival) Collaborative Group. Randomised trial of intravenous streptokinase, oral aspirin, both, or neither among 17,187 cases of suspected acute myocardial infarction: ISIS-2. Lancet 1988;2(8607):349–60.

[26] AIMS Trial Study Group. Effect of intravenous APSAC on mortality after acute myocardial infarction: preliminary report of a placebo-controlled clinical trial. Lancet 1988;1(8585): 545–9.

[27] Fibrinolytic Therapy Trialists' (FTT) Collaborative Group. Indications for fibrinolytic therapy in suspected acute myocardial infarction: collaborative overview of early mortality and major morbidity results from all randomised trials of more than 1000 patients. Lancet 1994; 343(8893):311–22. Erratum in: Lancet 1994;343(8899):742.

[28] Boersma E, Maas AC, Deckers JW, et al. Early thrombolytic treatment in acute myocardial infarction: reappraisal of the golden hour. Lancet 1996;348(9030):771–5.

[29] Morrison LJ, Verbeek PR, McDonald AC, et al. Mortality and prehospital thrombolysis for acute myocardial infarction: a meta-analysis. JAMA 2000;283(20):2686–92.

[30] GREAT Group. Feasibility, safety, and efficacy of domiciliary thrombolysis by general practitioners: Grampian region early anistreplase trial. BMJ 1992;305(6853):548–53.

[31] Kalla K, Christ G, Karnik R, et al. Vienna STEMI Registry Group. Implementation of guidelines improves the standard of care: the Viennese registry on reperfusion strategies in ST-elevation myocardial infarction (Vienna STEMI registry). Circulation 2006;113(20): 2398–405 [Epub 2006 May 15].

[32] Widimsky P, Budesinsky T, Vorac D, et al. 'PRAGUE' Study Group Investigators. Long distance transport for primary angioplasty vs immediate thrombolysis in acute myocardial infarction: final results of the randomized national multicentre trial—PRAGUE-2. Eur Heart J 2003;24(1):94–104.

[33] Bonnefoy E, Lapostolle F, Leizorovicz A, et al. Comparison of Angioplasty and Prehospital Thromboysis in Acute Myocardial Infarction study group. Primary angioplasty versus prehospital fibrinolysis in acute myocardial infarction: a randomised study. Lancet 2002; 360(9336):825–9.

[34] Gruppo Italiano per lo Studio della Sopravvivenza nell'Infarto Miocardico. GISSI-2: a factorial randomised trial of alteplase versus streptokinase and heparin versus no heparin among 12,490 patients with acute myocardial infarction. Lancet 1990;336(8707):65–71.

[35] ISIS-3 (Third International Study of Infarct Survival) Collaborative Group. ISIS-3: a randomised comparison of streptokinase vs tissue plasminogen activator vs anistreplase and of aspirin plus heparin vs aspirin alone among 41,299 cases of suspected acute myocardial infarction. Lancet 1992;339(8796):753–70.

[36] The GUSTO Angiographic Investigators. The effects of tissue plasminogen activator, streptokinase, or both on coronary-artery patency, ventricular function, and survival after acute myocardial infarction. N Engl J Med 1993;329(22):1615–22. Erratum in: N Engl J Med 1994;330(7):516.

[37] Assessment of the Safety and Efficacy of a New Thrombolytic Investigators. Single-bolus tenecteplase compared with front-loaded alteplase in acute myocardial infarction: the ASSENT-2 double-blind randomised trial. Lancet 1999;354(9180):716–22.

[38] The Global Use of Strategies to Open Occluded Coronary Arteries (GUSTO III) Investigators. A comparison of reteplase with alteplase for acute myocardial infarction. N Engl J Med 1997;337(16):1118–23.

[39] InTIME-II Investigators. Intravenous NPA for the treatment of infarcting myocardium early: InTIME-II, a double-blind comparison of single-bolus lanoteplase vs accelerated alteplase for the treatment of patients with acute myocardial infarction. Eur Heart J 2000; 21(24):2005–13.

[40] Antman EM, Giugliano RP, Gibson CM, et al. The TIMI 14 Investigators. Abciximab facilitates the rate and extent of thrombolysis: results of the thrombolysis in myocardial infarction (TIMI) 14 trial. Circulation 1999;99(21):2720–32.

[41] Strategies for Patency Enhancement in the Emergency Department (SPEED) Group. Trial of abciximab with and without low-dose reteplase for acute myocardial infarction. Circulation 2000;101(24):2788–94.

[42] Topol EJ, GUSTO V Investigators. Reperfusion therapy for acute myocardial infarction with fibrinolytic therapy or combination reduced fibrinolytic therapy and platelet glycoprotein IIb/IIIa inhibition: the GUSTO V randomised trial. Lancet 2001;357(9272):1905–14.

[43] Assessment of the Safety and Efficacy of a New Thrombolytic Regimen (ASSENT)-3 Investigators. Efficacy and safety of tenecteplase in combination with enoxaparin, abciximab, or unfractionated heparin: the ASSENT-3 randomised trial in acute myocardial infarction. Lancet 2001;358(9282):605–13.

[44] Sabatine MS, Cannon CP, Gibson CM, et al. CLARITY-TIMI 28 Investigators. Addition of clopidogrel to aspirin and fibrinolytic therapy for myocardial infarction with ST-segment elevation. N Engl J Med 2005;352(12):1179–89 [Epub 2005 Mar 9].

[45] Chen ZM, Jiang LX, Chen YP, et al, COMMIT (ClOpidogrel and Metoprolol in Myocardial Infarction Trial) collaborative group. Addition of clopidogrel to aspirin in 45,852 patients with acute myocardial infarction: randomised placebo-controlled trial. Lancet 2005; 366(9497):1607–21.

[46] Antman EM, Morrow DA, McCabe CH, et al. ExTRACT-TIMI 25 Investigators. Enoxaparin versus unfractionated heparin with fibrinolysis for ST-elevation myocardial infarction. N Engl J Med 2006;354(14):1477–88 [Epub 2006 Mar 14].

[47] Sabatine MS, Morrow DA, Montalescot G, et al. Clopidogrel as Adjunctive Reperfusion Therapy (CLARITY)-Thrombolysis in Myocardial Infarction (TIMI) 28 Investigators. Angiographic and clinical outcomes in patients receiving low-molecular-weight heparin versus unfractionated heparin in ST-elevation myocardial infarction treated with fibrinolytics in the CLARITY-TIMI 28 Trial. Circulation 2005;112(25):3846–54 [Epub 2005 Nov 15].

[48] Antman EM. Hirudin in acute myocardial infarction: safety report from the Thrombolysis and Thrombin Inhibition in Myocardial Infarction (TIMI) 9A Trial. Circulation 1994;90(4): 1624–30.

[49] Neuhaus KL, von Essen R, Tebbe U, et al. Safety observations from the pilot phase of the randomized r-Hirudin for Improvement of Thrombolysis (HIT-III) study: a study of the Arbeitsgemeinschaft Leitender Kardiologischer Krankenhausarzte (ALKK). Circulation 1994;90(4):1638–42.

[50] White H, Hirulog and Early Reperfusion or Occlusion (HERO)-2 Trial Investigators. Thrombin-specific anticoagulation with bivalirudin versus heparin in patients receiving fibrinolytic therapy for acute myocardial infarction: the HERO-2 randomised trial. Lancet 2001; 358(9296):1855–63.

[51] PRIME Investigators. Multicenter, dose-ranging study of efegatran sulfate versus heparin with thrombolysis for acute myocardial infarction: the Promotion of Reperfusion in Myocardial Infarction Evolution (PRIME) trial. Am Heart J 2002;143(1):95–105.

[52] Gore JM, Granger CB, Simoons ML, et al. Stroke after thrombolysis: mortality and functional outcomes in the GUSTO-I trial. Global Use of Strategies to Open Occluded Coronary Arteries. Circulation 1995;92(10):2811–8.

[53] Van de Werf F, Barron HV, Armstrong PW, et al. ASSENT-2 Investigators, Assessment of Safety and Efficacy of a New Thrombolytic. Incidence and predictors of bleeding events after fibrinolytic therapy with fibrin-specific agents: a comparison of TNK-tPA and rt-PA. Eur Heart J 2001;22(24):2253–61.

[54] Antman EM, Anbe DT, Armstrong PW, et al. American College of Cardiology, American Heart Association, Canadian Cardiovascular Society. ACC/AHA guidelines for the management of patients with ST-elevation myocardial infarction: executive summary. A report of the American College of Cardiology/American Heart Association Task Force on Practice Guidelines. J Am Coll Cardiol 2004;44(3):671–719. Erratum in J Am Coll Cardiol 2005; 45(8):1376.

[55] Ahmed S, Antman EM, Murphy SA, et al. Poor outcomes after fibrinolytic therapy for ST-segment elevation myocardial infarction: impact of age (a meta-analysis of a decade of trials). J Thromb Thrombolysis 2006;21(2):119–29.

[56] Thiemann DR, Coresh J, Schulman SP, et al. Lack of benefit for intravenous thrombolysis in patients with myocardial infarction who are older than 75 years. Circulation 2000;101(19): 2239–46.

[57] Stenestrand U, Wallentin L. Register of Information and Knowledge About Swedish Heart Intensive Care Admissions (RIKS-HIA). Fibrinolytic therapy in patients 75 years and older with ST-segment-elevation myocardial infarction: one-year follow-up of a large prospective cohort. Arch Intern Med 2003;163(8):965–71.

[58] Gruppo Italiano per lo Studio della Sopravvivenza nell'Infarto Miocardico. GISSI-3: effects of lisinopril and transdermal glyceryl trinitrate singly and together on 6-week mortality and ventricular function after acute myocardial infarction. Lancet 1994;343(8906): 1115–22.

[59] ISIS-4 (Fourth International Study of Infarct Survival) Collaborative Group. ISIS-4: a randomised factorial trial assessing early oral captopril, oral mononitrate, and intravenous magnesium sulphate in 58,050 patients with suspected acute myocardial infarction. Lancet 1995; 345(8951):669–85.

[60] First International Study of Infarct Survival Collaborative Group. Randomised trial of intravenous atenolol among 16 027 cases of suspected acute myocardial infarction: ISIS-1. Lancet 1986;2(8498):57–66.

[61] Roberts R, Rogers WJ, Mueller HS, et al. Immediate versus deferred beta-blockade following thrombolytic therapy in patients with acute myocardial infarction: results of the Thrombolysis in Myocardial Infarction (TIMI) II-B Study. Circulation 1991;83(2):422–37.

[62] Magnesium in Coronaries (MAGIC) Trial Investigators. Early administration of intravenous magnesium to high-risk patients with acute myocardial infarction in the Magnesium in Coronaries (MAGIC) Trial: a randomised controlled trial. Lancet 2002;360(9341): 1189–96.

[63] Swedberg K, Held P, Kjekshus J, et al. Effects of the early administration of enalapril on mortality in patients with acute myocardial infarction: results of the Cooperative New Scandinavian Enalapril Survival Study II (CONSENSUS II). N Engl J Med 1992;327(10): 678–84.

[64] Ambrosioni E, Borghi C, Magnani B. The Survival of Myocardial Infarction Long-Term Evaluation (SMILE) Study Investigators. The effect of the angiotensin-converting-enzyme inhibitor zofenopril on mortality and morbidity after anterior myocardial infarction. N Engl J Med 1995;332(2):80–5.

[65] Keeley EC, Boura JA, Grines CL. Comparison of primary and facilitated percutaneous coronary interventions for ST-elevation myocardial infarction: quantitative review of randomised trials. Lancet 2006;367(9510):579–88. Erratum in: Lancet 2006;367(9523):1656.

ELSEVIER
SAUNDERS

THE MEDICAL
CLINICS
OF NORTH AMERICA

Med Clin N Am 91 (2007) 639–655

Primary Percutaneous Coronary Intervention in Acute Myocardial Infarction

Kanwar P. Singh, MD[a],*, Robert A. Harrington, MD[b]

[a]Pat and Jim Calhoun Cardiovascular Center, University of Connecticut,
Farmington, CT 06030, USA
[b]Division of Cardiology and Duke Clinical Research Institute,
2400 Pratt St., Lower Level, Durham, NC 27705, USA

Primary percutaneous coronary intervention (PCI) has emerged as the preferred therapy for acute ST-segment elevation myocardial infarction (STEMI). Multiple randomized trials and a recent meta-analysis have shown that primary PCI lowers mortality, stroke, and recurrent myocardial infarction rates compared with fibrinolytic therapy, even when patients initially present to community centers and require transfer to centers with primary PCI capabilities. These findings are robust and seem consistent across multiple subgroups with high degrees of clinical risk. Research efforts to improve the availability and performance of primary PCI for STEMI address three main questions: (1) what is the optimal adjuvant medical regimen to improve the chances of medical reperfusion and hence facilitate primary PCI; (2) whether the performance of primary PCI is safe and feasible at centers without on-site surgical backup; and (3) how systems can be refined to decrease the time that patients spend awaiting primary PCI. This article summarizes the data relating to the performance, challenges, and future directions of primary PCI for STEMI, emphasizing current American College of Cardiology (ACC)/American Heart Association (AHA) guidelines for managing STEMI.

Meta-analyses comparing primary percutaneous coronary intervention and fibrinolysis

In 1997, Weaver and colleagues [1] reported a landmark meta-analysis of trials comparing primary angioplasty with intravenous fibrinolytic therapy

* Corresponding author.
  E-mail address: ksingh@uchc.edu (K.P. Singh).

0025-7125/07/$ - see front matter © 2007 Elsevier Inc. All rights reserved.
doi:10.1016/j.mcna.2007.03.008
medical.theclinics.com

for acute myocardial infarction. This analysis of 2606 patients found a 34% relative risk reduction for mortality at 30 days among patients treated with primary angioplasty (4.4% for patients treated with primary angioplasty versus 6.5% for patients treated with fibrinolytics; odds ratio [OR], 0.66; 95% confidence interval [CI], 0.46–0.94; $P = .02$). A subsequent meta-analysis reported by Keeley and colleagues [2] in 2003 described both short- and long-term outcomes among 7739 patients who had STEMI and were eligible to undergo fibrinolytic therapy studied in 23 randomized clinical trials of primary PCI, including stenting versus fibrinolytics. In this analysis, the performance of primary PCI for STEMI was associated with short-term (4–6 weeks) reductions in multiple key clinical end points, including death (7% versus 9%, $P = .0002$), nonfatal MI (3% versus 7%, $P < .0001$), recurrent ischemia (6% versus 21%, $P < .0001$), total stroke (1% versus 2%, $P = .0004$), and hemorrhagic stroke (0.05% versus 1%, $P < .0001$). The only clinical end point not favoring PCI was major hemorrhage, which was higher among patients treated with PCI (7% versus 5%, $P = .032$); these bleeding events were largely related to arterial access sites. Long-term findings, defined as 6 to 18 months follow-up, showed that short-term benefits of primary PCI are durable (Fig. 1).

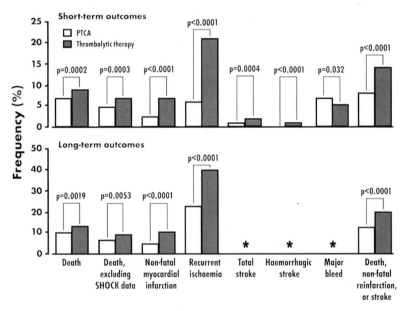

Fig. 1. Short- and long-term outcomes in patients who have STEMI treated with primary PCI or intravenous lysis. PCI, percutaneous coronary intervention; PTCA, percutaneous transluminal coronary angioplasty; STEMI, ST-elevation myocardial infarction. (*From* Keeley EC, Boura JA, Grines CL. Primary angioplasty versus intravenous thrombolytic therapy for acute myocardial infarction: a quantitative review of 23 randomized trials. Lancet 2003;361(9351): 13–20; with permission.)

Recognizing the potential for era-effect, the Keeley study also compared the results after breaking down the 23 studies into two groups: the first 10 trials included in the Weaver analysis versus the subsequent 13. Similar benefits with primary PCI were found. Furthermore, when stratified according to the type of fibrinolytic, benefits of primary PCI were similar regardless of whether or not medical reperfusion was fibrin-specific (Fig. 2). Additionally, the analysis of the five trials involving patient transfer for primary PCI found similar treatment benefits, despite a mean treatment delay of 39 minutes with PCI.

These data underpin the current ACC/AHA/Society for Coronary Angiography and Interventions (SCAI) 2005 Guidelines Update for Percutaneous Coronary Intervention, which assign a class I indication with level A evidence for the performance of primary PCI within 90 minutes of presentation and within 12 hours of symptom onset by skilled operators with experienced staff and an appropriate environment, including cardiac surgical backup [3].

Importance of timing of symptom onset

Observations from large datasets have shown that the timing of the onset of symptoms plays a critical role in determining the optimal strategy for reperfusion [4]. The Comparison of Angioplasty and Prehospital Thrombolysis in Acute Myocardial Infarction (CAPTIM) study was a randomized trial

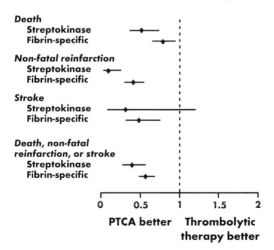

Fig. 2. Short-term outcomes among patients treated with primary PCI or fibrinolysis according to fibrin specificity. PCI, percutaneous coronary intervention; PTCA, percutaneous transluminal coronary angioplasty. (*From* Keeley EC, Boura JA, Grines CL. Primary angioplasty versus intravenous thrombolytic therapy for acute myocardial infarction: a quantitative review of 23 randomized trials. Lancet 2003;361(9351):13–20; with permission.)

comparing prehospital fibrinolysis and transfer to an interventional facility (with rescue PCI if needed) with primary PCI in patients who had STEMI. The overall study found no advantage in the primary end point of the 30-day incidence of death, nonfatal recurrent infarction, or disabling stroke for primary PCI. Randomization within 2 hours (n = 460) or 2 hours or more (n = 374) after symptom onset did not affect the primary treatment outcome. However, patients randomized within 2 hours of symptom onset strongly trended toward lower 30-day mortality with prehospital fibrinolysis compared with patients randomized to treatment with primary PCI (2.2% versus 5.7%, $P = .058$), whereas mortality was similar in patients randomized with a longer duration of symptoms (5.9% versus 3.7%, $P = .47$) [5]. Furthermore, cardiogenic shock, although rare, was less frequent with fibrinolytic therapy than with primary PCI among patients randomized within 2 hours of symptom onset (1.3% versus 5.3%, $P = .032$), whereas rates were similar in patients randomized later. This trial had a planned sample size of 1200 patients to detect the anticipated 5% absolute reduction of the primary end point with a two-sided α of 0.05 and β of 0.15 (85% power). Unfortunately, the trial was terminated because of poor patient recruitment. Funding was lost after 840 patients (70% of the intended sample size) were enrolled.

In the Primary Angioplasty in AMI Patients from General Community Hospitals Transported to PTCA Units versus Emergency Thrombolysis (PRAGUE)-2 study, 850 patients who had STEMI in the Czech Republic were randomized to transportation to the nearest hospital for local fibrinolysis or to the nearest center capable of primary PCI. Randomization-to-balloon time in the PCI group was 97 ± 27 minutes, and randomization-to-needle time in the fibrinolysis group was 12 ± 10 minutes. The primary end point— mortality at 30 days—using intention-to-treat analysis occurred in 10% of the fibrinolysis group compared with 6.8% in the PCI group ($P = .12$) [6]. Among the 299 patients randomized more than 3 hours after the onset of symptoms, the mortality of the fibrinolytic group was 15.3% compared with 6% in the PCI group ($P < .02$). This unexpected finding led the study's ethical committee to halt the trial. By contrast, patients randomized within 3 hours of symptom onset (n = 551) showed no difference in mortality whether treated with fibrinolysis or transfer for primary PCI (7.4% versus 7.3%, P value not reported).

Point estimates favored primary PCI in these studies' primary end points but failed to achieve statistical significance, perhaps partly because of their premature terminations before the full sample size was achieved. However, the studies are informative regarding the importance of the timing of symptom onset. These observations, and a systematic analysis of multiple randomized and nonrandomized trials by Gersh and colleagues [7], have suggested that, for patients who present within 3 hours of symptom onset with STEMI, a strategy of fibrinolysis may be a reasonable alternative to primary PCI unless balloon inflation can occur no more than 60 minutes after fibrinolysis could be administered (Fig. 3). Current ACC/AHA guidelines for the management of STEMI include this caveat to the performance of primary PCI with a class I recommendation with level B evidence [8].

The importance of door-to-balloon time

Shorter door-to-balloon times have been shown in multiple analyses to affect mortality [4], but this concept has not been without debate because of some conflicting data. For example, the Zwolle study group analyzed data on 1791 patients who underwent primary PCI from 1994 to 2001. In their analysis, no relationship was found between door-to-balloon time and mortality. Instead, symptom onset-to-balloon time was significantly associated with angiographically favorable outcomes and 1-year mortality. Using multivariate analysis, a symptom onset-to-balloon time of more than 4 hours was identified as an independent predictor of 1-year mortality [9].

By contrast, in a much larger recent cohort study of 29,222 STEMI patients treated with PCI within 6 hours of presentation at 395 hospitals that participated in the National Registry of Myocardial Infarction (NRMI)-3 and -4 from 1999 to 2002, longer door-to-balloon time was associated with increased in-hospital mortality (mortality rate of 3.0%, 4.2%, 5.7%, and 7.4% for door-to-balloon times of 90 minutes or less, 91 to 120 minutes, 121 to 150 minutes, and more than 150 minutes, respectively; P for trend <.01) [10]. When

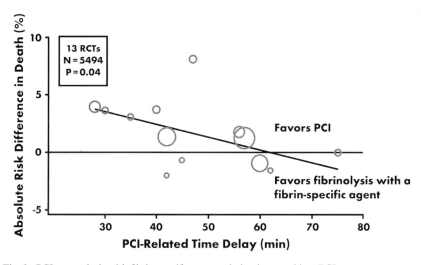

Fig. 3. PCI versus lysis with fibrin-specific agents: timing is everything. PCI, percutaneous coronary intervention; RCT, randomized controlled trial. (*From* Nallamothu BK, Antman EM, Bates ER. Primary percutaneous intervention versus fibrinolytic therapy in acute myocardial infarction: does the choice of fibrinolytic agent impact on the importance of time-to-treatment? Am J Cardiol 2004;94(6):772–4; with permission.)

adjusted for patient characteristics, patients who had door-to-balloon time of more than 90 minutes had increased mortality (OR, 1.42; 95% CI, 1.24–1.62) compared with those who had shorter door-to-balloon times. In categorical subgroup analyses, increasing mortality with longer door-to-balloon time was seen, regardless of symptom onset-to-door time (≤ 1 hour, > 1–2 hours, > 2 hours) and regardless of the presence or absence of high-risk factors. Although debate continues in the scientific community regarding the best treatment for STEMI, the push to shorten times—both from symptom onset to presentation and from door-to-balloon—makes intuitive sense and is well supported by evidence. Current ACC/AHA/SCAI guidelines recommend medical contact-to-balloon times less than 90 minutes with a class I indication with level B evidence [3,8].

Guidelines versus real-world practice

Unfortunately, STEMI care in the community continues to underperform relative to these standards. A recent analysis of more than 100,000 patients at more than 1000 hospitals in the NRMI-3 showed that few patients receive reperfusion therapy within the ACC/AHA recommended timelines [11]. In this retrospective observational study of data regarding STEMI care from 1999, only 46% of the patients in the fibrinolytic therapy cohort were treated within the recommended 30-minute door-to-needle time; only 35% of the patients in the PCI cohort were treated within the recommended 90-minute door-to-balloon time. Furthermore, improvements in these times over the subsequent 4-year study period were not statistically significant (door-to-needle: -0.01 min/y, 95% CI -0.24 to $+0.23$, $P > .9$; door-to-balloon: -0.57 min/y, 95% CI -1.24 to $+0.10$, $P = .09$). Only 33% (337 of 1015) of hospitals improved door-to-needle time by more than 1 min/y, and 26% (110 of 421) improved door-to-balloon time by more than 3 min/y. High annual PCI volume and location in New England were associated with significantly greater improvement in door-to-balloon time.

Concerted efforts are necessary to streamline logistics and reduce times at underperforming centers. Research into institutions that have successfully improved their systems of care can provide key lessons and models for the greater health care population [12].

Transfer for primary percutaneous coronary intervention

The enthusiasm for primary PCI and its attendant benefits over medical reperfusion have led to significant interest in the development of systems that allow community centers (or "spokes") to refer patients to regional tertiary care centers with primary PCI capability ("hubs"). Studies in European systems of care, such as those in the Netherlands, the Czech

Republic, and Denmark, have effectively shown that, despite inherent delays of up to 50 minutes, primary PCI imparts meaningful clinical benefits when compared with fibrinolysis [6,13,14]. Of these recent studies, the most compelling was the Danish Multicenter Randomized Study on Thrombolytic Therapy versus Acute Coronary Angioplasty in Acute Myocardial Infarction (DANAMI)-2 trial performed in Denmark, in which 1572 patients who had acute STEMI were randomized to undergo treatment with PCI or accelerated treatment with intravenous alteplase. Twenty-four spokes enrolled a total of 1129 patients, and 5 hubs enrolled a total of 443 patients. The primary end point was a composite of death, reinfarction, or disabling stroke at 30 days. Among patients presenting to spokes, the primary end point occurred in 8.5% of the patients in the PCI group compared with 14.2% of those in the fibrinolysis group ($P = .002$) [14]. The treatment effect was smaller but significant at hubs, where primary PCI did not require transfer (6.7% versus 12.3% primary end point for PCI versus fibrinolysis $P = .05$). Among all patients, the benefit was primarily driven by reduced rates of reinfarction (1.6% in the PCI arm versus 6.3% in the fibrinolysis group, $P < .001$). Point estimates favored PCI, but no statistically significant differences were observed in the rate of death (6.6% versus 7.8%, $P = .35$) or stroke (1.1% versus 2.0%, $P = .15$). Spoke-to-hub transfer required less than 2 hours in 96% of cases.

Subsequent meta-analyses of transfer for primary PCI have underscored its benefit compared with fibrinolysis. One study pooled 3750 patients from six trials of transfer for primary PCI. Using a combined primary study end point of death, recurrent myocardial infarction, or stroke, a 42% (95% CI 29–53%, $P < .001$) [15] reduction was seen in the transfer group compared with the fibrinolysis group. Individually, reinfarction was reduced by 68% (95% CI, 34–84%; $P < .001$), and stroke was reduced by 56% (95% CI, −5%–77%; $P = .015$). A trend toward reduction in all-cause mortality of 19% was seen (95% CI, −3%–36%; $P = .08$) with transfer for PCI.

Despite the beneficial features associated with transfer for primary PCI, studies evaluating transfer for primary PCI have not been executed successfully in the United States. After 39 months of enrollment, the promising Air Primary Angioplasty in Myocardial Infarction (AIR-PAMI) study was terminated prematurely because of slow patient accrual. In this study of high-risk STEMI, 138 patients (32% of anticipated sample size) were randomized to undergo primary PCI or fibrinolysis [16]. The Addressing the Value of Facilitated Angioplasty Compared with Eptifibatide Monotherapy in Acute Myocardial Infarction (ADVANCE MI) trial, another large primary PCI trial, was designed to randomize 5640 patients who had STEMI to undergo eptifibatide monotherapy or eptifibatide plus reduced-dose tenecteplase combination therapy before primary PCI. A subrandomization of enoxaparin or unfractionated heparin was planned in a 2×2 fashion. However, after enrollment of less than 3% of intended subjects over 11 months, the trial was discontinued for reasons unrelated to safety or efficacy [17].

Rather, sponsorship was terminated because the trial was believed not to be executable in its intended form. Some investigators noted that they perceived diametric pressures: enrollment requirements versus institutional efforts to shorten door-to-balloon times that may have been hampered by the delays associated with obtaining informed consent, randomization, and other vital protocol measures. Similar to the AIR-PAMI experience, patient accrual was slower than anticipated, resulting in premature termination. The ethical implications of premature termination of a trial for reasons other than achievement of a prespecified end point are considerable and have been discussed elsewhere [18]. However, given increasing financial pressures on hospitals and increased scrutiny from quality monitoring by reimbursement and accreditation agencies in the United States, clinical trials of facilitated primary PCI will need to be adapted to contemporary clinical practice with efficient consent and randomization processes.

How far away is the hub?

Conservative estimates of the percent of adults in the United States who have access to primary PCI centers are approximately 30%. However, a recent systematic review using data from the American Hospital Association Annual Survey and 2000 U.S. Census data on adults 18 years of age or older found that median distances to the closest PCI hospital were 11.3 (interquartile range [IQR] 5.7–28.5) minutes and 7.9 (IQR 3.5–22.4) miles. A total of 79% of the adult population lived within 60 minutes of a PCI hospital [19]. For those whose nearest facility does not have primary PCI, 74% would require additional transport times of less than 30 minutes if directly referred to a PCI hospital as opposed to a non-PCI hospital. Although these estimates varied substantially across urban, suburban, and rural regions, nearly 80% of Americans reside within 60 minutes of a primary PCI center. Such estimates, although encouraging, are only a part of the equation. Unfortunately, data from the NRMI 3/4 show that the median total door-to-balloon time for patients requiring transfer for primary PCI is 180 minutes, with only 4.2% achieving times less than 90 minutes [20]. Coordinated systems of care that enable and promote rapid interhospital transportation for tertiary care require more than short transport times.

In the authors' medical community in central North Carolina, primary PCI is available at a limited number of major medical centers. A large percentage of patients who have STEMI seen at Duke University Medical Center arrive from outlying facilities. In an effort to centralize and streamline STEMI care, referring physicians use a single hotline telephone number that generates a real-time conference call between the referring physician, the on-call cardiac care unit (CCU) attending physician, a CCU fellow, interventional team members, and the Duke Life Flight transport team. The method of reperfusion is chosen collectively based on the patient's clinical situation in combination with available transportation options and the anticipated transport-to-balloon times. This strategy has markedly simplified an otherwise unwieldy process and minimizes the logistical time delays to reperfusion.

Primary percutaneous coronary intervention without on-site surgical backup

The Atlantic Cardiovascular Patient Outcomes Research Team (C-PORT) study was designed to test the hypothesis that primary PCI is superior to fibrinolysis even when performed at centers with neither cardiac surgical backup nor extant PCI programs. In this study, 11 community centers in Maryland and Massachusetts were trained rigorously for 3-month periods to create new PCI programs around experienced operators. Fibrinolytic-eligible patients who had STEMI were randomized to undergo either accelerated tissue plasminogen activator or primary PCI. Between July 1996 and December 1999, 451 patients who had STEMI of less than 12 hours duration were included. The primary end point—the 6-month composite of death, recurrent myocardial infarction, or stroke— occurred in the PCI group less frequently than in the fibrinolysis group (10.7% versus 17.7%, $P = .03$) [21]. The combined end point was driven primarily by the incidence of recurrent myocardial infarction (5.3% versus 10.6%, $P = .04$). The trial was originally intended to include 2550 patients but was terminated early because of inadequate funding. The investigators concluded that, after an extensive development program, community centers can safely and effectively perform primary PCI without cardiac surgical backup. Furthermore, this program could benefit patients through reducing significant cardiovascular and cerebrovascular morbidity and mortality. Similar benefits were seen in the subsequent multicenter trial reported by Wharton and colleagues [22]. An ongoing registry called Atlantic C-PORT II is collecting data at numerous other sites in other states.

Despite these and other subsequent smaller-center experiences, current ACC/AHA/SCAI guidelines for the performance of PCI continue to classify primary PCI for STEMI without on-site surgical backup as a class III recommendation with level C evidence. However, the guidelines state that unsupported primary PCI might be considered under certain very specific (C-PORT–like) circumstances, such as performance of PCI by an experienced operator (defined as one who performs more than 75 interventions per year with at least 11 primary PCI cases) at a center performing more than 36 primary PCI cases per year with an experienced staff and 24 hour-per-day coverage; a complete array of interventional devices, including intra-aortic balloon counter pulsation; and the proven ability to transfer patients rapidly to nearby centers with cardiac surgery. Nevertheless, primary PCI performed even under these conditions without surgical backup is still given a class IIb recommendation with level B evidence. This recommendation is based on the rare but non-zero need for urgent cardiac backup, related to the discovery of coronary disease ill-suited to primary PCI or the occurrence of major complications during primary PCI that require surgical therapy (eg, dissection, perforation). The ACC/AHA/SCAI Writing Committee recommends concentrating skilled personnel in central tertiary health care settings rather than diluting resources and personnel into multiple freestanding primary PCI centers.

Adjuvant medical therapy in primary percutaneous coronary intervention and facilitated percutaneous coronary intervention

Facilitated primary PCI refers to the use of medical therapy to increase the likelihood of a patent infarct-related artery at acute angiography. The marriage of three key observations led to the concept of facilitated primary PCI: (1) time is myocardium—earlier reperfusion (medical or mechanical) leads to improved clinical outcomes; (2) although superior to fibrinolysis, primary PCI often takes longer than guidelines suggest; and (3) spontaneous reperfusion before definitive mechanical revascularization is an independent predictor of early and late survival, even when corrected for postprocedural flow [23].

Several trials have been performed to identify an optimal combination of medical therapies that would promote reperfusion during the attendant delays in performing primary PCI. The goal of these clinical trials is to determine the ideal combination of upstream medical adjuvant therapy for PCI. Candidate regimens have included full-dose fibrinolytic + PCI; reduced-dose fibrinolytic + glycoprotein receptor (GP) IIb/IIIa antagonists + PCI; and GP IIb/IIIa alone with PCI. Additional areas of investigation include the dosing and use of antithrombins, such as unfractionated heparin, low-molecular-weight heparins, and direct thrombin inhibitors, and synergistic antiplatelet therapy with thienopyridines.

Full-dose fibrinolysis

Several small clinical trials from the late 1980s and early 1990s suggested that facilitation with full-dose fibrinolysis was potentially harmful, but each had design and statistical limitations [24–27]. More recent developments in medical therapies have created new concepts in STEMI therapy. Efforts to improve pharmacologic reperfusion strategies resulted in discoveries about the central role of platelets, GP IIb/IIIa antagonists, and optimal (lower) unfractionated heparin dosing. Simultaneous improvements in interventional techniques, catheters, stents, and other devices expanded on balloon angioplasty to create the modern lesion-specific PCI approach in interventional cardiology. These parallel advances led investigators to reconsider the supposed incompatibility of fibrinolysis and primary PCI.

Unfortunately, despite these advances, it appears that full-dose fibrinolysis still cannot be recommended in the context of planned primary PCI. The recently published Assessment of the Safety and Efficacy of a New Thrombolytic Regimen (ASSENT)-4 PCI trial was a large randomized trial that showed that the use of full-dose tenecteplase (TNK) therapy before planned primary PCI was not beneficial. The study compared TNK-facilitated PCI with standard primary PCI in an open-label design study; the trial was halted on recommendation of the Data and Safety Monitoring Board after 33% of the planned 4000 patients were enrolled because an unacceptable excess of in-hospital mortality was observed in the facilitated PCI arm (6% versus 3%, $P = .0105$) [28].

Although angiographic outcomes seen on initial acute angiography were improved by full-dose tenecteplase, clinical outcomes, including death, worsened with this treatment strategy. These results illustrate the challenge in translating biomarker end points into clinical outcomes and show that reperfusion is a dynamic process that may not be adequately captured with a single "snapshot" view of the infarct-related artery obtained during acute angiography.

Glycoprotein IIb/IIIa antagonists

The use of platelet receptor glycoprotein IIb/IIIa antagonists has revolutionized the performance of PCI to reduce ischemic complications. Of the three intravenous formulations available, abciximab is the only GP IIb/IIIa antagonist supported by a significant body of evidence in acute MI. In a pooled analysis of 3266 patients, treatment with abciximab significantly reduced the 30-day composite end point of death, reinfarction, or ischemic or urgent target-vessel revascularization (TVR) (OR, 0.54; 95% CI, 0.40–0.72) [29], with trends toward reduced 30-day death and death or reinfarction, at the cost of an increased likelihood of major bleeding (OR, 1.74; 95% CI, 1.11–2.72). At 6 months, abciximab significantly reduced the occurrence of death, reinfarction, or any TVR (OR, 0.80; 95% CI, 0.67–0.97), and trends favored a reduction in mortality and the composite of death or reinfarction. The strength of these data supports the ACC/AHA class IIa recommendation with level B evidence for the use of abciximab during primary PCI. However, the use of eptifibatide or tirofiban is limited to class IIb support with level C evidence because of an absence of compelling prospective randomized evidence.

Combination therapy

Although primary PCI with full-dose fibrinolysis does not appear promising, reduced-dose fibrinolysis in combination with GP IIb/IIIa antagonists to facilitate primary PCI continues to be studied. To date, one randomized STEMI trial of GP IIb/IIIa blockade alone versus GP IIb/IIIa blockade + reduced-dose fibrinolysis with a planned immediate invasive strategy has been reported: the Bavarian Revascularization Alternatives (BRAVE) trial. This trial studied whether upstream combination therapy with reduced-dose fibrinolytics + GP IIb/IIIa blockade + primary PCI would result in smaller scintigraphic infarct size when compared with upstream GP IIb/IIIa blockade + primary PCI. Two hundred fifty-three patients who had acute STEMI were randomized to therapy with abciximab + PCI or abciximab + reduced-dose reteplase + PCI. Pre-PCI thrombolysis in myocardial infarction (TIMI) grade 3 flow was more common among patients treated with combination therapy (TIMI III flow 40% versus 18%, $P < .01$); however, scintigraphic infarct size was not reduced in the combination therapy arm versus the abciximab-alone arm (13% versus 11.5%, respectively, $P = .81$) [30]. Non-significant increases were seen in death/myocardial infarction (2.4% versus 1.6%), death/myocardial infarction /stroke (3.2% versus 1.6%), and major bleeding (5.6% versus 1.6%) with combination therapy. Subset analyses of patients who required transfer for primary PCI and those who had earlier times to revascularization showed no treatment differences.

The findings from the BRAVE trial should be interpreted cautiously because it was a small trial, significantly underpowered to show differences in clinical outcomes. Furthermore, end points such as infarct size with SPECT sestamibi scanning have not been proven to be reliable biomarkers to differentiate the clinical benefits of therapies for STEMI. Combination therapy with GP IIb/IIIa receptor blockade and fibrinolysis has been shown to improve surrogate markers such as angiographic flow patterns and ST-segment resolution in randomized clinical trials [31–34]. However, combination medical therapy without immediate PCI has not been shown to improve survival in two large studies [35,36]. Thus, the relationship between markers of reperfusion success and clinical outcomes such as mortality is uncertain. The risks and benefits of combination facilitated primary PCI are best studied in adequately powered, large-scale, definitive trials.

The Facilitated Intervention with Enhanced Reperfusion Speed to Stop Events (FINESSE) trial is the only ongoing large trial studying combination facilitated PCI for STEMI [37]. Three arms of therapy will be compared in a 1:1:1 fashion in 3000 patients: (1) early PCI after reduced-dose reteplase (5 units + 5 units) + abciximab bolus doses administered in the emergency department; (2) early PCI after abciximab bolus administered in the emergency department; and (3) primary PCI with abciximab initiated in the cardiac catheterization laboratory.

The primary efficacy end point of FINESSE is the composite of all-cause mortality and post-myocardial infarction complications within 90 days of randomization. Complications included in the end point are resuscitated ventricular fibrillation occurring more than 48 hours after randomization, rehospitalization or emergency department visit for congestive heart failure, and cardiogenic shock. This novel composite end point was chosen to reflect the physiologic hypothesis that combination medical therapy before PCI will result in earlier and improved reperfusion, leading to improved myocardial salvage, and, hence, decreased infarct size–dependent complications. Current ACC/AHA guidelines for facilitated PCI provide a cautious class IIb recommendation with level B evidence. However, the document does not distinguish between various regimens used for facilitation. Furthermore, at the 3005 guidelines publication, data from ASSENT-4 PCI were not yet available. Therefore, future recommendations will probably change to distinguish between the various types of facilitated PCI and will recommend against full-dose fibrinolysis when primary PCI is planned. The data from FINESSE will help to clarify the optimal way to use abciximab.

Bare metal stents versus drug-eluting stents in ST-segment elevation myocardial infarction

The usefulness of sirolimus and paclitaxel stents is clear among patients who have coronary disease. Multiple randomized controlled studies with these devices have shown improvements in long-term outcomes with regard to restenosis and associated TVR when compared with bare metal stents. However, their use in STEMI is presently off-label and not well described. Small registries have suggested that both sirolimus- and paclitaxel-eluting stents compare favorably with acute and long-term results with bare metal stents.

In one study of 306 consecutive patients who experienced STEMI who received sirolimus-eluting stents (SES) (n = 156) or bare metal stents (BMS) (n = 150), patients treated with SES had lower in-hospital (0.6% versus 5.3%, $P = .015$) and 6-month (1.9% versus 10.1%, $P = .003$) mortality rates [38]. At 6 months, patients who had SES were less likely to have target vessel revascularization (1.3% versus 8.1%, $P = .005$) and achieve the composite end point (death, myocardial infarction, TVR) (3.2% versus 16.1%, $P = .0001$). No subacute thrombosis or clinical restenosis occurred in the SES group. By multivariate discriminant analysis, stent type (SES versus BMS) was the most significant determinant of the 6-month composite end point ($P = .01$) and the need for target vessel revascularization ($P = .02$). Similarly, in a Canadian retrospective comparison of paclitaxel-eluting stents (PES) (n = 60) versus bare metal stents (n = 137) in consecutive patients who underwent primary or rescue PCI over a 1-year period, the PES cohort showed a 65% ($P = .02$) decrease in the combined end point of death, recurrent myocardial infarction, and target vessel revascularization at 1 year compared with the BMS group [39].

A Dutch study found no difference in the rates of major adverse cardiac events between two cohorts of SES (n = 186) and PES (n = 136) at 30 days and 1 year. At 30 days, the rate of all-cause mortality and reinfarction was similar between groups (6.5% versus 6.6% for SES and PES, respectively, $P = 1.0$) [40]. A significant difference in TVR favored SES, but this was lost at 1-year follow-up. One-year survival rates free of major adverse cardiac events were similar in the two groups (90.2% for SES and 85% for PES, $P = .16$).

Recently, the Single High Dose Bolus Tirofiban and Sirolimus Eluting Stent versus Abciximab and Bare Metal Stent in Myocardial Infarction (STRATEGY) phase II study comparing abciximab + BMS versus tirofiban + SES was reported. In this small study, 14 of 74 patients (19%; 95% CI 10%–28%) in the tirofiban plus SES group and 37 of 74 patients (50%; 95% CI, 44%–56%) in the abciximab plus BMS group reached the primary end point (death, myocardial infarction, stroke, or binary restenosis at 8 months), suggesting that a less-expensive GP IIb/IIIa antagonist with SES is a more efficacious and perhaps less expensive strategy than abciximab and BMS [41]. A follow-up phase III study, the Multicentre 2×2 Factorial Randomised Study Comparing Tirofiban Administered with the Single High-Dose Bolus versus Abciximab and Sirolimus Eluting Stent versus Bare Metal Stent in Acute Myocardial Infarction (MULTI-STRATEGY) trial with a planned enrollment of 600 patients is currently underway.

Despite the success of drug-eluting stents in reducing the risks for restenosis, concerns have arisen recently regarding late stent thrombosis; the balance of risk versus benefit requires further study.

Future directions

Ongoing research efforts seek to determine optimal ways to combine adjuvant medical therapy to lower bleeding risks while continuing to provide effective antiplatelet, antithrombin, and fibrinolytic activities. Novel approaches, such as anti-inflammatory and immune-modulatory agents, the use of myocardial and endothelial progenitor cells, or advanced analyses of individual metabolomic risk factors, will likely provide the largest advances in the field. From the standpoint of delivery of care, the implementation of established evidence-based interventions, such as rapid transfer for primary PCI with shortened delays to revascularization, is the main avenue to improve care [42].

Summary

Primary PCI is the preferred method of achieving durable reperfusion for patients who have STEMI. Current ACC/AHA guidelines promote door-to-balloon times of less than 90 minutes at well-equipped, high-volume centers, with procedures performed by high-volume operators and experienced support staff with ready access to surgical backup. These standards are supported by various strengths of evidence, but the achievement of these standards in real-world practice lags behind these goals. Ongoing research is needed to further improve patient outcomes through the use of optimal adjuvant therapies and improved systems of care to speed primary PCI in existing centers and extend it further into the community.

References

[1] Weaver WD, Simes RJ, Betriu A, et al. Comparison of primary coronary angioplasty and intravenous thrombolytic therapy for acute myocardial infarction: a quantitative review. JAMA 1997;278(23):2093–8.

[2] Keeley EC, Boura JA, Grines CL. Primary angioplasty versus intravenous thrombolytic therapy for acute myocardial infarction: a quantitative review of 23 randomised trials. Lancet 2003;361(9351):13–20.

[3] Smith SC Jr, Feldman TE, Hirshfeld JW Jr, et al. ACC/AHA/SCAI 2005 guideline update for percutaneous coronary intervention: a report of the American College of Cardiology/American Heart Association Task Force on Practice Guidelines (ACC/AHA/SCAI Writing Committee to Update the 2001 Guidelines for Percutaneous Coronary Intervention). Available at: http://www.acc.org/clinical/guidelines/percutaneous/update/index.pdf. Accessed June 10, 2006.

[4] Cannon CP, Gibson CM, Lambrew CT, et al. Relationship of symptom-onset-to-balloon time and door-to-balloon time with mortality in patients undergoing angioplasty for acute myocardial infarction. JAMA 2000;283(22):2941–7.

[5] Steg PG, Bonnefoy E, Chabaud S, et al. Comparison of Angioplasty and Prehospital Thrombolysis In acute Myocardial infarction (CAPTIM) Investigators. Impact of time to treatment on mortality after prehospital fibrinolysis or primary angioplasty: data from the CAPTIM randomized clinical trial. Circulation 2003;108(23):2851–6.

[6] Widimsky P, Budesinsky T, Vorac D, et al, for the 'PRAGUE' Study Group Investigators. Long distance transport for primary angioplasty vs immediate thrombolysis in acute myocardial infarction. Final results of the randomized national multicentre trial—PRAGUE-2. Eur Heart J 2003;24(1):94–104.

[7] Gersh BJ, Stone GW, White HD, et al. Pharmacological facilitation of primary percutaneous coronary intervention for acute myocardial infarction: is the slope of the curve the shape of the future? JAMA 2005;293(8):979–86.

[8] Antman EM, Anbe DT, Armstrong PW, et al. ACC/AHA guidelines for the management of patients with ST-elevation myocardial infarction: a report of the American College of Cardiology/American Heart Association Task Force on Practice Guidelines (Committee to revise the 1999 guidelines for the management of patients with acute myocardial infarction). 2004. Available at: http://www.acc.org/clinical/guidelines/stemi/exec_summ/index.pdf. Accessed June 28, 2006.

[9] De Luca G, Suryapranata H, Zijlstra F, et al, for the ZWOLLE Myocardial Infarction Study Group. Symptom-onset-to-balloon time and mortality in patients with acute myocardial infarction treated by primary angioplasty. J Am Coll Cardiol 2003;42(6):991–7.

[10] McNamara RL, Wang Y, Herrin J, et al, for the NRMI Investigators. Effect of door-to-balloon time on mortality in patients with ST-segment elevation myocardial infarction. J Am Coll Cardiol 2006;47(11):2180–6.

[11] McNamara RL, Herrin J, Bradley EH, et al, for the NRMI Investigators. Hospital improvement in time to reperfusion in patients with acute myocardial infarction, 1999 to 2002. J Am Coll Cardiol 2006;47(1):45–51.

[12] Bradley EH, Curry LA, Webster TR, et al. Achieving rapid door-to-balloon times: how top hospitals improve complex clinical systems. Circulation 2006;113(8):1079–85.

[13] Vermeer F, Oude Ophuis AJ, vd Berg EJ, et al. Prospective randomized comparison between thrombolysis, rescue PTCA, and primary PTCA in patients with extensive myocardial

infarction admitted to a hospital without PTCA facilities: a safety and feasibility study. Heart 1999;82(4):426–31.

[14] Andersen HR, Nielsen TT, Rasmussen K, et al, for the DANAMI-2 Investigators. A comparison of coronary angioplasty with fibrinolytic therapy in acute myocardial infarction. N Engl J Med 2003;349(8):733–42.

[15] Dalby M, Bouzamondo A, Lechat P, et al. Transfer for primary angioplasty versus immediate thrombolysis in acute myocardial infarction: a meta-analysis. Circulation 2003;108(15): 1809–14.

[16] Grines CL, Westerhausen DR, Grines L, et al, for the Air PAMI Study Group. A randomized trial of transfer for primary angioplasty versus on-site thrombolysis in patients with high-risk myocardial infarction: the Air Primary Angioplasty in Myocardial Infarction Study. J Am Coll Cardiol 2002;39(11):1713–9.

[17] ADVANCE MI Investigators. Facilitated percutaneous coronary intervention for acute ST-segment elevation myocardial infarction: results from the prematurely terminated ADdressing the value of facilitated ANgioplasty after combination therapy or eptifibatide monotherapy in acute myocardial infarction (ADVANCE MI) trial. Am Heart J 2005; 150(1):116–22.

[18] Psaty BM, Rennie D. Stopping medical research to save money: a broken pact with researchers and patients. JAMA 2003;289(16):2128–31.

[19] Nallamothu BK, Bates ER, Wang Y, et al. Driving times and distances to hospitals with percutaneous coronary intervention in the United States: implications for prehospital triage of patients with ST-elevation myocardial infarction. Circulation 2006;113(9):1189–95.

[20] Nallamothu BK, Bates ER, Herrin J, et al. Times to treatment in transfer patients undergoing primary percutaneous coronary intervention in the United States: National Registry of Myocardial Infarction (NRMI)-3/4 analysis. Circulation 2005;111(6):761–7.

[21] Aversano T, Aversano LT, Passamani E, et al, for the Atlantic Cardiovascular Patient Outcomes Research Team (C-PORT). Thrombolytic therapy vs. primary percutaneous coronary intervention for myocardial infarction in patients presenting to hospitals without on-site cardiac surgery: a randomized controlled trial. JAMA 2002;287(15):1943–51.

[22] Wharton TP Jr, Grines LL, Turco MA, et al. Primary angioplasty in acute myocardial infarction at hospitals with no surgery on-site (the PAMI-No SOS study) versus transfer to surgical centers for primary angioplasty. J Am Coll Cardiol 2004;43(11):1943–50.

[23] Stone GW, Cox D, Garcia E, et al. Normal flow (TIMI-3) before mechanical reperfusion therapy is an independent determinant of survival in acute myocardial infarction: analysis from the primary angioplasty in myocardial infarction trials. Circulation 2001;104(6): 636–41.

[24] O'Neill WW, Weintraub R, Grines CL, et al. A prospective, placebo-controlled, randomized trial of intravenous streptokinase and angioplasty versus lone angioplasty therapy of acute myocardial infarction. Circulation 1992;86(6):1710–7.

[25] Topol EJ, Califf RM, George BS, et al, for the Thrombolysis and Angioplasty in Acute Myocardial Infarction Study Group. A randomized trial of immediate vs. delayed elective angioplasty after intravenous tissue plasminogen activator in acute myocardial infarction. N Engl J Med 1987;317(10):581–8.

[26] Simoons ML, Arnold AE, Betriu A, et al, for the European Cooperative Study Group for recombinant Tissue-type Plasminogen Activator (rTPA). Thrombolysis with tissue plasminogen activator in acute myocardial infarction: no additional benefit from immediate percutaneous coronary angioplasty. Lancet 1988;1(8579):197–203.

[27] The TIMI Research Group. Immediate versus delayed catheterization and angioplasty following thrombolytic therapy for acute myocardial infarction. TIMI IIa results. JAMA 1988; 260(19):2849–58.

[28] Assessment of the Safety and Efficacy of a New Treatment Strategy with Percutaneous Coronary Intervention (ASSENT-4 PCI) investigators. Primary versus tenecteplase-facilitated

percutaneous coronary intervention in patients with ST-segment elevation acute myocardial infarction (ASSENT-4 PCI): randomised trial. Lancet 2006;367(9510):569–78.

[29] Kandzari DE, Hasselblad V, Tcheng JE, et al. Improved clinical outcomes with abciximab therapy in acute myocardial infarction: a systematic overview of randomized clinical trials. Am Heart J 2004;147(3):457–62.

[30] Kastrati A, Mehilli J, Schlotterbeck K, et al. Bavarian Reperfusion Alternatives Evaluation (BRAVE) Study Investigators. Early administration of reteplase plus abciximab vs abciximab alone in patients with acute myocardial infarction referred for percutaneous coronary intervention: a randomized controlled trial. JAMA 2004;291(8):947–54.

[31] Strategies for Patency Enhancement in the Emergency Department (SPEED) Group. Trial of abciximab with and without low-dose reteplase for acute myocardial infarction. Circulation 2000;101(24):2788–94.

[32] Antman EM, Giugliano RP, Gibson CM, et al, for the TIMI Investigators. Abciximab facilitates the rate and extent of thrombolysis: results of the Thrombolysis in Myocardial Infarction (TIMI) 14 trial. Circulation 1999;99(21):2720–32.

[33] Brener SJ, Zeymer U, Adgey J, et al, for the INTRO AMI Investigators. Eptifibatide and low-dose tissue plasminogen activator in acute myocardial infarction: the Integrilin and Low Dose Thrombolysis in Acute Myocardial Infarction (INTRO AMI) trial. J Am Coll Cardiol 2002;39(3):377–86.

[34] Giugliano RP, Roe MT, Harrington RA, et al, for the INTEGRITI Investigators. Combination reperfusion therapy with eptifibatide and reduced-dose tenecteplase for ST-elevation myocardial infarction: results of the integrilin and tenecteplase in acute myocardial infarction (INTEGRITI) phase II angiographic trial. J Am Coll Cardiol 2003;41(8):1251–60.

[35] The GUSTO Investigators. Reperfusion therapy for acute myocardial infarction with fibrinolytic therapy or combination reduced fibrinolytic therapy and platelet glycoprotein IIb/IIIa inhibition: the GUSTO V randomised trial. Lancet 2001;357(9272):1905–14.

[36] The ASSENT-3 Investigators. Efficacy and safety of tenecteplase in combination with enoxaparin, abciximab, or unfractionated heparin: the ASSENT-3 randomised trial in acute myocardial infarction. Lancet 2001;358(9282):605–13.

[37] Herrmann HC, Kelley MP, Ellis SG. Facilitated PCI: rationale and design of the FINESSE trial. J Invasive Cardiol 2001;13(suppl A):10A–5A.

[38] Newell MC, Henry CR, Sigakis CJ, et al. Comparison of safety and efficacy of sirolimus-eluting stents versus bare metal stents in patients with ST-segment elevation myocardial infarction. Am J Cardiol 2006;97(9):1299–302.

[39] Schwalm JD, Ahmad M, Velianou JL, et al. Primary and rescue percutaneous coronary intervention with paclitaxel-eluting stent implantation in ST-elevation myocardial infarction. Am J Cardiol 2006;97(9):1308–10.

[40] Hofma SH, Ong AT, Aoki J, et al. One year clinical follow up of paclitaxel eluting stents for acute myocardial infarction compared with sirolimus eluting stents. Heart 2005;91(9):1176–80.

[41] Valgimigli M, Percoco G, Malagutti P, et al, for the STRATEGY Investigators. Tirofiban and sirolimus-eluting stent versus abciximab and bare-metal stent for acute myocardial infarction: a randomized trial. JAMA 2005;293(17):2109–17.

[42] Rathore SS, Epstein AJ, Nallamothu BK, et al. Regionalization of ST-segment elevation acute coronary syndromes care: putting a national policy in proper perspective. J Am Coll Cardiol 2006;47(7):1346–9.

ELSEVIER
SAUNDERS

THE MEDICAL
CLINICS
OF NORTH AMERICA

Med Clin N Am 91 (2007) 657–681

The Use of Biomarkers for the Evaluation and Treatment of Patients with Acute Coronary Syndromes

Amy K. Saenger, PhD[a], Allan S. Jaffe, MD[a,b],*

[a]Department of Laboratory Medicine and Pathology, Mayo Clinic, Gonda Building-5th floor,
200 First Street SW, Rochester, MN 55905, USA
[b]Cardiovascular Division, Mayo Clinic, Gonda Building-5th floor,
200 First Street SW, Rochester, MN 55905, USA

The advent of inexpensive, highly accurate, and predictive markers of myocardial injury, inflammation, and hemodynamic stability has revolutionized the evaluation and treatment of patients who have acute coronary syndromes (ACSs). These blood biomarkers require small sample volumes, can be run expeditiously, and provide important information concerning the diagnosis, risk stratification, and treatment of these patients. To understand the use of these markers, one must have some knowledge about what elevations in these markers imply, how they have to be collected and measured to provide reliable information, when to suspect analytic confounds, and what the key values are that impart the diagnostic, prognostic, and therapeutic information. This article discusses these issues, emphasizing what clinicians must know for optimal test use, and then addresses the practical use of these markers in patients who have ACS.

Dr. Jaffe is a consultant and receives research support from Dade-Behring and Beckman-Coulter. He is or has been a consultant to many of the biomarker diagnostic companies, including Dade-Behring, Ortho Diagnostics, Beckman-Coulter, Liposcience, Pfizer, GSK, Bayer, Abbott, Biosite, Diadexus, and Roche.

* Corresponding author. Cardiovascular Division, Mayo Clinic, Gonda Building-5th floor, 200 First Street SW, Rochester, MN 55905.

E-mail address: jaffe.allan@mayo.edu (A.S. Jaffe).

Biochemistry and measurement of relevant cardiac markers for use in patients who have acute coronary syndromes

Cardiac troponin

The troponin complex is located on the thin filament of striated muscle, along with actin and tropomyosin. Three unique genes encode the troponin subunits for Ca^{2+} binding (TnC), inhibition (TnI), and tropomyosin-binding (TnT). TnI and TnT have different isoforms expressed in smooth and skeletal muscle that are encoded by separate genes, and thus have differing amino acid sequences [1]. In contrast, TnC has identical amino acid sequences in skeletal and cardiac tissues, thus rendering it a less-specific cardiac biomarker. Some fetal isoforms of cardiac TnT are expressed in damaged skeletal muscle, causing questions about the specificity of first-generation troponin T assays. Changes to subsequent generations of the assay have rendered this issue obsolete. Thus, **detectable release of cardiac TnI (cTnI) or TnT (cTnT) indicates some degree of cardiac injury** [2]. It is hypothesized that, upon myocyte injury, uncomplexed fragments of troponins (23.5–33.5 kd), which constitute 3% to 5% of the troponin in a cell and are believed to reside in the cytosol, are released into the bloodstream first [3,4]. Progression of necrosis then leads to release of the remaining troponin bound to contractile units. Differences in the release of free versus bound units of troponin are important determinants of the early sensitivity of troponin assays because some antibodies may detect these fragments better than others.

Using contemporary sensitive assays and the cutoff values suggested by the American College of Cardiology/European Society of Cardiology (ACC/ESC) guidelines groups, troponin levels start to rise 2 to 3 hours after the onset of chest discomfort. **Thus, in upwards of 80% of patients, a definitive diagnosis can be made in 2 to 3 hours** [5]. For that reason, recent studies suggest that previously touted "rapidly rising" markers that lack specificity, such as myoglobin, creatine kinase (CK) isoforms, and fatty acid–binding protein, are no longer needed [6,7]. Values of CK-MB and cTn generally peak within 24 hours, or even earlier when reperfusion therapies are effective.

In 2000, the ESC/ACC consensus group recommended that the 99th percentile of a reference control population be used as the diagnostic cutoff, after even minor elevations of troponin were shown to be clearly of prognostic importance [8]. As assay sensitivity improves, **using the 99th percentile of a normal population clearly improves the sensitivity of detection of patients at risk** [9,10]. Furthermore, increased assay sensitivity leads to more patient diagnoses. For example, many of the ACS studies have used cTnT. However, when comparing the sensitivity of cTnT with the contemporary highly sensitive assays used in the Global Utilization of Strategies To open Occluded arteries (GUSTO)-IV substudy [11], additional patients at risk are detected with greater accuracy. In the example cited, the increase was 11%; and individuals identified in this cohort benefited from the aggressive therapies previously shown to provide an improved prognosis in patients who had elevations of cTn. Therefore, the use of insensitive assays should be discouraged. Furthermore, the use of the 10% coefficient of variability (CV) as a cutoff value, which was initially proposed to reduce analytic false-positive results, clearly detects fewer patients at risk [12]. More importantly, clinicians often assumed this value was the upper limit of normal and ignored values between the 99th percentile and the 10% CV value. However, awareness of the problems of poor assay precision at lower values (eg, between the 99th percentile and the 10% CV value) is important, but the 10% CV value should not be used as a cutoff for evaluating patients who may have ACS.

Very recent data indicate that some minor elevations of troponin can occur from structural cardiac disease alone [13–17]. The best example of this phenomenon occurs in patients who have renal failures. Although troponin is a marker of a poor prognosis in this population, the fact that this group exists suggests the need to distinguish these elevations from those indicative of acute events. **The presence of a rising pattern of values over time is therefore crucial to detecting patients who have acute problems** [18]. The use of a rising pattern has been validated in the initial assessment of patients who have ACS [5], detecting reinfarction [19], and evaluating those who have renal failure [20]. ESC/ACC and American Heart Association (AHA) guidelines recommend serial measurements at presentation and again at 6–9–12 hours [8,21], but recent data suggest that an additional sample taken at 2 to 3 hours will identify up to 80% of those who will eventually experience elevations in troponin [5]. In an occasional high-risk patient whose values are initially normal, even subsequent values may be valuable. Without a history suggestive of ischemia and with no new ischemic ECG changes, the lack of troponin elevation (presuming a contemporary high-sensitivity assay) during a 6- to 12-hour observation period effectively excludes a diagnosis of acute myocardial infarction and the 30-day event rate in these patients is near zero [22]. Unfortunately, studies using insensitive assays or high cutoff values are abundant in the clinical literature to tout the use of other markers [23], resulting in confusion among clinicians about this critical issue. **Troponin can remain elevated up to 10 to 14 days after an event,** helping to diagnose patients who have delayed seeking treatment. Nonetheless, re-elevations are easily seen, allowing reinfarction to be diagnosed unambiguously [19].

Most troponin assays rely on monoclonal antibodies (MAbs), with a capture MAb to bind the troponin and another labeled MAb to measure the amount of troponin bound to the capture MAb. A calibration curve is then used to calculate the troponin concentration. The International Federation of Clinical Chemistry Committee on Standardization of Markers of Cardiac Damage (IFCC-SMCD) has developed quality specifications for cardiac troponin assays [24]. All guideline groups suggest that assays unable to provide published information concerning antibody specificity, calibration, sample dilution, assay specificity, and documentation of preanalytic factors from peer-reviewed publications should be used cautiously, if at all [8,25]. However, assay heterogeneity is an important consideration when evaluating troponin levels. The form of troponin detected by the assay can vary and a large number of possible combinations of troponin complexes and post-translational modifications to the protein can alter one assay's specificity and sensitivity versus another. In addition, patients who have ACS can release different complexes of troponin. The primary degradation sites for cTnT and cTnI are the C- and N-terminal sequences. Therefore, assays that have antibodies directed toward the central portion of the molecule will have greater relative increases in concentration over time and a longer duration of elevation [26]. In contrast, antibodies directed toward the more unstable C- and N-terminal portions of troponin fragments will have a limited window of detection. Recently, antibodies (or the so-called "interfering factor") have been reported against the central epitopes used by many assays, which can, in a very small percentage of patients, lead to false-negative results [27,28].

One of the major issues facing troponin measurements is in the lack of standardization of cTnI assays. Measurement of cTnI using various commercial assays currently available can yield results that differ up to 30-fold. **Thus, values obtained with one assay cannot be directly extrapolated to other assays.** The key values for the assays available in the United States are provided in Table 1 (update troponin assay information is available on the IFCC Web site.)

The American Association for Clinical Chemistry (AACC) has established a Troponin I Standardization Committee [29], which has developed standard reference material that improves the variability between assays, but complete standardization is not likely to occur because of differences in the epitopes targeted by the various antibodies.

Preanalytic and analytic problems can also influence any assay, although for most contemporary cTn assays, the frequency of these problems is slight. Interferences can be caused by heterophilic or human antianimal antibodies [30,31]. The presence of fibrin strands in serum can cause errors in many immunoassay systems [32]. Icteric or hemolyzed samples may also cause inaccuracy in immunoassays based on fluorimetric detection of the signal. False-negative results, although much less common than false-positive results, have been documented and a small percentage of the population is known to possess troponin autoantibodies [27,28]. On suspicion of false-positive or false-negative results, communication with the laboratory is essential, and in almost all instances techniques are available to clarify the result.

Fundamental to interpreting cTn levels, primarily in patients who have possible ACS, is the appreciation that many other acute processes beyond ischemic heart disease can cause elevations in cTn. **Thus, elevated values of**

Table 1
Cardiac troponin assays

Assay	Low-density lipoprotein	99th Percentile	WHO-ROC Cutoff	10%[a] CV
Abbott				
ARCH	0.009	0.012	0.3	0.032
AxSYM *ADV*	0.02	0.04	0.4	0.16
i-STAT	0.02	0.08 (WB)	ND	0.1
Bayer				
Centaur	0.02	0.1	1.0	0.35
Ultra	0.006	0.04	0.9	0.03
Beckman Accu	0.01	0.04	0.5	0.06
Biosite Triage	0.05	<0.05	0.4	0.5
Biomerieux Vds	0.001	0.01	0.16	0.11
Dade				
RxL	0.04	0.07	0.6–1.5	0.14
CS	0.03	0.07	0.6–1.5	0.06
DPC Immulite	0.1	0.2	1.0	0.6
MKI Pathfast	0.006	0.01	0.06	0.06
Ortho				
Vitros	0.02	0.08	0.4	0.12
ES (R&D)	0.012	0.032	NA	0.053
Response	0.03	<0.03 (WB)	ND	0.21
Roche				
Elecsys	0.01	<0.01	0.03	0.03
Reader	0.05	<0.05 (WB)	0.1	ND
Tosoh AIA	0.06	0.06	0.31–0.64	0.06

Abbreviations: CV, coefficient of variability; NA, not applicable; ND, not done; WB, whole blood; WHO-ROC, World Health Organization and Receiver Operator Curve value predicated on previous CKMB standard.

[a] Per manufacture.

cTn indicate acute cardiac injury, but not its cause. Box 1 provides a partial list of other situations where cTn can be elevated. (For those in green italics, at least some information suggests prognostic significance when the elevations occur.)

Brain natriuretic peptide

The suspicion that the heart is an endocrine function was raised approximately 50 years ago when it was shown that dilation of cardiac atria produced natriuresis [33]. Subsequently, intracellular granules were found in atrial myocytes resembling those found in endocrine cells through electron microscopy and, in 1981, extracts of atrial tissue were injected into rats, inducing rapid natriuresis and diuresis [34]. The active factor was termed atrial natriuretic peptide (ANP), a 28 amino-acid peptide. In 1988, an ANP-like natriuretic peptide was isolated from the porcine brain, and given the name *brain natriuretic peptide* (BNP) [35]. It is now well accepted that most circulating forms of BNP originate from the ventricular myocardium,

---

Box 1. Elevations of troponins without overt ischemic heart disease

Trauma, including contusion, ablation, pacing, implantable cardioverter defibrillator firings including atrial defibrillators, cardioversion, endomyocardial biopsy, cardiac surgery, after interventional closure of atrial septal defects
Congestive heart failure, acute and chronic
Aortic valve disease and hypertrophic obstructive cardiomyopathy with significant left ventricular hypertrophy
Hypertension
Hypotension, often with arrhythmias
Postoperative noncardiac surgery patients who seem to do well
Renal failure
Critically ill patients, especially those who have diabetes, respiratory failure, gastrointestinal bleeding, sepsis
Drug toxicity (eg, doxorubicin, 5-fluorouracil, trastuzumab, snake venoms, carbon monoxide poisoning)
Hypothyroidism
Abnormalities in coronary vasomotion, including coronary vasospasm
Apical ballooning syndrome
Inflammatory diseases (eg, myocarditis, parvovirus B19, Kawasaki disease, sarcoid, smallpox vaccination, or myocardial extension of bacterial endocarditis)
Patients who have undergone PCI who appear to be uncomplicated
Pulmonary embolism, severe pulmonary hypertension
Sepsis
Burns, especially if total body surface area is more than 30%
Infiltrative diseases including amyloidosis, hemochromatosis, sarcoidosis and scleroderma
Acute neurologic disease, including cerebrovascular accidents, subarachnoid bleeds
Rhabdomyolysis with cardiac injury
Transplant vasculopathy
Vital exhaustion

---

and therefore it is now clear that BNP should best be referred to as *B-type natriuretic peptide* [36]. In contrast to ANP, most BNP is not stored in granules but requires the stimulation of RNA and transcription to be produced. It is also clear now that ANP and BNP belong to a class of natriuretic factors inclusive of C-type natriuretic peptide (CNP), dendroaspis natriuretic peptide, and urodilantin. In addition to atrial and ventricular cardiomyo-cytes, recent data suggest that other cell types, such as cardiac fibroblasts, can produce BNP [37].

BNP release and synthesis are activated by diastolic ventricular stretch [38]. Thus, BNP is stimulated in a broad spectrum of cardiovascular disease, in-cluding systolic and diastolic left ventricular dysfunction, acute coronary syndromes, stable coronary heart disease, valvular heart disease, acute and chronic right ventricular failure, and left and right ventricular hypertro-phy secondary to arterial or pulmonary hypertension. Experts hypothesize that BNP release is a compensatory mechanism in response to these stimuli to cardiac stretch. However, BNP expression and release also can also be stimulated by a variety of endocrine, paracrine, and autocrine factors that are initiated in heart failure, including norepinephrine, angiotensin II, gluco-corticoids, and proinflammatory cytokines.

BNP is a cyclic 32–amino acid polypeptide that is released as pro-BNP, a 108–amino acid precursor prohormone that is then believed to be cleaved enzymatically into its active form. The proteolytic enzymes responsible for this cleavage are still being elucidated, but are likely to be corin, furin, or perhaps both. Pro-BNP is cleaved into a biologically active C-terminal frag-ment (BNP) and a larger amino acid N-terminal fragment (NT-proBNP). BNP, NT-proBNP fragments, degradation fragments, and intact pro-BNP 1-108 are all found circulating in human plasma. Recent data suggest that pro-BNP may be the predominant circulating natriuretic peptide (NP) form [39–41]. Circulating levels of BNP and NT-proBNP differ, partly because of the slightly longer half-life of NT-proBNP (21 minutes versus 60–120 minutes, respectively). Concentrations of NT-proBNP are approxi-mately 20 times greater than those of BNP, but this ratio increases when renal dysfunction is present. Clearance of NPs is achieved through binding to NP receptors or through proteolysis. Renal excretion is an important clearance mechanism for NT-proBNP. Mechanistic details regarding BNP clearance are difficult to elucidate because the kidneys secrete and reabsorb BNP. Data comparing healthy individuals with those who have diagnosed heart failure show a shift in the ratio of the concentrations of BNP to NT-proBNP, suggesting that this ratio may be important in the future.

Commercially available assays to measure either BNP or NT-proBNP are immunometric sandwich assays, incorporating two MAbs that bind to dif-ferent epitopes of the antigen to be detected (ie, either BNP or NT-proBNP). BNP and NT-proBNP assays are available on either fully automated ana-lyzers or as a point-of-care whole blood assay (Fig. 1). All available BNP assays detect BNP fragments without significant cross-reactivity to related peptides (ANP, CNP, urodilantin, NT-proANP, NT-proCNP, and frag-ments) or other peptide hormones. As with troponin assays, clinicians must recognize the differences between BNP assays and that the reported BNP concentrations will differ depending on the testing platform used [42–44]. Each test must be validated separately, and reference intervals

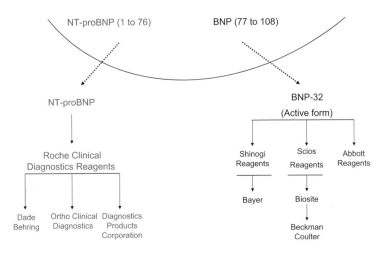

Fig. 1. Assays that are available and under development for measuring BNP and NT-proBNP.

and decision limits derived from clinical studies are valid only for the particular assay studied and should not be extrapolated to include other BNP assays. Similar to BNP assays, NT-proBNP assays do not exhibit cross-reactivity with other NP fragments and seem somewhat less sensitive to pro-BNP. Only one assay exists for NT-proBNP, reducing the issues of comparability that occur with BNP assays.

Most studies divide BNP and NT-proBNP values into tertiles or quartiles for evaluation, and thus the optimal cutoff value varies among studies. Morrow and colleagues [45] have propagated values of more than 80 ng/mL for patients who have ACS. However, this value is likely to change depending on the population studied and the assay used. In addition, various studies have garnered values at different times, ranging from time of presentation to 40 hours after admission. **This issue of proper cutoff values has been a major impediment to comparing results across studies and in promulgating the use of BNP values clinically** [46].

BNP and NT-proBNP levels are higher in women and increase with age in both genders [42,47,48]. This variation according to age and gender may be mediated partially by the development of mild renal impairment, left ventricular hypertrophy, or abnormal systolic and diastolic cardiac function with age. Thus, age- and gender-specific reference intervals should be used to interpret BNP and NT-proBNP values, as opposed to a single cutoff value. Obesity also has been observed to cause decreases in BNP and NT-proBNP concentrations in individuals who have heart failure and those who do not, perhaps because of an attenuation of BNP release or an increase in clearance [49]. Values for both BNP and NT-proBNP rise in patients experiencing renal failure as the degree of renal failure increases, although the increases are far greater for NT-proBNP than BNP [50,51].

Sample collection plays an important role in reporting accurate BNP and NT-proBNP values, and is the greatest cause of incorrect results. In comparison, analytic causes of false results are relatively rare. Samples for the measurement of BNP must be collected in ethylenediaminetetraacetic acid and assayed immediately. These samples degrade if not stored at $-70°C$. NT-proBNP is far more stable and, if refrigerated, is stable for days. If samples are stored at $-70°C$, they are stable even longer. Quality specifications are now available for BNP and NT-proBNP assays [52], and assays without published results of the recommended specifications should be used cautiously or avoided. Some of the original BNP assays lacked precision but, overall, the analytic variability is small compared with biologic variability. **Biologic variability is sufficiently high that values should change by a minimum of 50%, and ideally 100%, to ensure certain changes in a given patient are above biologic variability.** Certain assays are more susceptible to analytic interferences, and these interferences are similar to those mentioned with troponin assays.

C-reactive protein

Although historically regarded as a structural disease, atherosclerotic coronary artery disease is now widely appreciated as an inflammatory process. C-reactive protein was first described in 1930, when it was found to be able to bind to the C-polysaccharide on the cell wall of *Streptococcus pneumoniae*. It was shown to be a protein in 1941, and given the name *CRP*. CRP is an acute-phase reactant and is a sensitive systemic marker of inflammation and tissue damage. It is one of the most consistently increased and fastest-reacting acute-phase proteins with a half-life of 19 hours, suggesting it is part of the innate immune response. In atherosclerotic disease, these increases occur in response to cardiac necrosis and are believed to be mediated through increases in interleukin (IL)-6 [53]. Thus, values for risk stratification must be obtained very early after presentation (before the acute increases occur) or after 4 to 6 weeks, when the elevations related to necrosis have resolved, as shown in the Pravastatin or Atorvastatin Evaluation and Infection Therapy (PROVE-IT) trial [54]. **If obtained early, CRP values are believed to possibly reflect the magnitude of the unstable inflammatory state that exists, and thus be related to subsequent cardiovascular events.** Invasive studies have elegantly documented [55] that this inflammatory increase in patients who have ACS represents a systemic diathesis that is not solely related to the infarct-related blood vessel involved in the acute event. In highly inflammatory diseases such as ACS, it is now clear that, in addition to rises in CRP, high circulating levels of CRP are a risk factor for coronary artery disease. CRP binds selectively to low-density lipoprotein (LDL), especially oxidized and enzyme-modified LDL, and can be deposited in atherosclerotic plaques where it has a range of proinflammatory properties that could potentially contribute to the pathogenesis, progression, and complications of atheroma [56].

In the mid-1990s, immunoassays for CRP became more sensitive and showed that patients presenting with low-level increases of CRP were at substantially higher risk for future coronary events than those in the normal population. The emphasis in cardiovascular medicine on high-sensitivity CRP (hs-CRP) does not imply that what is being measured is different from CRP; rather, the sensitivity refers to the lower detection limit of the assay procedures being used. Increases in CRP concentration are associated with future coronary events in apparently healthy individuals, regardless of gender, and patients who have ACS [57]. Current AHA/Centers for Disease Control and Prevention (CDC) guidelines specify cut-points for clinical interpretation, with CRP concentrations less than 1 mg/L associated with low risk, 1 to 3 mg/L with average risk, and more than 3 mg/L with high risk [58]. Several studies have also shown that CRP results are additive with LDL concentrations in predicting an individual's risk for coronary heart disease during primary prevention [59]. Therefore, the AHA/CDC panel recommends that LDL values be combined with CRP results in an algorithm for risk assessment of heart disease.

More than 30 methods are commercially available for CRP measurement and, as with troponin and BNP, performance varies depending on the method used. Studies using different assays have had significant discrepancies between results, thus, standardization will be necessary in the near future [58]. The CDC is identifying a suitable reference material, similar to the undertaking performed with cTnI assays. Most studies performed with CRP show no or little relationship between age or ethnicity and serum concentrations of CRP, and gender or ethnic-specific cut points for CRP are currently not advocated. **However, recent data from the Mayo Clinic [60] and the Dallas Heart study [61] suggest that gender and racial differences exist that should be taken into account.** Physiologic conditions and lifestyle behaviors, such as smoking, obesity, exercise, and alcohol use, are all known to affect CRP concentrations. Elevations are associated with increased body mass index and cigarette smoking, whereas moderate alcohol intake lowers CRP.

Creatine Kinase-MB

CK is found in heart muscle, skeletal muscle, and the brain. It is composed of M and B subunits that form CK-BB, CK-MB, and CK-MM. CK-MB has higher specificity for the myocardium because the concentration in myocytes is arguably much greater. Serial CK-MB measurements were the gold standard for many years and, when measured by mass assay, have a modest sensitivity and reasonable specificity for evaluating patients who have ACS [62]. However, CK-MB is much less sensitive than troponin, rises more slowly given contemporary assays, has less sensitive cutoff values, and is sufficient in skeletal muscle to actually impair specificity in some cases. For example, in evaluating patients experiencing chest pain, roughly

10% will have elevated values of CK-MB but normal troponin values [62]. These patients do extremely well and very likely most, if not all, of these elevations are not caused by cardiac abnormalities. Thus, little is gained by using both assays and the cost increase can be substantial. Thus, we **do not recommend using CK-MB in patients who have ACS unless cTn values are not available.** Whenever CK-MB is used, gender-specific ranges should be used [62]. Some may still rely on CK-MB to diagnose reinfarction, but the data for troponin suggest it is equivalent [19]. **Recent data suggest that, when the baseline troponin is used for risk stratification in patients undergoing percutaneous coronary intervention, neither elevation in CK-MB nor troponin retain any prognostic importance** [63]. These findings are important to the analysis of trials such as the Invasive Versus Conservative Treatment in Unstable Coronary Syndrome (ICTUS) trial [64].

Myoglobin, creatine kinase isoforms, and fatty acid–binding protein

Each of these markers has been touted as more rapidly rising than others and thus of potential use in excluding myocardial injury in patients who present with chest discomfort. However, most studies suggesting that approach used either insensitive troponin assays or higher cutoff values than recommended; the recent paper regarding fatty acid–binding protein [65] is a good example. **With sensitive contemporary assays for troponin and the cutoff values suggested, these markers no longer add value** [6]. In addition, all of these markers lack sensitivity for the myocardium, making false-positives widespread.

Emerging cardiac biomarkers

Historically, biochemical markers have not only contributed to a better understanding of the underlying pathophysiological mechanisms of ACS but also improved the evaluation of patients who have suspected ACS. Diagnosis of ACS relies heavily on biomarkers only increased after necrosis. For this reason, intense research continues into the development and clinical investigation of these sensitive biomarkers that do not depend on the presence of irreversible myocardial damage. Several cardiac biomarkers are emerging that have great potential for detecting ACS before myocardial necrosis occurs, namely myeloperoxidase, pregnancy-associated plasma protein A (PAPP-A), placental growth factor (PlGF), and soluble CD40 ligand [66].

Myeloperoxidase (MPO) is a hemoprotein abundantly expressed in neutrophils and secreted during their activation, including across the coronary sinus [55]. MPO is hypothesized to participate in the initiation and progression of cardiovascular diseases through the oxidative modification of LDL, considered to be a key event in atherogenesis promotion. MPO was shown to predict early risk for myocardial infarction and the risk for other major adverse cardiac events in patients who had chest pain in the ensuing 30-day and 6-month periods [67,68]. Unfortunately, either single samples or high cutoff values for troponin were used in these studies.

PAPP-A is a zinc-binding matrix metalloproteinase first identified in the serum of pregnant women. PAPP-A degrades insulin-like growth factor–binding protein (IGFBP)-4 and -5, releasing insulin-like growth factor (IGF), which seems to be a growth modulator in local proliferative response to tissue [69]. Therefore, PAPP-A probably has an important role in not only the progression of atherosclerosis but also the development of restenosis after coronary interventions. In a study by Bayes-Genis and colleagues [70], circulating PAPP-A concentrations more than 10 mU/L allowed patients who had ACS to be identified with a sensitivity of 89.2% and a specificity of 81.3%. Concentrations of PAPP-A were also correlated with free IGF-1 and CRP but not cTnI or CK-MB. In another study of more than 200 serial patients who had ACS, PAPP-A levels were shown to be a strong independent predictor of ischemic cardiac events and the need for revascularization in patients presenting with suspected myocardial infarction but who remain troponin–negative, albeit with an insensitive cutoff value for troponin [71]. PAPP-A remains a promising biomarker for risk stratification in patients who have ACS, but further validation studies are required using larger cohorts.

PlGF belongs to the family of vascular endothelial growth factors. It stimulates vascular smooth muscle growth, recruits macrophages into atherosclerotic lesions, up-regulates tumor necrosis factor α, enhances production of tissue factor, and stimulates pathologic angiogenesis. These processes are known contributors to plaque progression and destabilization. Although data from the c7E3 Fab Anti Platelet Therapy in Unstable Refractory Angina (CAPTURE) trial established PlGF as a novel, powerful, independent prognostic determinant of clinical outcome in patients who have ACS [72,73], only one sample was available and high cutoff values were used for cardiac troponin.

CD40 is expressed on various immune cells within atherosclerotic lesions, including endothelial cells, smooth muscle cells, and monocytes/macrophages, whereas CD40L is largely expressed on CD4+ T cells and activated platelets. Experiments in hyperlipidemic mice have shown that the size of coronary plaques and their inflammatory cell content can be decreased by using an inhibitory antibody against CD40L. In addition to the immunoregulatory properties by CD40–CD40L interaction, evidence suggests that tissue factor, the initiator of blood coagulation, is up-regulated through CD40 ligation by activated lymphocytes and platelets. Membrane-bound CD40L may be proteolytically cleaved to form soluble CD40L (sCD40L). This form is present in the circulation and probably has similar activities in vivo in the membrane-bound form. Although the source of sCD40L in blood is still not fully elucidated, the general opinion is that activated platelets are the most important source. Two recent studies have evaluated the potential value of sCD40L as a predictor of adverse cardiovascular events. Data suggest that sCD40L is an independent predictor of risk, and is associated with an increased risk for death and recurrent ischemic events [74,75]. Chronic elevations may be caused by the shedding of the protein into the plasma from the unstable atherosclerotic plaque. Again, further studies are required using multiple samples and the recommended contemporary cutoff values for contemporary troponin assays.

Clinical use of biomarkers for the detection and guidance of treatment of patients who have acute coronary syndromes

Patients who have ACSs present in a variety of ways, with higher and lower risk profiles. The interpretation of increases in cardiac biomarkers depends critically on the patient subset being evaluated. Accordingly, the following sections will be divided by risk category.

High- and intermediate-risk patients

Patients who present with high-risk ACS also represent a heterogeneous group. They include patients who have ST-elevation ACSs and those who have non–ST-elevation ACSs.

Those with ST-segment elevation ACSs (see Chapter 5) do not require the acute use of biomarkers for either diagnosis or guidance of treatment. Efforts are usually oriented toward the most prompt reperfusion possible with minimal delay, and therefore waiting for biomarker testing results is inappropriate. In some patients for whom diagnosis is uncertain, troponin measurements may be helpful, and although physicians usually would not wait for biomarker results, substantial information suggests that these values help define prognosis. In patients who have an ST-elevation myocardial infarction, an elevated troponin is a potent adverse prognostic marker [76–79], probably partly because biomarkers of myocardial necrosis, such as troponin, take time to become elevated. Therefore patients who have biomarker elevations are, as a group, probably those who present late after the onset of symptoms.

It is well known that the rapidity with which reperfusion therapies are applied is an important factor in the eventual success of therapy and the prognosis of patients. Thus, later treatment should be associated with less successful reperfusion, less myocardial salvage, a larger infarct size, and a more adverse prognosis [80]. Therefore, unsurprisingly, multiple studies have confirmed that patients who have elevated troponin levels at presentation are less apt to experience rapid reperfusion from thrombolytic agents and undergo successful primary PCI than those who have no elevations. For example, one study showed that patients who had no elevations of biomarkers had a 96% success rate with primary PCI, whereas only 76% of those who had elevations achieved Thrombolysis in Myocardial Infarction (TIMI) grade 3 flow postprocedure [79].

In studies attempting to correct for the time from acute infarction onset to treatment, the negative prognostic impact of elevations in troponin persists despite correction [81]. The lack of correspondence between elevations in cardiac biomarkers and time from onset is also observed in patients who present with so-called "aborted infarction" where biomarker release is modest (usually defined as two times the CK value) [82,83]. Regardless of the mechanism, an elevated troponin at the time of treatment defines a group of patients who are less apt to establish normal coronary perfusion, more apt to have congestive heart failure and shock, and those are prone to subsequent mortality [76]. Data in patients who have inferior infarction suggest that primary stenting may obviate some of this effect [84], but this concept has not been tested prospectively in a trial. Clinically, if an early troponin elevation is seen, aggressive adjunctive therapy may be considered to improve coronary perfusion.

Most patients present with non–ST-elevation ACSs. Those who have ST-segment changes are at higher risk than those who have T-wave inversion or normal ECGs [85]. Some data suggest that individuals with ST-segment change have more procoagulant activity, probably reflecting the severity of the underlying coronary artery disease [86]. Those who have normal or near-normal ECGs are at low risk, and more appropriately would be considered for ruling out acute myocardial infarction rather than being unstable coronary ischemia [87]. Therefore, these patients must be considered as different subsets.

In patients who have high or intermediate risk (see the article by Singh in this issue), elevations in cardiac biomarkers should be sought assiduously. Some studies use only the first sample on presentation, because the mean time to presentation for many patients who have ACSs is prolonged (eg, up to 13 hours in Essence and Tactics TIMI 18) [88]. However, values on admission and 6 to 9 hours later are essential to optimize the use of troponin, because some patients who have non–ST-segment elevation myocardial infarctions do present shortly after the onset of symptoms [22]. Elevations of troponin above the 99th percentile of the normal range, assuming a highly sensitive contemporary assay, are diagnostic of cardiac injury and therefore fulfill criteria provided by the ESC/ACC for the diagnosis of acute non–ST-segment elevation myocardial infarction [8,89]. Criteria with troponin are far more sensitive than those used previously based on CK-MB, but individuals who meet these criteria are similar to those who met previous criteria for non–ST-segment elevation myocardial infarction using CK-MB [90–92]. These patients tend to have recurrent events that cause their long-term prognosis to be equivalent to that of patients who have ST-segment elevation AMI. In some studies, patients with only troponin elevations have a worse outcome than those who have troponin and CK-MB elevations. This may be caused by a lack of recognition of these patients' risk and thus the undertreatment [93]. In most studies, individuals who have troponin elevations alone have a similar, although slightly better, prognosis [91,92].

Earlier studies using insensitive assays first elaborated this principle [22] but, despite improved assay sensitivity, patients who have elevated troponin and an acute presentation are clearly at substantially greater risk than those who have no elevations [11]. The number of patients at risk who do not have elevations varies depending on the sensitivity of the troponin assay used to make the triage. Therefore, physicians are strongly advised to know the specific troponin assay used at their institution and its sensitivity.

The reasons for associating elevated troponin with an adverse risk after an acute presentation with ischemic heart disease are well defined. The anatomy of patients who have elevated troponin is substantially worse than those who do not have elevations [94–97]. The frequency of triple vessel disease, asymmetric stenoses, evidence of procoagulant activity, poor TIMI flow, and blush grades have been well described in these individuals (Fig. 2). Disease that manifests cardiac damage should be expected to be more severe than disease that does not. These anatomic correlates establish the framework for the subsequent therapeutic impact of some more aggressive interventions. In individuals whose troponin elevations are associated with more acute lesions, many of which are known to be thrombogenic, agents such as low molecular weight heparin, which has been shown to be more efficacious than unfractionated heparin, and IIB/IIIA platelet antagonists will be beneficial [98,99].

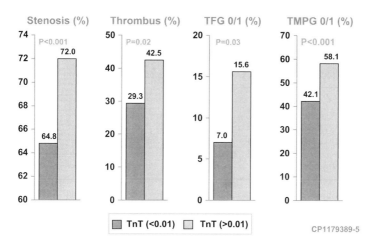

Fig. 2. Relationship of troponin elevations and coronary anatomy in patients who have ACS. TFG, TIMI Flow grade; TMPG, TIMI myocardial perfusion grade. (*Data from* Wong G, Morrow D, Murphy S, et al. Elevations in troponin T and I are associated with abnormal tissue level perfusion: a TACTICS-TIMI 18 substudy. Circulation 2002;106:202–7.)

Most studies suggest that triage using troponin is critical. Patients who have elevations benefit from these adjunctive agents, predominantly with a reduction in recurrent ischemic events, whereas those who have no elevations do not [98–102]. Questions have recently arisen as to whether the concomitant use of clopidogrel might obviate some benefits of these other interventions. However, clopidogrel and IIB/IIIA agents currently seem to be positively synergistic [103]. Equally important are patients who have no troponin elevations, assuming good assays and appropriate cutoff values are used, who do not benefit from the use of IIB/IIIA agents and low molecular weight heparin. However, this is not so for clopidogrel [104]. In addition, consistent with the coronary angiographic data presented earlier, patients who have elevated troponin benefit from an early invasive interventional strategy [105,106]. The response to these interventions result in reduced mortality and less recurrent myocardial infarction (Fig. 3). The time range defined as early varies substantially and is much shorter in studies performed in the United States [105] compared with those in Europe [106]. Nonetheless, intervention during hospitalization is suggested for those who present with ACSs, are at high or intermediate risk, and have elevated troponin values. Obviously, subsequent to the acute treatment, therapy with statin agents, beta blockers, and agents designed to improve secondary prevention is clearly indicated.

Biomarkers such as CRP and BNP can be used synergistically with troponin [45,57,107]. Patients who have elevated troponins often have more adverse hemodynamic profiles, and therefore the constellation of elevated troponin and elevated BNP is frequent [45,107]. Thus, elevations in BNP define a group that has worse hemodynamics and thus a worse prognosis. In

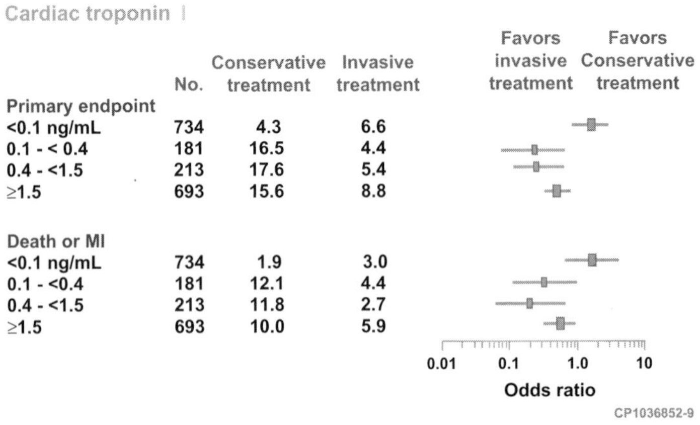

Fig. 3. Data from TACTICS-TIMI 18 showing that patients who have any elevation of troponin benefit from an invasive strategy. (*From* Morrow DA, Cannon CP, Rifai N, et al. Ability of minor elevations of troponins I and T to predict benefit from an early invasive strategy in patients with unstable angina and non-ST elevation myocardial infarction: results from a randomized trial. JAMA 2001;286:2405; with permission.)

addition, elevated CRP in association with an elevated troponin has a worse prognosis, perhaps because it identifies individuals who have more extensive unstable coronary heart disease. Both CRP and BNP seem to help predict subsequent mortality but not recurrent infarction, which is best predicted by troponin [45,57,107].

Elevation of a given marker could be a marker of fatal ischemic events rather than nonfatal ischemic events. An elevated CRP not only identifies additional patients who may not have elevations in troponin but particularly identifies those who have adverse cardiovascular risk after discharge. Thus, troponin tends to provide a more immediate risk assessment, whereas CRP provides a somewhat later evaluation. Recent data from the PROVE-IT trial [54] indicate that, despite lipid-lowering effects of statin agents, elevations of CRP that persisted despite therapy were still highly prognostic (Fig. 4). Perhaps the proper synthesis of these data is to rely on troponin during hospitalization and then assay CRP after 6 weeks to detect patients who may be at longer-term risk.

Whether subsequent treatment of elevations in CRP and BNP would be beneficial is unclear. For BNP, synergism regarding prognosis also exists. However, whereas troponin allows therapeutic strategies to be triaged and identifies individuals most apt to benefit from aggressive anticoagulation and intervention, the present data suggest that elevations of BNP and CRP cannot be used to define therapeutic options, except in the women discussed later and one recent paper by James and colleagues [108], which suggests the benefit of an invasive strategy in these patients.

Patients who have normal troponins but elevations of CRP and BNP seem to have a higher risk than those who have no elevations, especially with women (Fig. 5) [109]. Some studies suggest that women may be somewhat less prone to have elevated troponins and particularly will benefit

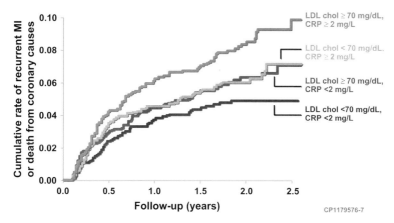

Fig. 4. Data from PROVE-IT suggesting the importance of elevations of CRP late after the acute event. (*From* Ridker P, Cannon C, Morrow D, et al. C-reactive protein levels and outcomes after statin therapy. N Engl J Med 2005;352:26; with permission.)

TACTICS-TIMI 18

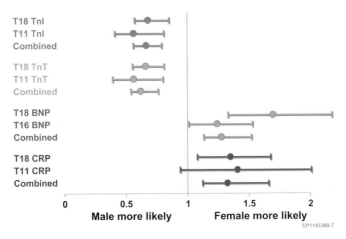

Fig. 5. Frequency of elevated CRP, BNP, and troponin in patients who have ACS in TIMI 18. (*From* Wiviott SD, Cannon CP, Morrow DA, et al. Differential expression of cardiac biomarkers by gender in patients with unstable angina/non-ST-elevation myocardial infarction: a TACTICS-TIMI 18 (Treat Angina with Aggrastat and determine Cost of Therapy with an Invasive or Conservative Strategy-Thrombolysis In Myocardial Infarction 18) substudy. Circulation 2004;109:583; with permission.)

from lower recommended threshold levels. In a recent epidemiologic study, Roger and colleagues [92] showed that most new diagnoses of myocardial infarction in response to the new standards using sensitive contemporary assays and sensitive cutoff values occurred in women. In addition, when individuals who have normal troponins are evaluated on admission, as in the Treat Angina with Aggrastat and Determine Cost of Therapy with an Invasive or Conservative Strategy) TACTICS-TIMI 18 study (unfortunately, a subsequent troponin was not available), women seem less likely to have troponin elevations than men [109], although they often have elevations of BNP and CRP. One report [109] showed that women who had elevations of either marker with normal troponin values on admission (serial values were not available) experienced benefit from an invasive strategy. In the absence of elevations of any markers, the response to an invasive strategy was not favorable. Men, who tended to have more elevations of troponin and less of CRP and BNP, experienced a good response with elevations of troponin and a null response with no troponin elevations.

High-risk patients who have elevations of troponin often undergo PCI. When PCI is performed in the setting of an elevated baseline troponin, further elevations in biomarkers after PCI should not be used to infer additional damage caused by the procedure [63]. In these circumstances, recent data suggest baseline, and not postprocedural, troponin predicts risk. These data also apply to the use of CK-MB [63,64].

Low-risk patients

Patients at low risk to rule in or rule out acute myocardial infarction are well triaged using troponin. Again, sensitive, contemporary assays and appropriate cutoff values are essential. When used, 80% of patients can be diagnosed (the rule-in group) in 2 to 3 hours. Total ascertainment takes at least 6 hours [5]. In most studies, patients who have normal troponin values are at extremely low risk; and experience no events over a 30-day period [22]. Those who have elevations are at substantially higher risk even if the elevations are modest (Fig. 6) [22,110]. Some of the elevations in patients who are "low risk" may not be caused by acute coronary disease, but perhaps by chronic heart disease, renal dysfunction, myocarditis, pulmonary embolism, and various other potential causes. Nonetheless, in patients who present with chest discomfort, an elevated troponin is associated with a substantial increase in the risk for coronary artery disease defined angiographically.

In one study [87] that used a higher cTnT value than recommended, 90% of patients who had minor elevations in troponin in this low-risk group (minimal or absent ECG changes) had significant coronary artery disease which, in two thirds, was double or triple vessel disease. In contrast, in those who had "normal values" according to this study, only 23% had coronary artery disease using angiography and, in only 12%, it was more than single-vessel disease. In addition, individuals who had elevations had significantly more adverse events over the 1-year follow-up period than those who had no

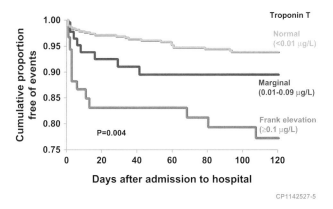

Fig. 6. Events in patients seen in the emergency department. Those who had even minor elevations of troponin had an adverse prognosis. Note excellent prognosis in those with normal values. (*From* Henrikson C, Howell E, Bush D, et al. Prognostic usefulness of marginal troponin T elevation. Am J Cardiol 2004;93:278; with permission.)

elevations. Fortunately, most of the events were recurrent angina or myocardial infarctions and not sudden cardiac death. However, some did not have coronary disease and therefore one must remember that other potential causes for elevations exist, as delineated in Box 1. A specific therapeutic strategy predicated on troponin in low-risk groups who rule in has not yet been determined. One could argue, based on the data presented for patients who present with ACSs, that some patients included in the earlier trials may have been at low risk and that the same principles should apply.

Unfortunately, a specific data analysis examining that issue has not been accomplished. Nonetheless, acute (a rising pattern) elevations in troponin indicate cardiac injury and, when patients present with chest discomfort, admission and evaluation are mandatory [5,18]. **These principles should guide the care of in-patients who also have renal failure. These individuals may have modest elevations in troponin at baseline, which are prognostically significant [14,111], but when they present acutely, either with a low- or a high-risk story, elevations of troponin are highly prognostic [20,112]. Patients who have renal failure do even more poorly that those who do not. Similar principles will probably apply as assays become more sensitive, but more elevations that are related to structural heart disease will also be detected, making criteria based on rising pattern critical [18].**

References

[1] Christenson R, Azzazy H. Biochemical markers of the acute coronary syndrome. Clin Chem 1998;44:1855–64.

[2] Jaffe A. Elevations in cardiac troponin measurements: false false-positives: the real truth. Cardiovasc Toxicol 2001;1:87–92.

[3] Adams J 3rd, Schechtman K, Landt Y, et al. Comparable detection of acute myocardial infarction by creatine kinase MB isoenzyme and cardiac troponin I. Clin Chem 1994;40: 1291–5.

[4] Katus H, Remppis A, Scheffold T, et al. Intracellular compartmentation of cardiac troponin T and its release kinetics in patients with reperfused and nonreperfused myocardial infarction. Am J Cardiol 1991;67:1360–7.

[5] MacRae A, Kavsak P, Lustig V, et al. Assessing the requirement for the 6-hour interval between specimens in the American heart association classification of myocardial infarction in epidemiology and clinical research studies. Clin Chem 2006;52:812–8.

[6] Eggers K, Oldgren J, Nordenskjold A, et al. Diagnostic value of serial measurement of cardiac markers in patients with chest pain: limited value of adding myoglobin to troponin I for exclusion of myocardial infarction. Am Heart J 2004;148:574–81.

[7] Ilva T, Eriksson S, Lund J, et al. Improved early risk stratification and diagnosis of myocardial infarction, using a novel troponin I assay concept. Eur J Clin Invest 2005;35:112–6.

[8] Alpert J, Thygesen K, Antman E, et al. Myocardial infarction redefined-a consensus document of The Joint European Society of Cardiology/American College of Cardiology Committee for the redefinition of myocardial infarction. J Am Coll Cardiol 2000;36:959–69.

[9] James S, Armstrong P, Califf R, et al. Troponin T levels and risk of 30-day outcomes in patients with the acute coronary syndrome: prospective verification in the GUSTO-IV trial. Am J Med 2003;115:178–84.

[10] James S, Flodin M, Johnston N, et al. The antibody configurations of cardiac troponin I assays may determine their clinical performance. Clin Chem 2006;52:832–7.

[11] James S, Lindback J, Tilly J, et al. Troponin-T and N-terminal pro-B-type natriuretic peptide predict mortality benefit from coronary revascularization in acute coronary syndromes: s GUSTO-IV Substudy. J Am Coll Cardiol 2006;48:1146–54.

[12] Apple F, Wu A, Jaffe A. European Society of Cardiology and American College of Cardiology guidelines for redefinition of myocardial infarction: how to use existing assays clinically and for clinical trials. Am Heart J 2002;144:981–6.

[13] Zethelius B, Johnston N, Venge P. Troponin I as a predictor of coronary heart disease and mortality in 70-year-old men. Circulation 2006;113:1071–8.

[14] Apple F, Murakami M, Pearce L, et al. Predictive value of cardiac troponin I and T for subsequent death in end-stage renal disease. Circulation 2002;106:2941–5.

[15] Schulz O, Sigusch H. Impact of an exercise-induced increase in cardiac troponin I in chronic heart failure secondary to ischemic or idiopathic dilated cardiomyopathy. Am J Cardiol 2002;90:547–50.

[16] Schulz O, Kirpal K, Stein J, et al. Importance of low concentrations of cardiac troponins. Clin Chem 2006;52:1614–5.

[17] Wallace T, Abdullah S, Drazner M, et al. Prevalence and determinants of troponin T elevation in the general population. Circulation 2006;113:1958–65.

[18] Jaffe A . Chasing troponin, how low can you go if you can see the rise? J Am Coll Cardiol 2006;48:1763–4.

[19] Apple F, Murakami M. Cardiac troponin and creatine kinase MB monitoring during in-hospital myocardial reinfarction. Clin Chem 2005;51:460–3.

[20] Ie EH, Klootwijk PJ, Weimar W, et al. Significance of acute versus chronic troponin T elevation in dialysis patients. Nephron Clin Pract 2004;98:87–92.

[21] Luepker R, Apple F, Christenson R, et al. Case definition for acute coronary heart disease in epidemiology and clinical research studies: a statement from the AHA Council on Epidemiology and Prevention; the European Society of Cardiology Working Group on Epidemiology and Prevention; Centers for Disease Control and Prevention; and the National Heart, Lung, and Blood Institute. Circulation 2003;108:2543–9.

[22] Hamm C, Goldmann B, Heeschen C, et al. Emergency room triage of patients with acute chest pain by means of rapid testing for cardiac troponin T or Troponin I. N Engl J Med 1997;337:1648–53.

[23] Jaffe A, Katus H. Acute coronary syndrome biomarkers: the need for more adequate reporting. Circulation 2004;110:104–6.

[24] Panteghini M, Gerhardt W, Apple F, et al. Quality specifications for cardiac troponin assays. Clin Chem Lab Med 2001;39:174–8.

[25] Jaffe AS, Ravkilde J, Roberts R, et al. It's time for a change to a troponin standard. Circulation 2000;102:1216–20.

[26] Katruka A. Antibody selection strategies in cardiac troponin assay. In: Wu AHB, editor. Cardiac markers. 2nd edition. Totowa (NJ): Humana Press Inc.; 2003. p. 173–86.

[27] Eriksson S, Halenius H, Pulkki K, et al. Negative interference in cardiac troponin I immunoassays by circulating troponin autoantibodies. Clin Chem 2005;51:839–47.

[28] Eriksson S, Hellman J, Pettersson K. Autoantibodies against cardiac troponins. N Engl J Med 2005;352:98–100.

[29] Christenson R, Duh S, Apple F, et al. Standardization of cardiac Troponin I assays: round robin of ren candidate reference materials. Clin Chem 2001;47:431–7.

[30] Kricka L. Human anti-animal antibody interferences in immunological assays. Clin Chem 1999;45:942–56.

[31] Fitzmaurice T, Brown C, Rifai N, et al. False increase of cardiac troponin I with heterophilic antibodies. Clin Chem 1998;44:2212–4.

[32] Kazmierczak S, Sekhon H, Richards C. False-positive troponin I measured with the Abbott AxSYM attributed to fibrin interference. Int J Cardiol 2005;101:27–31.

[33] Kisch B. Electron microscopy of the atrium of the heart. I. Guinea pig. Exp Med Surg 1956;114.

[34] Debold A, Borenstein H, Veress A, et al. A rapid and potent natriuretic response to atrial myocardial extract in rats. Life Sci 1981;28.

[35] Sudoh T, Kangawa K, Minamino N, et al. A new natriuretic peptide in porcine brain. Nature 1988;332:78–81.

[36] Mukoyama M, Nakao K, Hosoda K, et al. Brain natriuretic peptide as a novel cardiac hormone in humans: evidence for an exquisite dual natriuretic peptide system, atrial natriuretic peptide and brain natriuretic peptide. J Clin Invest 1991;87:1402–12.

[37] Tsuruda T, Boerrigter G, Huntley B, et al. Brain natriuretic peptide is produced in cardiac fibroblasts and induces matrix metalloproteinases. Circ Res 2002;91:1127–34.

[38] Iwanaga Y, Nishi I, Furuichi S, et al. B-Type natriuretic peptide strongly reflects diastolic wall stress in patients with chronic heart failure. J Am Coll Cardiol 2006;47:742–8.

[39] Hawkridge A, Heublein D, Bergen H, et al. Quantitative mass spectral evidence for the absence of circulating brain natriuretic peptide (BNP-32) in severe human heart failure. Proc Nation Ac Sciences 2005;102:17442–7.

[40] Giuliani I, Rieunier F, Larue C, et al. Assay for measurement of intact B-type natriuretic peptide prohormone in blood. Clin Chem 2006;52:1054–61.

[41] Schellenberger U, O'Rear J, Guzzetta A, et al. The precursor to B-type natriuretic peptide is an O-linked glycoprotein. Arch Biochem Biophys 2006;451:160–6.

[42] Wu A, Packer M, Smith A, et al. Analytical and clinical evaluation of the Bayer ADVIA centaur automated B-type natriuretic peptide assay in patients with heart failure: a Multisite Study. Clin Chem 2004;50:867–73.

[43] Hammerer-Lercher A, Ludwig W, Falkensammer G, et al. Natriuretic peptides as markers of mild forms of left ventricular dysfunction: effects of assays in patients with heart failure: a multisite study. Clin Chem 2004;50:1174–83.

[44] Sorti S, Prontera C, Emdin M, et al. Analytical performance and clinical results of a fully automated MEIA system for BNP assay: comparison with a POCT method. Clin Chem Lab Med 2004;42:1178–85.

[45] Morrow D, deLemos J, Blazing M, et al. Prognostic value of serial B-type natriuretic peptide testing during follow-up of patients with unstable coronary artery disease. JAMA 2005; 294:2866–71.

[46] Jaffe AS, Babuin L, Apple FS. Biomarkers in acute cardiac disease: the present and the future. J Am Coll Cardiol 2006;48:1–11.

[47] Yeo K, Wu A, Apple F, et al. Multicenter evaluation of the Roche NT-proBNP assay and comparison to the Biosite Triage BNP assay. Clin Chim Acta 2003;338:107–15.

[48] Raymond I, Groenning B, Hildebrandt P, et al. The influence of age, sex, and other variables on the plasma level of NT-proBNP in a large sample of the general population. Heart 2003;89:745–51.

[49] Krauser D, Lloyd-Jones D, Chae C, et al. Effect of body mass index on natriuretic peptide levels in patients with acute congestive heart failure: a ProBNP Investigation of Dyspnea in the Emergency Department (PRIDE) substudy. Am Heart J 2004;149:744–50.

[50] Luchner A, Hengstenberg C, Lowel H, et al. N-terminal pro-brain natriuretic peptide after myocardial infarction-a marker of cardio-renal dysfunction. Hypertension 2002;39: 99–104.

[51] McCullough P, Duc P, Omland T, et al. BNP and renal function in the diagnosis of heart failure: an analysis from the breathing not properly multinational study. Am J Kidney Dis 2003;41:571–9.

[52] Apple F, Panteghini M, Ravkilde J, et al. Quality specifications for B-type natriuretic peptide assays. Clin Chem 2005;51:486–93.

[53] Rader D. Inflammatory markers of coronary risk. N Engl J Med 2000;343:1179–82.

[54] Ridker P, Cannon C, Morrow D, et al. C-reactive protein levels and outcomes after statin therapy. N Engl J Med 2005;352:20–8.

[55] Buffon A, Biasucci L, Liuzzo G, et al. Widespread coronary inflammation in unstable angina. N Engl J Med 2002;347:5–12.

[56] Hansson G, Libby P. The immune response in atherosclerosis: a double-edged sword. Immunology 2006;6:508–19.

[57] James S, Armstrong P, Barnathan E, et al. Troponin and C-reactive protein have different relations to subsequent mortality and myocardial infarction after acute coronary syndrome: a GUSTO-IV substudy. J Am Coll Cardiol 2003;41:916–24.

[58] Myers G, Rifai N, Tracy R, et al. CDC/AHA workshop on markers of inflammation and cardiovascular disease: application to clinical and public health practice: report from the laboratory science discussion group. Circulation 2004;110:545–9.

[59] Pai J, Pischon T, Ma J, et al. Inflammatory markers and the risk of coronary heart disease in men and women. N Engl J Med 2004;351:2599–610.

[60] McConnell J, Branum E, Ballman C, et al. Gender differences in C-reactive protein concentrations—confirmation with two sensitive methods. Clin Chem Lab Med 2002;40:56–9.

[61] Khera A, McGuire D, Murphy S, et al. Race and gender differences in C-reactive protein levels. J Am Coll Cardiol 2005;46:464–9.

[62] Lin JC, Apple FS, Murakami MM, et al. Rates of positive cardiac troponin I and creatine kinase MB mass among patients hospitalized for suspected acute coronary syndromes. Clin Chem 2004;50:333–8.

[63] Miller W, Garratt K, Burritt M, et al. Baseline troponin level: key to understanding the importance of post-PCI troponin elevations. Eur Heart J 2006;27:1061–9.

[64] de Winter R, Windhausen F, Cornel J, et al. Early invasive versus selectively invasive management for acute coronary syndromes. N Engl J Med 2005;353:1095–104.

[65] O'Donoghue M, deLemos J, Morrow D, et al. Prognostic utility of heart-type fatty acid binding protein in patients with acute coronary syndromes. Circulation 2006;114:550–7.

[66] Apple F, Wu A, Mair J, et al. Future biomarkers for detection of ischemia and risk stratification in acute coronary syndrome. Clin Chem 2005;51:810–24.

[67] Baldus S, Heeschen C, Meinertz T, et al. Myeloperoxidase serum levels predict risk in patients with acute coronary syndromes. Circulation 2003;108:1140–5.

[68] Brennan M, Penn M, Van Lente F, et al. Prognostic value of myeloperoxidase in patients with chest pain. N Engl J Med 2003;349:1595–604.

[69] Bayes-Genis A, Conover C, Schwartz R, et al. The insulin-like growth factor axis: a review of atherosclerosis and restenosis. Circ Res 2000;86:125–30.

[70] Bayes-Genis A, Conover C, Overgaard M, et al. Pregnancy-associated plasma protein A as a marker of acute coronary syndromes. N Engl J Med 2001;345:1022–9.

[71] Lund J, Qin Q, Ilva T, et al. Circulating pregnancy-associated plasma protein A predicts outcome in patients with acute coronary syndrome but no troponin I elevation. Circulation 2003;108:1924–6.

[72] Heeschen C, Dimmeler S, Fichtlscherer S, et al. Prognostic value of placental growth factor in patients with acute chest pain. JAMA 2004;291:435–41.

[73] Lenderink T, Heeschen C, Fichtlscherer S, et al. Elevated placental growth factor levels are associated with adverse outcomes at four-year follow-up in patients with acute coronary syndromes. J Am Coll Cardiol 2006;47:307–11.

[74] Heeschen C, Dimmeler S, Hamm C, et al. Soluble CD40 ligand in acute coronary syndromes. N Engl J Med 2003;348:1104–11.

[75] Varo N, deLemos J, Libby P, et al. Soluble CD40L risk prediction after acute coronary syndromes. Circulation 2003;108:1049–52.

[76] Ohman E, Armstrong P, Christenson R, et al. Cardiac troponin T levels for risk stratification in acute myocardial ischemia. GUSTO IIA Investigators. N Engl J Med 1996;335:1333–41.

[77] Newby L, Christenson R, Ohman E, et al. Value of serial troponin T measures for early and late risk stratification in patients with acute coronary syndromes. The GUSTO-IIa investigators. Circulation 1998;98:1853–9.

[78] Giannitsis E, Muller-Bardorff M, Lehrke S, et al. Admission troponin T level predicts clinical outcomes, TIMI flow, and myocardial tissue perfusion after primary percutaneous intervention for acute ST-segment elevation myocardial infarction. Circulation 2001;104:630–5.

[79] Matetzky S, Sharir T, Domingo M, et al. Elevated troponin I level on admission is associated with adverse outcome of primary angioplasty in acute myocardial infarction. Circulation 2000;102:1611–6.

[80] Gersh B, Stone G, White H, et al. Pharmacological facilitation of primary percutaneous coronary intervention for acute myocardial infarction: is the slope of the curve the shape of the future? JAMA 2005;293:979–86.

[81] Ohman E, Armstrong P, White H, et al. Risk stratification with a point-of-care cardiac troponin T test in acute myocardial infarction. Am J Cardiol 1999;84:1281–6.

[82] Taher T, Fu Y, Wagner G, et al. Aborted myocardial infarction in patients with ST-segment elevation: insights from the assessment of the safety and efficacy of a new thrombolytic regimen-3 trial electrocardiographic substudy. J Am Coll Cardiol 2004;44:38–43.

[83] Lamfers E, Hooghoudt T, Uppelschoten A, et al. Effect of prehospital thrombolysis on aborting acute myocardial infarction. Am J Cardiol 1999;84:928–30.

[84] Giannitsis E, Lehrke S, Wiegand U, et al. Risk stratification in patients with inferior acute myocardial infarction treated by percutaneous coronary interventions: the role of admission troponin T. Circulation 2000;102:2038–44.

[85] Ottani F, Galvani M, Nicolini F, et al. Elevated cardiac troponin levels predict the risk of adverse outcomes in patients with acute coronary syndromes. Am Heart J 2000;140:917–27.

[86] Eisenberg P, Kenzora J, Sobel B, et al. Relation between ST segment shifts during ischemia and thrombin activity in patients with unstable angina. J Am Coll Cardiol 1991;18:898–903.

[87] deFilippi C, Tocchi M, Parmar R, et al. Cardiac troponin T in chest pain unit patients without ischemic electrocardiographic changes: angiographic correlates and long-term clinical outcomes. J Am Coll Cardiol 2000;35:1827–34.

[88] deLemos J, Morrow D, Gibson M, et al. The prognostic value of serum myoglobin in patients with non–ST-segment elevation acute coronary syndromes: results from the TIMI 11B and TACTICS-TIMI 18 studies. J Am Coll Cardiol 2002;40:238–44.

[89] The Joint European Society of Cardiology/American College of Cardiology Committee. Myocardial infarction redefined—a consensus document of the Joint European Society of Cardiology/American College of Cardiology Committee for the Redefinition of Myocardial Infarction. Eur Heart J 2000;21:1502–13.

[90] Bursi F, Babuin L, Barbieri A, et al. Vascular surgery patients: perioperative and long-term risk according to the ACC/AHA guidelines, the additive role of post-operative troponin elevation. Eur Heart J 2005;26:2448–56.

[91] Kavsak PA, MacRae AR, Palomaki GE, et al. Health outcomes categorized by current and previous definitions of acute myocardial infarction in an unselected cohort of troponin-naïve emergency department patients. Clin Chem 2006;52:2028–35.

[92] Roger V, Killian J, Weston S, et al. Redefinition of myocardial infarction: prospective evaluation in the community. Circulation 2006;114:790–7.

[93] Salomaa V, Koukkunen H, Ketonen M, et al. A new definition for myocardial infarction: what difference does it make? Eur Heart J 2005;26:1719–25.

[94] Lindahl B, Diderholm E, Lagerqvist B, et al. Mechanisms behind the prognostic value of troponin T in unstable coronary artery disease: a FRISC II substudy. J Am Coll Cardiol 2001;38:979–86.

[95] Heeschen C, van Den Brand M, Hamm C, et al. Angiographic findings in patients with refractory unstable angina according to troponin T status. Circulation 1999;100:1509–14.

[96] Okamatsu K, Takano M, Sakai S, et al. Elevated troponin T Levels and lesion characteristics in non–ST-elevation acute coronary syndromes. Circulation 2004;109:465–70.

[97] Wong G, Morrow D, Murphy S, et al. Elevations in troponin T and I are associated with abnormal tissue level perfusion: a TACTICS-TIMI 18 substudy. Circulation 2002;106: 202–7.

[98] Hamm C, Heeschen C, Vahanian A, et al. Benefit of abciximab in patients with refractory unstable angina in relation to serum troponin T levels. N Engl J Med 1999;340:1623–9.

[99] Newby L, Ohman E, Christenson R, et al. Benefit of glycoprotein IIb/IIIa Inhibition in patients with acute coronary syndromes and troponin T–positive status: the PARAGON-B Troponin T substudy. Circulation 2001;103:2891–6.

[100] Lindahl B, Venge P, Wallentin L. Troponin T identifies patients with unstable coronary artery disease who benefit from long-term antithrombotic protection. Fragmin in Unstable Coronary Artery Disease (FRISC) Study Group. J Am Coll Cardiol 1997;29:43–8.

[101] Morrow D, Antman E, Tanasijevic M, et al. Cardiac troponin I for stratification of early outcomes and the efficacy of enoxaparin in unstable angina: a TIMI-11B substudy. J Am Coll Cardiol 2000;36:1812–7.

[102] Heeschen C, Hamm C, Goldmann B, et al. Troponin concentrations for stratification of patients with acute coronary syndromes in relation to therapeutic efficacy of tirofiban. Lancet 1999;354:1757–62.

[103] Kastrati A, Mehilli J, Neumann F, et al. Abciximab in patients with acute coronary syndromes undergoing percutaneous coronary intervention after clopidogrel pretreatment: the ISAR-REACT 2 Randomized Trial. JAMA 2006;295:1531–8.

[104] The Clopidogrel in Unstable Angina to Prevent Recurrent Events Trial Investigators. Effects of clopidogrel in addition to aspirin in patients with acute coronary syndromes without ST-segment elevation. N Engl J Med 2001;345:494–502.

[105] Morrow DA, Cannon CP, Rifai N, et al. Ability of minor elevations of troponins I and T to predict benefit from an early invasive strategy in patients with unstable angina and non-ST elevation myocardial infarction: results from a randomized trial. JAMA 2001;286:2405–12.

[106] F Ragmin and Fast Revascularisation during InStability in Coronary artery disease Investigators. Invasive compared with non-invasive treatment in unstable coronary-artery disease: FRISC II prospective randomized multicenter study. Lancet 1999;354:708–15.

[107] Heeschen C, Hamm C, Mitrovic V, et al. for the platelet receptor inhibition in ischemic syndrome management (PRISM) investigators. N-terminal pro–B-type natriuretic peptide levels for dynamic risk stratification of patients with acute coronary syndromes. Circulation 2004;110:3206–12.

[108] James S, Lindahl B, Timmer J, et al. Usefulness of biomarkers for predicting long-term mortality in patients with diabetes mellitus and non-ST-elevation acute coronary syndromes (a GUSTO IV substudy). Am J Cardiol 2006;97:167–72.

[109] Wiviott SD, Cannon CP, Morrow DA, et al. Differential expression of cardiac biomarkers by gender in patients with unstable angina/non-ST-elevation myocardial infarction: a TAC-TICS-TIMI 18 (Treat Angina with Aggrastat and determine Cost of Therapy with an Invasive or Conservative Strategy-Thrombolysis In Myocardial Infarction 18) substudy. Circulation 2004;109:580–6.

[110] Henrikson C, Howell E, Bush D, et al. Prognostic usefulness of marginal troponin T elevation. Am J Cardiol 2004;93:275–9.

[111] deFilippi C, Wasserman S, Rosanio S, et al. Cardiac troponin T and C-reactive protein for predicting prognosis, coronary atherosclerosis, and cardiomyopathy in patients undergoing long-term hemodialysis. JAMA 2003;290:353–9.

[112] Aviles R, Askari A, Lindahl B, et al. Troponin T levels in patients with acute coronary syndromes, with or without renal dysfunction. N Engl J Med 2002;346:2047–52.

THE MEDICAL
CLINICS
OF NORTH AMERICA

ELSEVIER
SAUNDERS

Med Clin N Am 91 (2007) 683–700

Management of non–ST-Segment Elevation Myocardial Infarction

Stephen E. Van Horn, Jr., MD, Calin V. Maniu, MD*

Division of Cardiology, Medical University of South Carolina, 135 Rutledge Avenue, Suite 1201, P.O. Box 250592, Charleston, SC 29425, USA

In the United States, 1.2 million people experience acute coronary syndromes (ACS) annually, and non–ST-segment elevation myocardial infarction (NSTEMI) represent a significant proportion of these events [1]. NSTEMI is distinguished from unstable angina by the finding of elevated serum levels of cardiac biomarkers. Patients presenting with NSTEMI have a high risk of future cardiovascular events—their mortality at 1 year equals or exceeds that of patients presenting with ST-segment elevation myocardial infarctions (MI) [2]. This is caused part by the presence of multivessel disease and a greater risk of residual ischemia. This article presents an up-to-date overview of the management options currently available for patients who have NSTEMI. The majority of literature does approach NSTEMI as part of the wider encompassing non-ST-segment elevation acute coronary syndrome (NSTEACS), and there are very few publications that exclusively or specifically discuss management of NSTEMI. Unless specified otherwise, all the management recommendations in this article are based on the current American College of Cardiology/American Heart Association (ACC/AHA) guideline update for the management of patients who have unstable angina and NSTEMI [3]. The ACC/AHA guidelines recommendations use a customary classification:

Class I, conditions for which there is evidence or general agreement that a given procedure or treatment is useful and effective

Class II, conditions for which there is conflicting evidence or divergence of opinion about the usefulness and efficacy of a procedure or treatment

---

* Corresponding author.
E-mail address: maniuc@musc.edu (C.V. Maniu).

0025-7125/07/$ - see front matter © 2007 Elsevier Inc. All rights reserved.
doi:10.1016/j.mcna.2007.02.008   *medical.theclinics.com*

Class IIa, weight of evidence and opinion are in favor of usefulness
and efficacy

Class IIb, usefulness and efficacy are less well-established by evidence
and opinion

Class III, conditions for which there is evidence or general agreement that
the procedure or treatment is not useful and effective, and in some
cases may be harmful.

Risk stratification

Patients who have NSTEACS present on a relatively wide spectrum of
risk for "hard" cardiovascular outcomes (death or MI). Features that
have been associated with poorer prognosis are accelerating chest pain in
the previous 48 hours, prolonged angina at rest, signs of heart failure, new
or worsening mitral regurgitation murmur, age greater than 75 years, hemodynamic or arrhythmic instability, ST-segment deviation (≥ 0.5 mm), and
elevation of cardiac biomarkers. (Please also refer to the article by Singh
in this issue.)

Several risk-predictive models have been devised that allow for classification of these patients in different risk categories, thus allowing for tailoring
of the aggressiveness of therapeutic interventions. The most validated and
commonly used method is the Thrombolysis in Myocardial Infarction
(TIMI) risk score that combines age, ECG changes, clinical characteristics,
and cardiac biomarkers. A higher score predicts a higher chance of recurrent
cardiovascular event [4].

Elevation of cardiac biomarkers (especially cardiac troponins)—the hall-
mark of NSTEMI—has been shown to be one of the most powerful single
factors associated with worse outcomes in patients who have NSTEACS
[5,6]. (Please also refer to the article by Jaffe and colleagues in this issue.)

Thus patients who have NSTEMI are included in the high-risk subgroup
of patients presenting with NSTEACS. Several studies have shown that troponin status can be used to guide antithrombotic and interventional therapies [7,8]; however, troponin elevations have been reported in patients who
do not have a clear history suggestive of myocardial ischemia [9], in which
case they may not be diagnostic for ACS.

Management

Patients who have suspected ACS with prolonged chest discomfort at
rest, hemodynamic instability, or recent syncope or presyncope should be
immediately referred to an emergency department or specialized chest
pain center. Their initial management should include a rapid assessment including history, ECG (within 10 minutes), and obtaining biomarkers of cardiac injury (preferably cardiac troponin). Once the diagnosis of NSTEMI
has been established, aggressive therapy is begun, with the goal of relieving

ischemic pain and preventing adverse outcomes such as death or recurrent MI.

Antiplatelet therapy

Aspirin

Aspirin irreversibly inhibits cyclooxygenase-1 within platelets and prevents the formation of thromboxane A2, thus diminishing platelet aggregation. Aspirin has been shown to reduce by 50% the incidence of death and non-fatal MI in several trials and a large meta-analysis [10–12]. Higher doses of aspirin do not provide greater benefit, but appear to be associated with a higher incidence of side effects (bleeding, gastrointestinal side effects). With low-dose aspirin, the full antithrombotic effect takes up to 2 days to manifest, whereas with standard doses the effect comes on within hours. Thus the ACC/AHA guidelines recommend an initial dose of 160 to 325 mg nonenteric formulation to be given, followed by 75 to 325 mg/day of an enteric or nonenteric formulation that should be continued indefinitely. A syndrome of "aspirin-resistance" has emerged recently, described as a relative failure to inhibit platelet aggregation, or the development of a clinical event while on aspirin therapy. Currently there are no prospective data demonstrating that aspirin resistance is clinically relevant, however, or that a biomarker or specific platelet function test can reliably predict aspirin resistance and that this test is tied to clinical outcome [13].

Thienopyridines

The thienopyridines, ticlopidine and clopidogrel, are adenosine diphosphate antagonists that inhibit platelet activation. The antiplatelet effects are irreversible, but take several days to become clinically manifest in the absence of a loading dose. Because their antiplatelet mechanism is different from that of aspirin, the combination exerts an additive effect. Although ticlopidine was the initial agent studied, clopidogrel is currently the preferred thienopyridine because of a more rapid onset of action and a more favorable safety profile. Based on the result of the CAPRIE (clopidogrel versus aspirin in patients at risk of ischaemic events) study [14], clopidogrel should be administered to patients unable to take aspirin because of hypersensitivity or major gastrointestinal contraindication. This trial enrolled 19,185 patients who had known atherosclerotic vascular disease. When compared with aspirin, clopidogrel resulted in a 9% relative risk reduction in adverse cardiovascular events (vascular death, MI, or ischemic stroke) without an increase in bleeding [14]. Clopidogrel should be added to aspirin as part of the initial medical management of NSTEMI. This Class I recommendation is based upon the CURE (clopidogrel in unstable angina to prevent recurrent events) trial [15], which enrolled 12,562 patients. Patients receiving aspirin and clopidogrel (300 mg loading dose followed by 75 mg daily) for 3 to 12 months (mean 9 months) had a 20% relative risk reduction in the primary combined end point of cardiovascular death, nonfatal MI, or stroke when compared with patients receiving aspirin only. Clopidogrel therapy was associated with a 1% absolute risk increase of major bleeding [15]. In the observational substudy of the CURE trial, which included 2658 patients who underwent percutaneous coronary intervention (PCI), clopidogrel therapy was associated with a relative risk reduction of 30% of the composite end point of cardiovascular death and MI [16]. The excess bleeding in the CURE trial was noted in patients on higher doses of aspirin or who underwent coronary artery bypass graft (CABG) surgery within 5 days of discontinuation of clopidogrel [15]. Further support for addition of clopidogrel to aspirin comes from subgroup analysis of the CREDO (clopidogrel for reduction of events during observation) trial [17]. Out of the 2116 patients enrolled in CREDO, about two thirds presented with ACS. Pretreatment with clopidogrel before PCI and continuation of clopidogrel therapy for 1 year after PCI resulted in a trend for reduction of the composite end point of death, stroke, and MI at 1 year. Although addition of clopidogrel to aspirin appears to have an important role in patients who have NSTEMI, a couple of issues are not completely resolved. The ACC/AHA guidelines recommend initiation of clopidogrel in addition to aspirin as soon as possible for patients in whom an early noninvasive approach is planned. The timing for starting clopidogrel for patients undergoing an early invasive approach is not well-defined because there is an absence of solid data in the literature addressing this specific issue. The concern regarding CABG-related bleeding occasionally results in delaying the administration of clopidogrel in patients undergoing early (within 24–36 hours of admission) coronary angiography until is clear that CABG will not be scheduled within the next several days. The authors' opinion is that for patients who have NSTEMI and who are receiving intravenous glycoprotein IIb/IIIa antagonists (which result in more powerful but more easily reversible antiplatelet effects than clopidogrel) this strategy is reasonable. For centers that do not perform very early angiography routinely for NSTEMI patients, the balance of potential risks and benefits of initiating clopidogrel before angiography needs to be considered on an individual basis [18]. If clopidogrel has been initiated and patients are scheduled to undergo CABG, clopidogrel should be withheld for at least 5 days if possible. The second issue is with regard to duration of the clopidogrel treatment. It is not entirely clear how long clopidogrel therapy should be maintained. Based on the CURE and CREDO trials, the ACC/AHA guidelines recommend that clopidogrel should be continued for at least 1 month and up to 9 months after NSTEMI. The CHARISMA (clopidogrel for high atherothrombotic risk and ischemic stabilization, management, and avoidance) trial [19] enrolled 15,603 subjects to test the hypothesis that long-term treatment with a combination of clopidogrel and aspirin would provide greater protection against cardiovascular events than aspirin alone in a broad population of patients at risk [19]. After a median of 28 months of follow-up, overall the trial showed that combination therapy was not more effective than aspirin alone. Although further extension of the duration of clopidogrel therapy can be considered on an individual basis for patients at very high risk of ischemic events (ie, recurrent ACS presentations in spite of otherwise optimal medical therapy), this is not supported as a general recommendation based on the currently available data.

Glycoprotein IIb/IIIa antagonists

When platelets are activated, the glycoprotein IIb/IIIa receptors on the platelet surface undergo conformational changes, increasing their affinity for binding fibrinogen, which is the final pathway in platelet aggregation. Glycoprotein IIb/IIIa antagonists prevent platelet aggregation, resulting in a potent antithrombotic effect. Abciximab, eptifibatide and tirofiban are the three glycoprotein IIb/IIIa antagonists approved for use in NSTEMI. They possess significantly different pharmacokinetic and pharmacodynamic properties [20].

The ACC/AHA recommendations are based on the results of several trials that tested the various glycoprotein IIb/IIIa antagonists in patients undergoing PCI and in patients who had NSTEACS. The CAPTURE (c7E3 fab antiplatelet therapy in unstable refractory angina) trial enrolled 1265 patients who had unstable angina scheduled to undergo PCI, and showed that administration of abciximab resulted in a 30% relative risk reduction of the primary outcome (death, MI, or urgent revascularization) at 30 days [21]. The PRISM-PLUS (platelet receptor inhibition in ischemic syndrome management in patients limited by unstable signs and symptoms) trial enrolled 1530 patients who had NSTEACS, and showed that administration of tirofiban resulted in a 30% relative risk reduction of the primary end point (death, MI, refractory ischemia) at 7 days [22]. Thirty percent of patients in PRISM-PLUS underwent PCI. The PURSUIT (platelet glycoprotein IIb/IIIa in unstable angina: receptor suppression using integrilin therapy) trial enrolled 9461 patients who had NSTEACS, and showed that administration of eptifibatide resulted in a 10% relative risk reduction of death and MI at 30 days [23]. Thirteen percent of patients in PURSUIT underwent PCI.

Based on these results, in patients who have NSTEMI managed with an early invasive strategy, administration of glycoprotein IIb/IIIa antagonists in addition to aspirin and heparin received a Class I indication in the ACC/AHA guidelines. Because there were no definitive data on the safety and efficacy of quadruple therapy (adding glycoprotein IIb/IIIa antagonist to a combination of aspirin, clopidogrel, and heparin) in patients who have NSTEACS undergoing an early invasive strategy at the time of writing of the current ACC/AHA guidelines, this combination received only a Class IIa indication. A subsequently published trial, the ISAR-REACT 2 (intracoronary stenting and antithrombotic regimen: rapid early action for coronary treatment 2) study, enrolled 2022 patients who had NSTEACS undergoing PCI. Administration of abciximab in addition to aspirin, clopidogrel, and heparin resulted in a 25% relative risk reduction of the composite end point (death, MI, and urgent target vessel revascularization) at 30 days, with the benefit confined to the patients presenting with elevated troponin levels. This was accomplished without an increased risk of bleeding [24].

Administration of glycoprotein IIb/IIIa antagonists in patients who have NSTEACS and for whom an invasive strategy is not scheduled is more controversial. A meta-analysis of glycoprotein IIb/IIIa antagonists in all randomized, placebo-controlled trials of this strategy pooled together 31,402 patients and showed a 1% absolute risk reduction of the incidence of death or MI at 30 days, but also a 1% absolute risk increase of major bleeding [25]. Subgroup analysis showed that the benefit of the ischemic end point was confined to patients who actually underwent coronary revascularization within 30 days (38% of patients) and those who had elevated troponin levels. The GUSTO IV-ACS (global use of strategies to open occluded coronary arteries IV–acute coronary syndrome) trial specifically studied 7800 patients presenting with NSTEACS who were not planned to undergo early revascularization. No benefit was noted from the abciximab administration, even in the subgroup of patients who had elevated troponin levels [26]. Based on the available evidence, the ACC/AHA guidelines gave abciximab a Class III indication for use in patients who have NSTEMI in whom PCI is not planned. In NSTEMI patients for whom an early invasive strategy is not planned, tirofiban and eptifibatide are given a Class IIa recommendation. These medications should not be administered to low risk, troponin-negative patients in whom PCI is not planned.

Several trials have tested the effect of oral glycoprotein IIb/IIIa antagonists in non–ST-segment elevation ACS [27,28]. The results were very disappointing, with an increased risk of bleeding and mortality associated with the use of these agents.

Anticoagulant therapy

Several anticoagulants have been studied as add-on therapy to aspirin in the treatment of non–ST-segment elevation ACS.

Unfractionated heparin

The anticoagulant effect of heparin is accomplished by accelerating the action of the proteolytic enzyme antithrombin that inactivates Factors IIa, IXa, and Xa, and prevents thrombus formation [29]. Several trials have demonstrated an incremental benefit from adding unfractionated heparin (UFH) to aspirin over aspirin alone [12,30–33]. In a meta-analysis involving six trials [34], the relative risk reduction of the end point of death and MI was 33%. The ACC/AHA guidelines state that patients who present with NSTEMI should be treated with heparin unless a contraindication exists. UFH has poor bioavailability and marked variability in anticoagulant response among patients. The anticoagulant effect of UFH requires monitoring with the activated partial thromboplastin time. Its use has been associated with a rare but dangerous complication, autoimmune heparin-induced thrombocytopenia with thrombosis. Most of the trials of UFH in NSTEACS have continued therapy for 2 to 5 days. The optimal duration of therapy is not well-established.

Low molecular weight heparins

Low molecular weight heparins (LMWH) inhibit thrombin and Factor Xa with relatively more potent activity of catalyzing the inactivation of Factor Xa than thrombin. LMWH offer the advantages of increased bioavailability, lower rates of heparin-associated thrombocytopenia, and more predictable anticoagulant effect, with once or twice a day subcutaneous dosing, usually obviating the need for laboratory monitoring of their anticoagulant activity. There are several LMWH available on the market, but the agent that has been more extensively studied for patients who have NSTEACS is enoxaparin. The FRISC (fragmin during instability in coronary artery disease) study compared dalteparin or placebo for 6 days and then for 35 to 45 days, and found a 63% risk reduction in death or MI during the first 6 days [35]. The ESSENCE (efficacy and safety of subcutaneous enoxaparin in non-Q-wave coronary events) trial compared UFH and enoxaparin in 3171 patients. The primary end point (death, MI or recurrent angina at 14 days) was significantly lower in the patients assigned to enoxaparin without an increase in major bleeding [36]. In the TIMI 11B (throbolysis in myocardial infarction 11B) trial, which enrolled 3910 patients, enoxaparin therapy was associated with a 15% relative risk reduction in the rate of death, MI, or urgent revascularization at 43 days compared with UFH [37]. This occurred at the expense of a doubling of the risk of major bleeding, which was incurred mainly in the 5 weeks of outpatient therapy. The ACC/AHA guidelines give a Class I recommendation for using UFH or LMWH in patients who have NSTEACS, whereas a Class IIa recommendation is given for the preference of enoxaparin over UFH in patients who do not have renal failure and for whom CABG is not planned within 24 hours. A concern for dosing of enoxaparin surrounds severe obesity, because of the unpredictable levels of absorption in these patients and renal insufficiency (creatinine clearance <60 mL/min) requiring measurement of anti-Xa levels, a laboratory marker of anticoagulant activity. Many practitioners have been reluctant to use LMWH (especially if coronary angiography with PCI is planned) because of concerns of reduced efficacy, increased bleeding, and inability to monitor anticoagulation in the catheterization laboratory.

Two large trials published after the ACC/AHA guidelines have provided more information about some of these contentious issues. In the A to Z (Aggrastat to Zocor) study, 3987 patients were randomized to receive UFH or enoxaparin in addition to aspirin and tirofiban. The primary outcome (7 day composite of death, MI, and refractory ischemia) was similar in both groups, but major bleeding appeared to be more common with enoxaparin [38]. In the SYNERGY (superior yield of the new strategy of enoxaparin, revascularization and glycoprotein IIb/IIIa inhibitors) trial, 10,027 high-risk patients undergoing an early invasive strategy were randomized to receive UFH or enoxaparin. The incidence of the primary outcome (30-day death or MI) was similar between the groups, but patients treated with enoxaparin had a higher incidence of major bleeding [39]. A systematic overview of all six randomized trials comparing enoxaparin and UFH in NSTEACS included 21,946 patients, and found that there was a 9% relative risk reduction in the combined end point of death or MI at 30 days for enoxaparin versus UFH. This analysis found no significant difference in major bleeding at seven days [40]. Enoxaparin provided consistent benefit for patients managed with an early conservative strategy, and the authors' opinion is that enoxaparin should be the anticoagulant of choice for this type of patients. For patients managed with an early invasive strategy, UFH or enoxaparin are both good options. A permanent dialog should be maintained among emergency departments, coronary care units, and cardiac catheterization laboratories so as to avoid in-hospital changes in the type of anticoagulant administered, because this has been associated with an increased incidence of adverse events in the SYNERGY trial [39].

Direct thrombin inhibitors

Direct thrombin inhibitors (DTI) specifically block-soluble and clot-bound thrombin, without the need for a cofactor such as antithrombin. Hirudin, bivalirudin, and argatroban are the three parenteral DTI approved by the US Food and Drug Administration. Hirudin was compared with UFH in the GUSTO IIb (global use of strategies to open occluded coronary arteries IIb) (8011 patients who had NSTEACS) [41] and OASIS-2 (organization to assess strategies for ischemic syndromes 2) (10,141 patients who had NSTEACS) [42] trials, and has shown trends toward benefit, but there was no statistically significant reduction in the trials' primary end points. Despite its promise, further development of hirudin is unlikely. Bivalirudin is a synthetic version of hirudin with a shorter half-life. In contrast to hirudin, its major route of clearance is degradation by endogenous peptidases. It has been studied and approved mainly as an anticoagulant for PCI. The ACUITY (acute catheterization and urgent intervention triage strategy) trial [43] was presented at the 2006 ACC Annual Scientific Sessions. It evaluated treatment with heparin plus glycoprotein IIb/IIIa inhibition compared with bivalirudin with or without glycoprotein IIb/IIIa inhibition among 13,000 patients who had NSTEACS. It appears that bivalirudin alone was associated with a reduction in the net clinical benefit end point (death, MI, unplanned revascularization for ischemia, and major bleeding at 30 days) compared with UFH/enoxaparin plus glycoprotein IIb/IIIa inhibitors [43]. Argatroban is approved for treatment of heparin-induced thrombocytopenia, and has not been extensively studied in ACS. None of the DTI has received a recommendation in the ACC/AHA guidelines for management of NSTEACS.

New anticoagulants

Several drugs are currently being tested that would provide alternatives for the current anticoagulants, with the goal of preserving or enhancing the ischemic benefits without an increase in bleeding. The most promising and more extensively studied agent is fondaparinux, a synthetic pentasaccharide that selectively binds antithrombin and causes rapid and predictable inhibition of factor Xa. Fondaparinux was compared with enoxaparin in the OASIS-5 (organization to assess strategies for ischemic syndrome 5) trial, which enrolled 20,178 patients who had NSTEACS. The primary end point (death, MI, or refractory ischemia at 9 days) was similar between the groups, but fondaparinux was associated with a substantial reduction in major bleeding [44]. It is likely that these data will be incorporated into the next ACC/AHA guidelines for NSTEACS.

Anti-ischemic therapy

Nitrates

Nitrates are known to reduce myocardial oxygen demand while improving myocardial oxygen delivery. Although there is a lack of randomized, placebo-controlled clinical trial data on their effectiveness for symptomatic relief or reduction in cardiac events, nitrates have a Class I recommendation for patients who have NSTEMI, based on extensive, although uncontrolled, clinical observations. If symptoms are not relieved by repeated sublingual nitroglycerin administration and the initiation of intravenous beta-blockers, an intravenous nitroglycerin infusion is recommended (in the absence of contraindications). Intravenous nitroglycerin can be titrated, depending on symptoms and blood pressure response, up to a commonly used maximum dose of 200 mcg per minute. Attempts to wean the drip should be made in the absence of ischemic symptoms, and converting to oral or topical nitrates should be pursued.

Morphine sulfate

When symptoms are not immediately relieved by sublingual nitroglycerin or acute pulmonary congestion is present, intravenous morphine sulfate is a Class I recommendation for patients who have NSTEMI. It can be used repeatedly when symptoms recur despite adequate anti-ischemic therapy, with careful monitoring of the blood pressure, because it can induce hypotension, especially when administered along with intravenous nitroglycerin. No randomized trials have defined the contribution of morphine to the initial therapeutic schedule or its optimal administration schedule.

Beta-adrenergic blockers

Beta-adrenergic blockers have a Class I recommendation in NSTEMI because they decrease cardiac work and myocardial oxygen demand. Slowing of the heart rate provides a longer duration of diastole, allowing for more coronary blood flow. Beta blockers should be started early in the management of NSTEMI in the absence of contraindications (marked first-degree atrioventricular [AV] block, any form of second- or third-degree AV block in the absence of a pacemaker, marked sinus bradycardia, hypotension, history of asthma, or severe LV dysfunction with congestive heart failure). If concern exists about the administration of beta blockers, a low dose of a beta-1 selective agent should be used as first-line therapy. There is no evidence that any member of this class of agents is more effective than another. The doses are up-titrated to reach a target resting heart rate of 50 to 60 beats per minute, unless a limiting side effect is reached. The evidence for the use of beta blockers is based on limited randomized trials in NSTEACS [45]; however, the significant reductions in mortality or morbidity seen in large randomized trials for other types of coronary artery disease (ST-segment elevation MI, stable angina, heart failure) make a compelling indication for use of these agents in the absence of contraindications.

Calcium channel blockers

Calcium channel blockers (CCB) reduce cell transmembrane inward calcium flux, which inhibits myocardial and vascular smooth muscle contraction. Some CCB also slow sinus node impulse formation and atrioventricular conduction. Their use in NSTEMI is based on the variable combination of decreased myocardial oxygen demand (because of decreased afterload, contractility, and heart rate) and improved myocardial blood flow (coronary dilatation and slowing of the heart rate). The immediate-release dihydropyridine CCB should be avoided in the absence of adequate beta blockade, because they have been shown to increase the risk for MI or recurrent angina [46,47]. Verapamil and diltiazem have been studied more extensively in NSTEACS and there is no suggestion of harm, with some trials suggesting an actual benefit [48–51]. The ACC/AHA guidelines give oral long-acting CCB a Class IIa indication for recurrent ischemia in the absence of contraindications and when beta-blockers and nitrates are fully used. Class IIb indications are for extended-release, non-dihydropyridine CCB instead of beta-blockers, and immediate-release dihydropyridine CCB in the presence of beta-blockers.

Lipid-lowering therapy

There have been several randomized trials studying the timing and intensity of lipid-lowering therapy in the setting of ACS. The MIRACL (myocardial ischemia reduction with aggressive cholesterol lowering) trial randomized 3086 patients to high-dose atorvastatin versus placebo. The treatment arm was associated with a 16% relative risk reduction of the primary composite end point (death, MI, cardiac arrest, or recurrent symptomatic ischemia) after 16 weeks [52]. The Z phase of the A to Z trial randomized 4487 patients presenting with ACS (60% NSTEACS) to an early intensive versus a delayed conservative simvastatin strategy. The early intensive strategy showed a trend toward a decrease in the primary composite end point (cardiovascular death, MI, readmission for ACS, and stroke) but this did not reach statistical significance [53]. A meta-analysis that included 12 studies involving 13,024 patients who had ACS, and comparing statin therapy to placebo or "usual care," showed that there was no difference between the strategies when assessing the composite end point of death, MI, and stroke up to 4 months [54]. In the PROVE IT-TIMI 22 (pravastatin or atorvastatin evaluation and infection therapy-thrombolysis in myocardial infarction 22) trial, atorvastatin 80 mg was compared with pravastatin 40 mg in 4162 patients presenting with ACS (two thirds NSTEACS). The more intensive regimen resulted in a 16% relative risk reduction in the primary composite end point (death, MI, unstable angina requiring rehospitalization, revascularization, and stroke) at a mean follow-up of 24 months [55]. Patients in whom lipid-lowering therapy is initiated in the hospital are much more likely to be on such therapy at later time. The ACC/AHA guidelines give a Class I recommendation for initiation of statin therapy in patients who have LDL cholesterol greater than 130 mg/dL or low-density lipoprotein (LDL) cholesterol greater than 100 mg/dL after diet. Starting a statin 24 to 96 hours after admission for LDL greater than 100 mg/dL is given a Class IIa indication.

Other medical therapy

Angiotensin converting enzyme inhibitors (ACEI) have not been specifically studied in patients who have NSTEMI; however, ACEI have been shown to reduce mortality in patients who have acute ST segment elevation MI, or who have recent MI and left-ventricular systolic dysfunction, in diabetic patients who have left-ventricular systolic dysfunction, and in a broad spectrum of patients who have high-risk CAD [56–59]. Therefore the ACC/AHA guidelines for hospital care recommend as a Class IIa indication the use of ACEI in all patients post-ACS. Angiotensin II receptor blockers can be used as an alternative to ACEI in patients intolerant to ACEI.

Early invasive versus early conservative strategies

Although all patients who have NSTEMI need to receive appropriate medical therapy, the decision regarding the strategy for pursuing coronary angiography and revascularization (if appropriate) is a very important issue that needs to be addressed early on at presentation. In the early invasive strategy, all patients who have no clinically obvious contraindications undergo coronary angiography followed by angiographically driven revascularization (percutaneous or surgical). The early conservative strategy consists of aggressive medical therapy for all patients, whereas coronary angiography is reserved only for patients who have recurrent ischemia (angina at rest or with minimal activity, or dynamic ST segment changes) or high-risk features during the stress test performed while the patient receives optimal medical therapy. Several trials have compared these two strategies.

The two early trials comparing an early invasive versus a conservative strategy, the TIMI IIIB (thrombolysis in myocardial infarction IIIB) [60] and VANQWISH (veterans affairs non-Q-wave infarction strategies in hospital) [61] trials, did not demonstrate benefit from an invasive approach. In fact the VANQWISH trial showed an excess of deaths and MI with the invasive strategy. The results were related to a high mortality rate associated with CABG. These trials were performed before routine use of stents for PCI.

More recent trials have suggested that the early invasive strategy is superior. In the FRISC-II trial, 2457 patients who had NSTEACS were enrolled. The early invasive strategy was associated with a reduction in the rate of death and MI at 6 months and 1 year, along with reduced anginal symptoms and reduced hospital admissions [62]. The TACTICS-TIMI 18 (treat angina with aggrastat and determine cost of therapy with an invasive or conservative strategy–thrombolysis in myocardial infarction 18) trial enrolled 2200 patients who presented with NSTEACS, and showed that the composite end point of death, MI, or rehospitalization for ACS at 6 months was reduced with an early invasive strategy. The beneficial effects were observed in medium- and high- risk patients [63]. The RITA-3 (randomized intervention trial of unstable angina 3) trial randomized 1810 patients who presented with NSTEACS, and found a decreased rate of the composite end point of death, MI, or refractory angina compared with conservative therapy at 4 months. The differences found in this trial were mainly caused by the large reduction in refractory angina [64]. The ISAR-COOL (intracoronary stenting with antithrombotic regimen cooling-off) trial tested the hypothesis that prolonged antithrombotic pretreatment is beneficial before PCI in patients presenting with NSTEACS. The study enrolled 410 patients who were randomized to prolonged antithrombotic pretreatment before PCI or early PCI. Deferral of PCI did not improve outcomes when compared with immediate PCI with intense antiplatelet therapy [65]. A meta-analysis of seven trials including 9212 patients showed that the early invasive strategy is superior to the selectively invasive strategy in reducing death, MI, severe angina, and rehospitalization during long-term follow-up, but that lower risk patients who had negative baseline biomarker levels did not derive any benefit [66].

The current ACC/AHA guidelines recommend an early invasive strategy if patients have high risk criteria, including elevated troponin (ie, NSTEMI), new ST-segment depression, recurrent angina with heart failure or angina at rest, left ventricular dysfunction, hemodynamic instability, sustained ventricular tachycardia, prior PCI within 6 months, or prior CABG, but a decision to proceed with an invasive procedure must be made on a patient-to-patient basis.

Since the current ACC/AHA guidelines have been issued, the results of another study testing the two strategies for invasive evaluation in patients who have NSTEACS have been published. The ICTUS (invasive versus conservative treatment in unstable coronary syndromes) trial enrolled 1200 patients who had elevated troponin levels and who were treated with state-of-the-art medical therapy. The composite end point (death, MI, or rehospitalization for angina) at 1 year was not different between the two strategies [67]. Although there has been debate regarding the ICTUS trial results and their applicability to the clinical practice in the United States, it is likely that these new findings will be incorporated in the upcoming ACC/AHA guidelines.

Long-term risk factor modification

Education about the patient's clinical condition should begin upon admission. Specific instructions have to be provided for smoking cessation, and consideration of referral to a smoking cessation program should be given. Patients who have NSTEMI must be counseled on achieving and maintaining optimal weight, daily exercise, and diet, along with referral to an outpatient cardiac rehabilitation program. Diabetics need strict glycemic control (target hemoglobin A_1C < 7%). Aggressive LDL lowering is recommended with statin and diet. If high-density lipoprotein (HDL) is less than 40 mg/dL and triglycerides are over 200 mg/dL, a fibrate or niacin should be considered. For long-term medical therapy, the ACC/AHA guidelines give ACEI a Class I recommendation for ACS patients who have heart failure, left ventricular dysfunction (EF < 40%), hypertension, or diabetes. Hypertension should also be adequately controlled.

Special groups

Women

Women who have ACS present more frequently with atypical symptoms, and the ECG is less reliable as a first-line diagnostic tool. Women present more frequently with NSTEACS, whereas men more often have ACS with ST-segment elevation [68,69]. The FRISC II [62] and RITA 3 [64] trials discourage an early invasive management for women; however, TACTICS-TIMI 18 showed that women who have elevated troponins benefit from early interventions [63]. Complication rates during PCI are higher in women than in men. In the CURE trial [70], high-risk women who had NSTEACS underwent less coronary angiography and revascularization compared with men, and although they did not have a higher incidence of cardiovascular death, recurrent MI, or stroke, they suffered an increased rate of refractory ischemia and rehospitalization [70]. The ACC/AHA guidelines recommend that women be managed in a similar manner to men.

Elderly patients

Elderly patients are more likely to present with NSTEACS and have substantial in-hospital mortality, yet they are markedly less intensively treated and investigated than the younger patients [71,72]. Older age among patients who have ACS is associated with worse baseline characteristics, fewer invasive procedures, and worse outcome [73]. Elderly patients who have ACS are usually sicker on admission and have a worse outcome, but a subgroup selected for angiography and possible revascularization had similar outcomes to the younger cohort [74]. The TACTICS-TIMI 18 trial showed that there is a benefit associated with an early invasive strategy in the elderly, with a significant decrease in death and MI at the expense of an increased risk of major bleeding [75]. Age impacts use of guidelines-recommended care for newer agents and early in-hospital care. Further improvements in outcomes for elderly patients by optimizing the safe and early use of therapies are likely [76]. The ACC/AHA guidelines recommend that decisions on management of elderly patients who have NSTEMI should take into consideration their general medical condition, mental state, and overall life expectancy from their comorbid conditions. Intensive medical and interventional management can be undertaken, but with close observation for adverse effects of these therapies that are more frequent in this special population.

Summary

NSTEMI is a major cause of cardiovascular morbidity and mortality in the United States. It represents the highest risk category of NSTEACS, for which timely diagnosis and appropriate therapy are paramount to improve the outcomes. Evidence-based treatment, with combination of antiplatelet and anticoagulant therapy, and with serious consideration of early coronary angiography and revascularization, along with anti-ischemic therapy, is the mainstay of management for NSTEMI. Aggressive risk-factor control after the acute event is imperative for secondary prevention of cardiovascular events. Applying in practice the ACC/AHA guideline recommendations results in improved outcomes.

References

[1] American Heart Association. Heart disease and stroke statistics—2005 update. Dallas (TX): American Heart Association; 2005.
[2] Armstrong PW, Fu Y, Chang W-C, et al. Acute coronary syndromes in the GUSTO-IIb trial: prognostic insights and impact of recurrent ischemia. Circulation 1998;98:1860–8.
[3] Braunwald E, Antman EM, Beasley JW, et al. ACC/AHA 2002 guideline update for the management of patients with unstable angina and non-ST-segment elevation myocardial infarction—summary article: a report of the American College of Cardiology/American Heart Association Task Force on Practice Guidelines (Committee on the Management of Patients With Unstable Angina) 2002. Available at: http://www.acc.org/clinicalguidelines/unstable/unstable.pdf. Accessed April 19, 2007.
[4] Antman EM, Cohen M, Bernik PJLM, et al. The TIMI risk score for unstable angina/non-ST elevation MI. JAMA 2000;284:835–42.
[5] Ohman EM, Armstrong PW, Christenson RH, et al. Cardiac troponin T levels for risk stratification in acute myocardial ischemia. N Engl J Med 1996;335:1333–41.

[6] Antman EM, Tanasijevic MJ, Thompson B, et al. Cardiac troponin I levels to predict the risk of mortality in patients with acute coronary syndromes. N Engl J Med 1996;335:1342–9.

[7] Morrow DA, Cannon CP, Rifai N, et al. Ability of minor elevations of troponins I and T to predict benefit from an early invasive strategy in patients with unstable angina and non-ST elevation myocardial infarction: results from a randomized trial. JAMA 2001;286:2405–12.

[8] Morrow DA, Antman EM, Tanasijevic M, et al. Cardiac troponin I for stratification of early outcomes and the efficacy of enoxaparin in unstable angina: a TIMI-11B substudy. J Am Coll Cardiol 2000;36:1812–7.

[9] Fleming SM, O'Byrne L, Finn J, et al. False-positive cardiac troponin I in a routine clinical population. Am J Cardiol 2002;89:1212–5.

[10] Lewis HD, Davis JW, Archibald DG, et al. Protective effects of aspirin against acute myocardial infarction and death in men with unstable angina. Results of a Veterans Administration cooperative study. N Engl J Med 1983;309:396–403.

[11] Theroux P, Ouimet H, McCans J, et al. Aspirin, heparin, or both to treat acute unstable angina. N Engl J Med 1988;319:1105–11.

[12] Antithrombotic Trialists' Collaboration. Collaborative meta-analysis of randomised trials of antiplatelet therapy for prevention of death, myocardial infarction, and stroke in high risk patients. BMJ 2002;324:71–86.

[13] Freedman JE. The aspirin resistance controversy: clinical entity or platelet heterogeneity? Circulation 2006;113:2865–7.

[14] CAPRIE Steering Committee. A randomised, blinded, trial of clopidogrel versus aspirin in patients at risk of ischaemic events (CAPRIE). Lancet 1996;348:1329–39.

[15] The Clopidogrel in Unstable Angina to Prevent Recurrent Events Trial Investigators. Effects of clopidogrel in addition to aspirin in patients with acute coronary syndromes without ST-segment elevation. N Engl J Med 2001;345:494–502.

[16] Mehta SR, Yusuf S, Peters RJ, et al. Effects of pretreatment with clopidogrel and aspirin followed by long-term therapy in patients undergoing percutaneous coronary intervention: the PCI-CURE study. Lancet 2001;358:527–33.

[17] Steinhubl SR, Berger PB, Mann JT 3rd, et al. Early and sustained dual oral antiplatelet therapy following percutaneous coronary intervention: a randomized controlled trial. JAMA 2002;288:2411–20.

[18] Fox KAA, Mehta SR, Peters R, et al. Benefits and risks of the combination of clopidogrel and aspirin in patients undergoing surgical revascularization for non–ST-elevation acute coronary syndrome: the Clopidogrel in Unstable angina to prevent Recurrent ischemic Events (CURE) Trial. Circulation 2004;110:1202–8.

[19] Bhatt DL, Fox KAA, Hacke W, et al. Clopidogrel and aspirin versus aspirin alone for the prevention of atherothrombotic events. N Engl J Med 2006;354:1706–17.

[20] Topol EJ, Byzova TV, Plow EF. Platelet GPIIb-IIIa blockers. Lancet 1999;353:227–31.

[21] The CAPTURE investigators. Randomised placebo-controlled trial of abciximab before and during coronary intervention in refractory unstable angina: the CAPTURE study. Lancet 1997;349:1429–35.

[22] The Platelet Receptor Inhibition in Ischemic Syndrome Management in Patients Limited by Unstable Signs and Symptoms (PRISM-PLUS) Study Investigators. Inhibition of the platelet glycoprotein IIb/IIIa receptor with tirofiban in unstable angina and non–Q-wave myocardial infarction. N Engl J Med 1998;338:1488–97.

[23] The PURSUIT Trial Investigators. Inhibition of platelet glycoprotein IIb/IIIa with eptifibatide in patients with acute coronary syndromes. N Engl J Med 1998;339:436–43.

[24] Kastrati A, Mehilli J, Neumann FJ, et al. Abciximab in patients with acute coronary syndromes undergoing percutaneous coronary intervention after clopidogrel pretreatment: the ISAR-REACT 2 randomized trial. JAMA 2006;295:1531–8.

[25] Boersma E, Harrington RA, Moliterno DJ, et al. Platelet glycoprotein IIb/IIIa inhibitors in acute coronary syndromes: a meta-analysis of all major randomised clinical trials. Lancet 2002;359:189–98.

[26] The GUSTO IV-ACS Investigators. Effect of glycoprotein IIb/IIIa receptor blocker abciximab on outcome in patients with acute coronary syndromes without early coronary revascularisation: the GUSTO IV-ACS randomised trial. Lancet 2001;357:1915–24.

[27] The SYMPHONY Investigators. Comparison of sibrafiban with aspirin for prevention of cardiovascular events after acute coronary syndromes: a randomised trial. Lancet 2000; 355:337–45.

[28] Second SYMPHONY Investigators. Randomized trial of aspirin, sibrafiban, or both for secondary prevention after acute coronary syndromes. Circulation 2001;103:1727–33.

[29] Hirsh J. Heparin. N Engl J Med 1991;324:1565–74.

[30] The Risk Group. Risk of myocardial infarction and death during treatment with low dose aspirin and intravenous heparin in men with unstable coronary artery disease. Lancet 1990;336:827–30.

[31] Cohen M, Adams PC, Parry G, et al. Combination antithrombotic therapy in unstable rest angina and non–Q-wave infarction in non prior aspirin users. Primary end points analysis from the ATACS trial. Antithrombotic Therapy in Acute Coronary Syndromes Research Group. Circulation 1994;89:81–8.

[32] Theroux P, Waters D, Qiu S, et al. Aspirin versus heparin to prevent myocardial infarction during the acute phase of unstable angina. Circulation 1993;88:2045–8.

[33] Holdright D, Patel D, Cunningham D, et al. Comparison of the effect of heparin and aspirin versus aspirin alone on transient myocardial ischemia and in-hospital prognosis in patients with unstable angina. J Am Coll Cardiol 1994;24:39–45.

[34] Oler A, Whooley MA, Oler J, et al. Adding heparin to aspirin reduces the incidence of myocardial infarction and death in patients with unstable angina. A meta-analysis. JAMA 1996; 276:811–5.

[35] Fragmin during Instability in Coronary Artery Disease (FRISC) study group. Low-molecular-weight heparin during instability in coronary artery disease. Lancet 1996;347:561–8.

[36] Cohen M, Demers C, Gurfinkel EP, et al. A comparison of low-molecular-weight heparin with unfractionated heparin for unstable coronary artery disease. N Engl J Med 1997;337: 447–52.

[37] Antman EM, McCabe CH, Gurfinkel EP, et al. Enoxaparin prevents death and cardiac ischemic events in unstable angina/non–Q-wave myocardial infarction: results of the Thrombolysis in Myocardial Infarction (TIMI) 11B trial. Circulation 1999;100:1593–601.

[38] Blazing MA, de Lemos JA, White HD, et al. Safety and efficacy of enoxaparin vs. unfractionated heparin in patients with non–ST-segment elevation acute coronary syndromes who receive tirofiban and aspirin: a randomized controlled trial. JAMA 2004;292:55–64.

[39] Fergusson JJ, Califf RM, Antman EM, et al. Enoxaparin vs. unfractionated heparin in high-risk patients with non–ST-segment elevation acute coronary syndromes managed with an intended early invasive strategy: primary results of the SYNERGY randomized trial. JAMA 2004;292:45–54.

[40] Petersen JL, Mahaffey KW, Hasselblad V, et al. Efficacy and bleeding complications among patients randomized to enoxaparin or unfractionated heparin for antithrombin therapy in non–ST-segment elevation acute coronary syndromes: a systematic overview. JAMA 2004;292:89–96.

[41] The Global Use of Strategies to Open Occluded Coronary Arteries (GUSTO) IIb investigators. A comparison of recombinant hirudin with heparin for the treatment of acute coronary syndromes. N Engl J Med 1996;335:775–82.

[42] Organization to Assess Strategies for Ischemic Syndromes (OASIS-2) investigators. Effects of recombinant hirudin (lepirudin) compared with heparin on death, myocardial infarction, refractory angina, and revascularisation procedures in patients with acute myocardial ischaemia without ST elevation: a randomized trial. Lancet 1999;353:429–38.

[43] Stone GW, Bertrand ME, Moses JW, et al. Routine upstream initiation vs. deferred selective use of glycoprotein IIb/IIIa inhibitors in acute coronary syndromes: the ACUITY timing trial. JAMA 2007;297(6):591–602.

[44] The Fifth Organization to Assess Strategies in Acute Ischemic Syndromes investigators. Comparison of fondaparinux and enoxaparin in acute coronary syndromes. N Engl J Med 2006;354:1464–76.

[45] Yusuf S, Wittes J, Friedman L. Overview of results of randomized clinical trials in heart disease. II. Unstable angina, heart failure, primary prevention with aspirin, and risk factor modification. JAMA 1988;260:2259–63.

[46] Furberg CD, Psaty BM, Meyer JV. Nifedipine dose-related increase in mortality in patients with coronary heart disease. Circulation 1995;92:1326–31.

[47] Lubsen J, Tijssen JG. Efficacy of nifedipine and metoprolol in the early treatment of unstable angina in the coronary care unit: findings from the Holland Interuniversity Nifedipine/metoprolol Trial (HINT). Am J Cardiol 1987;60:18A–25A.

[48] Gibson RS, Boden WE, Theroux P, et al. Diltiazem and reinfarction in patients with non–Q-wave myocardial infarction. Results of a double-blind, randomized, multicenter trial. N Engl J Med 1986;315:423–9.

[49] Boden WE, Krone RJ, Kleiger RE, et al. Electrocardiographic subset analysis of diltiazem administration on long-term outcome after acute myocardial infarction. The Multicenter Diltiazem Post-Infarction Trial Research Group. Am J Cardiol 1991;67: 335–42.

[50] The Danish Study Group on Verapamil in Myocardial Infarction. Verapamil in acute myocardial infarction. Eur Heart J 1984;5:516–28.

[51] Pepine CJ, Faich G, Makuch R. Verapamil use in patients with cardiovascular disease: an overview of randomized trials. Clin Cardiol 1998;21:633–41.

[52] Schwartz GG, Olsson AG, Ezekowitz MD, et al. Effects of atorvastatin on early recurrent ischemic events in acute coronary syndromes. The MIRACL study: a randomized controlled trial. JAMA 2001;285:1711–8.

[53] de Lemos JA, Blazing MA, Wiviott SD, et al. Early intensive vs. a delayed conservative simvastatin strategy in patients with acute coronary syndromes: phase Z of the A to Z Trial. JAMA 2004;292:1307–16.

[54] Briel M, Schwartz GG, Thompson PL, et al. Effects of early treatment with statins on short-term clinical outcomes in acute coronary syndromes: a meta-analysis of randomized controlled trials. JAMA 2006;295:2046–56.

[55] Cannon CP, Braunwald E, McCabe CH, et al. Intensive versus moderate lipid lowering with statins after acute coronary syndromes. N Engl J Med 2004;350:1495–504.

[56] Yusuf S, Pepine CJ, Garces C, et al. Effect of enalapril on myocardial infarction and unstable angina in patients with low ejection fraction. Lancet 1992;340:1173–8.

[57] ACE Inhibitor Myocardial Infarction Collaborative Group. Indications for ACE inhibitors in the early treatment of acute myocardial infarction. Systematic overview of individual data from 100,000 patients in randomized trials. Circulation 1998;97: 2202–12.

[58] The Heart Outcomes Prevention Evaluation Study Investigators. Effects of an angiotensin converting enzyme inhibitor, ramipril, on cardiovascular events in high-risk patients. N Engl J Med 2000;342:145–53.

[59] The EURopean trial On reduction of cardiac events with Perindopril in stable coronary Artery disease Investigators. Efficacy of perindopril in reduction of cardiovascular events among patients with stable coronary artery disease: randomised, double-blind, placebo-controlled, multicentre trial (the EUROPA study). Lancet 2003;362:782–8.

[60] The TIMI IIIB Investigators. Effects of tissue plasminogen activator and a comparison of early invasive and conservative strategies in unstable angina and non–Q-wave myocardial infarction: results of the TIMI IIIB trial. Thrombolysis in myocardial ischemia. Circulation 1994;89:1545–56.

[61] Boden WE, O'Rourke RA, Crawford MH, et al. Outcomes in patients with acute non–Q-wave myocardial infarction randomly assigned to an invasive as compared with a conservative management strategy. N Engl J Med 1998;338:1785–92.

[62] FRagmin and Fast Revascularisation during InStability in Coronary artery disease Investigators. Invasive compared with non-invasive treatment in unstable coronary-artery disease: FRISC II prospective randomised multicentre study. Lancet 1999;354:708–15.

[63] Cannon CP, Weintraub WS, Demopoulos LA, et al. Comparison of early invasive and conservative strategies in patients with unstable coronary syndromes treated with the glycoprotein IIb/IIIa inhibitor tirofiban. N Engl J Med 2001;344:1879–87.

[64] Fox KA, Poole-Wilson P, Clayton TC, et al. 5-year outcome of an interventional strategy in non–ST-elevation acute coronary syndrome: the British Heart Foundation RITA 3 randomised trial. Lancet 2005;366:914–20.

[65] Neumann FJ, Kastrati A, Pogatsa-Murray G, et al. Evaluation of prolonged antithrombotic pretreatment ("cooling-off" strategy) before intervention in patients with unstable coronary syndromes: a randomized controlled trial. JAMA 2003;290:1593–9.

[66] Mehta SR, Cannon CP, Fox KA, et al. Routine vs. selective invasive strategies in patients with acute coronary syndromes: a collaborative meta-analysis of randomized trials. JAMA 2005;293:2908–17.

[67] de Winter RJ, Windhausen F, Cornel JH, et al. Early invasive versus selectively invasive management for acute coronary syndromes. N Engl J Med 2005;353:1095–104.

[68] Hochman JS, Tamis JE, Thompson TD, et al. Sex, clinical presentation, and outcome in patients with acute coronary syndromes. N Engl J Med 1999;341:226–32.

[69] Hochman JS, McCabe CH, Stone PH, et al. Outcome and profile of women and men presenting with acute coronary syndromes: a report from TIMI IIIB. J Am Coll Cardiol 1997;30: 141–8.

[70] Anand SS, Xie CC, Mehta SR, et al. Differences in the management and prognosis of men and women who suffer from acute coronary syndromes. J Am Coll Cardiol 2005; 46:1845–51.

[71] Rosengren A, Wallentin L, Simoons M, et al. Age, clinical presentation, and outcome of acute coronary syndromes in the Euroheart acute coronary syndrome survey. Eur Heart J 2006;27:789–95.

[72] De Servi S, Cavallini C, Dellavalle A, et al. Non–ST-elevation acute coronary syndrome in the elderly: treatment strategies and 30-day outcome. Am Heart J 2004;147:830–6.

[73] Hasdai D, Holmes DR Jr, Criger DA, et al. Age and outcome after acute coronary syndromes without persistent ST-segment elevation. Am Heart J 2000;139:858–66.

[74] Halon DA, Adawi S, Dobrecky-Mery I, et al. Importance of increasing age on the presentation and outcome of acute coronary syndromes in elderly patients. J Am Coll Cardiol 2004; 43:346–52.

[75] Bach RG, Cannon CP, Weintraub WS, et al. The effect of routine, early invasive management on outcome for elderly patients with non–ST-segment elevation acute coronary syndromes. Ann Intern Med 2004;141:186–95.

[76] Alexander KP, Roe MT, Chen AY, et al. Evolution in cardiovascular care for elderly patients with non–ST-segment elevation acute coronary syndromes: results from the CRUSADE national quality improvement initiative. J Am Coll Cardiol 2005;46:1479–87.

THE MEDICAL
CLINICS
OF NORTH AMERICA

Med Clin N Am 91 (2007) 701–712

Pathophysiology of Cardiogenic Shock Complicating Acute Myocardial Infarction

Eve D. Aymong, MD, MSc, FRCPC[a,b,*],
Krishnan Ramanathan, MB, ChB,
FRACP, FRCPC[a,b,c],
Christopher E. Buller, MD, FRCPC, FACC[a,b,c]

[a]*University of British Columbia, Vancouver, BC, Canada*
[b]*Division of Cardiology, University of British Columbia, 1081 Burrard Street,*
Room 474A, St. Paul's Hospital, Vancouver, BC, Canada V6Z 1Y6
[c]*Gordon and Leslie Diamond Health Care Centre, Level 9, Cardiology,*
2775 Laurel Street, Vancouver, BC, Canada V5Z 1M9

Cardiogenic shock complicating acute myocardial infarction (MI) remains a significant clinical problem despite advances in reperfusion therapy. Current estimates of the incidence of cardiogenic shock complicating MI remain stable at approximately 7% [1,2]. This devastating complication results in most early post-MI mortality [3].

Diagnostic criteria of cardiogenic shock

Cardiogenic shock is clinically defined as a state of end-organ dysfunction caused by hypoperfusion secondary to low cardiac output with associated hypotension, classically defined as a systolic blood pressure less than 90 mm Hg. Hypoperfusion can affect any organ system; those most prone to ischemia are the kidney and brain, resulting in decreased level of consciousness, cool extremities, and decreased urine output. Other hemodynamic criteria of cardiogenic shock, as shown in Box 1, include decreased cardiac index (<2.2 L/min/m^2) and elevated left ventricular filling pressures (pulmonary capillary wedge pressure or left ventricular end diastolic pressure >15 mm Hg) [4]. Evidence of presumed cardiogenic pulmonary edema is used as a surrogate for increased left ventricular filling pressure in the

---

* Corresponding author.
E-mail address: eaymong@providencehealth.bc.ca (E.D. Aymong).

doi:10.1016/j.mcna.2007.03.006
medical.theclinics.com

Box 1. Diagnostic criteria of cardiogenic shock

Clinical criteria
Systolic blood pressure <90 mm Hg
Evidence of hypoperfusion
   Cool, clammy periphery
   Decreased urine output
   Decreased level of consciousness

Hemodynamic criteria
Left ventricular end diastolic pressure or pulmonary capillary
   wedge pressure >15 mm Hg
Cardiac index <2.2 L/min/m^2

Data from Hochman JS, Sleeper LA, Webb JG, et al. Early revascularization in acute myocardial infarction complicated by cardiogenic shock. SHOCK Investigators. Should We Emergently Revascularize Occluded Coronaries for Cardiogenic Shock. N Engl J Med 1999;341(9):625–34.

---

absence of direct measurement of pulmonary capillary wedge pressure or left ventricular end diastolic pressure.

Any cut point of patient hemodynamics (ie, blood pressure or cardiac index) is obviously artificial and patient care must be guided on an individual basis. In addition, interventions to treat patients who have complicated myocardial infarction such as inotropes and intra-aortic balloon counter-pulsation can cloud these arbitrary cut points.

Classical paradigm of cardiogenic shock

The progressive downward spiral that describes the clinical deterioration of patients who have cardiogenic shock is portrayed in Fig. 1. The essential feature is that decreased coronary blood flow results in decreased cardiac output. This decrease in cardiac output leads to hypotension and progressively more cardiac ischemia and dysfunction. The resulting stuttering ischemia and infarction eventually results in left ventricular failure and death.

Fundamentals of myocardial physiology

To fully appreciate the pathophysiology that leads to cardiogenic shock, the fundamental aspects of normal cardiac function must be understood.

The heart is an obligate aerobic organ and can tolerate only minimal decreases in oxygen supply. The myocardial oxygen consumption of the normally contracting heart muscle is between 8 and 15 mL/min/100 g compared with 1.5 mL/min/100 g in the noncontracting heart. Even in its basal,

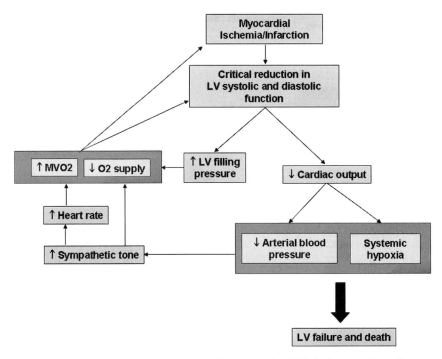

Fig. 1. The classic paradigm of progressive left ventricular (LV) dysfunction in cardiogenic shock. Consequences of progressive ischemia and infarction result in continually worsening hemodynamics and eventually left ventricular failure and death. MVO_2, myocardial oxygen consumption. (*From* Ganz P, Braunwald E. Coronary blood flow and myocardial ischemia. In: Braunwald E, editor. Heart disease. A textbook of cardiovascular medicine. 5th edition. Philadelphia: WB Saunders; 1997. p. 1161–84; with permission.)

noncontracting state, it extracts two to three times more oxygen than other organs.

Total myocardial oxygen consumption, or demand, is known as MVO_2. On a per-gram basis, this is determined by ventricular wall tension (wall stress), heart rate, and contractility (Fig. 2). Laplace's law approximates wall tension as follows:

Wall stress $= (P \times r)/2h$, where P is the transmural pressure,

r is the radius of the left ventricle, and

h is the thickness of the ventricular wall

Coronary blood flow, primarily a diastolic phenomenon, is an obvious requirement for myocardial oxygen supply. Diastolic coronary blood flow is directly proportional to perfusion pressure (which can be approximated by mean aortic diastolic pressure minus mean left ventricular diastolic

a.   MVO2   α   •Heart rate
               •Contractility
               •Wall stress

b.   Wall stress α $\dfrac{P \times r}{2h}$

c.   Coronary   α $\dfrac{\text{Perfusion pressure}}{\text{Coronary vascular resistance}}$
      blood flow

Fig. 2. Myocardial oxygen balance. (*A*) On a per-gram basis, MVO$_2$ is determined by heart rate, contractility, and ventricular wall tension (wall stress). (*B*) Wall stress is approximated by LaPlace's law, where *P* is left ventricular pressure, *r* is left ventricular radius, and *h* is left ventricular wall thickness. (*C*) Two of the primary determinants of coronary blood flow are depicted.

pressure) and is inversely proportional to coronary vascular resistance. In diastole, coronary vascular resistance is modulated primarily by complicated intrinsic effectors of vascular tone. In the presence of epicardial coronary stenoses and endothelial dysfunction that exists with ischemic heart disease, the compensatory mechanisms for maintenance of coronary flow are altered. Myocardial perfusion and coronary blood flow, especially of the subendocardium, occur predominantly in diastole [5].

Continuum of myocardial ischemia leading to dysfunction

Within seconds of loss of coronary blood flow, heart muscle becomes ischemic and myocardial mechanics are abruptly altered, resulting in both systolic and diastolic dysfunction. This process occurs before actual myocardial cell death as a result of acute oxygen debt. As ischemia progresses, the myocardium becomes stunned and will not immediately respond to reperfusion. If injury progresses, myocytes die and infarction ensues.

Although patients who experience cardiogenic shock have significant areas of dead myocardium, it is crucial to recognize that stunned or hibernating myocardium may play a significant role in the ongoing left ventricular dysfunction [6–8]. This fact is particularly important in understanding the fundamental role of complete revascularization in these patients [9].

Myocardial dysfunction can occur with viable tissue. Myocardial stunning causes myocardial dysfunction resulting from ischemic injury without myocardial necrosis or cell death [6–9]. It is defined as postischemic myocardial dysfunction with eventual return of normal contractile activity. Of course, whether myocardium will return to normal function is impossible to determine and stunning can last for hours to weeks.

Stunned myocardium occurs when myocardium has been reperfused and is still viable, yet displays ongoing dysfunction. Several mechanisms described for stunning include oxidative stress, reactive oxygen species formation, and altered calcium homeostasis with increased intracellular calcium [10]. Stunned myocardium may take days to fully recover. Experimental evidence suggests that this stunned muscle will respond to inotropic therapy, which remains a cornerstone of therapy for cardiogenic shock [11].

Distinct from myocardial stunning is hibernating myocardium [12]. Hibernating myocardium exists when myocardial perfusion is chronically reduced but basal function is intact. As the term implies, the muscle is sleeping to conserve energy. Hibernation results in both systolic and diastolic dysfunction that can be reversed through restoration of coronary blood flow with either percutaneous coronary intervention or coronary artery bypass grafting [13,14].

Hibernating myocardium may also contribute to the severity of left ventricular dysfunction in patients who have cardiogenic shock. This muscle is viable but in a state of persistent dysfunction because of chronically decreased blood flow. This fact may be important in acute myocardial dysfunction during MI, because hibernating myocardium cannot be recruited to become hypercontractile to preserve cardiac output. Although complete revascularization is ideal, hibernating myocardium may also be at risk for reperfusion injury through oxygen free radicals and increased cytosolic calcium release [12–14].

Compensatory responses to myocardial infarction

In the SHOCK (SHould we emergently revascularize Occluded Coronaries in cardiogenic shocK?) registry, the median time from MI symptoms to shock onset was 6.2 hours although the interquartile range was broad, from 1.7 to 20.1 hours [15]. These data indicate variability in the rate of full-blown shock onset after the initial ischemic insult. Vasoconstriction from falling cardiac output is believed to be the major compensatory mechanism. Patients in this "preshock" phase have low cardiac output and evidence of low organ perfusion but a falsely reassuring preserved systolic blood pressure.

Other compensatory responses to MI and falling cardiac output result in increased MVO_2. In response to stress and decrease in cardiac output, heart rate increases. In addition, noninfarcted myocardium is recruited to preserve forward output and contractility increases. As myocytes die, the left ventricle dilates acutely to preserve stroke volume and wall thickness decreases. Finally, diastolic relaxation is impaired in addition to systolic dysfunction, and left ventricular pressure increases. All of these features lead to increased MVO_2 (see Fig. 2). In the setting of cardiogenic shock, these mechanisms perpetuate the cycle of inadequate oxygen delivery and further ischemia ensues, as illustrated in Fig. 1.

Extent of atherosclerosis and myocardial infarction

Cardiogenic shock complicating acute MI is caused by predominant left ventricular failure in 80% of cases [16,17]. In the remaining 20%, shock results from right ventricular infarction or mechanical complications of MI, including ventricular septal rupture, acute mitral regurgitation, and free wall rupture. In patients who have predominantly left ventricular failure, extensive necrosis is evident and involves more than 40% of the left ventricle on autopsy [18]. Early pathologic studies of fatal cases of cardiogenic shock predating modern reperfusion showed the frequent occurrence of multiple acute and subacute infarctions of varying ages remote from the primary infarct. This evidence supports the concept that patients who have multivessel coronary artery disease who develop shock are prone to demand driven infarcts in remote coronary territories [19].

In many patients, acute occlusion of the left anterior descending artery is the culprit lesion and, in two thirds of all patients, multivessel disease is present [20]. The inciting clinical event leading to shock may not be a massive MI secondary to a single arterial occlusion, but the result of multiple small MIs with the final myocardial insult leading to a sudden loss of critical functioning myocardial mass [19,20].

Cardiogenic shock is a recognized complication in patients presenting with the full spectrum of acute coronary syndromes. The incidence of cardiogenic shock is more common in patients presenting with ECG evidence of ST elevation, occurring in between 4.2% and 7.2% of those who have ST-elevation MI undergoing thrombolytic therapy. It has also been described in up to 2.9% of patients who have other forms of acute coronary syndromes [21].

Infarct expansion and reinfarction have been identified as important risk factors for development of shock in STEMI and nonSTEMI. In settings of low coronary blood flow, thrombus may propagate to involve side branches and increase infarct size. MI is a hypercoagulable clinical state, and reocclusion of recanalized arteries leading to reinfarction can occur in up to 20% of patients undergoing thrombolytic therapy and 2% of patients post-percutaneous coronary intervention. Patients who experience reinfarction have significantly increased chance of developing cardiogenic shock [22,23].

When multivessel coronary artery disease is present, the ability of the unaffected myocardium to be recruited to preserve left ventricular function is impaired. This loss of compensatory hypercontractility in remote myocardium results in the inability to maintain cardiac output, possibly leading to progressive ischemia in territories remote from the initial infarct and contributing to the progressive deterioration in function.

The vicious cycle of diminished myocardial blood flow during shock

As a result of MI, left ventricular diastolic pressure increases. Subendo-cardial myocardial perfusion occurs almost solely during diastole, and is dependent on the pressure difference between aortic diastolic pressure and left ventricular cavity pressure. In cardiogenic shock, aortic pressure decreases and left ventricular pressure increases, leading to decreased coronary perfusion and progressive ischemia. Intra-aortic balloon counterpulsation may help coronary perfusion through increasing aortic diastolic pressure and should be used in patients who have cardiogenic shock [24].

To increase cardiac output, the heart rate increases, thereby increasing myocardial oxygen consumption directly and affecting coronary perfusion. As heart rate increases, the time spent in diastole decreases. The time for tissue perfusion decreases resulting in further ischemia of the subendocardium. The wavefront of ischemia results in eventual global dysfunction, and the spiral deterioration continues.

Cellular contribution to the continuum of deterioration

During acute MI, heart muscle dies. Cell death is predominantly caused by myonecrosis and lysosomal activation caused by ischemia. However, apoptosis, or programmed cell death, may play an important role in infarct extension, especially in the border zone adjacent to infarcted muscle [25–28].

Mitochondria are the powerhouses of the cardiac cells, generating energy in the form of adenosine triphosphate (ATP) to enable myocardial contraction, relaxation, and ion fluxes. In ischemia, the cardiomyocytes' ATP production is reduced by almost 99% [29]. Mitochondria are particularly sensitive to ischemia, reperfusion, and the generation of reactive oxygen species [30]. Several studies have shown that mitochondrial respiratory activity is impaired in the mitochondria of noninfarcted myocardium, and that this is associated with declining pump function. Free radical production may also be associated with alterations in mitochondrial function. Alterations in mitochondrial DNA production may be important in the development of cardiogenic shock post-MI [28–30].

In ischemia and infarction, hypoxia-inducible factor 1 (HIF-1) alpha is generated by the mitochondria to sense myocardial oxygenation. In response to low levels of myocardial oxygen, HIF-1 alpha is up-regulated, which may be an important mechanism for inducing a state of hibernation in the peri-infarct border zone [31].

Circulating mediators: the inflammatory paradigm

It is perplexing that some patients develop cardiogenic shock despite modestly sized risk territories, relative preservation of ejection fraction, and timely reperfusion therapy. In clinical studies of reperfusion therapy, cardiogenic shock occurs in up to 5% to 8% of patients after successful thrombolysis and 2% to 5% of patients who undergo successful primary angioplasty [22,23]. In the randomized SHOCK trial of patients who experienced confirmed cardiogenic shock, the average ejection fraction was 31% using left ventriculogram or echocardiogram [32]. Similar systolic impairment is seen in uncomplicated MI and routinely observed in the stable heart failure population. In addition, survivors of cardiogenic shock have good functional status at follow-up [33]. Together, these observations suggest a reversible and temporary component to cardiogenic shock, which has led researchers to seek other mechanisms beyond the classic paradigm of progressive myocardial ischemia and dysfunction.

Observational evidence supports the hypothesis that inflammatory cytokines are responsible for the vasodilation and inappropriately low systemic vascular resistance seen in patients who had cardiogenic shock despite successful revascularization [34]. Many patients then develop a systemic inflammatory response syndrome (SIRS) that is similar to that in patients who have sepsis and other shock syndromes. For instance, patients who have cardiogenic shock have similar levels of interleukin (IL)-6 as those who have septic shock. IL-6 is prognostically linked to the development of multisystem organ failure and mortality in these patients [35]. Alterations in many other cytokines have been observed, including IL-1 and tumor necrosis factor α [36]. Although IL-6 is recognized as a myocardial depressant, the exact mechanism through which IL-6 exerts its negative effects is undergoing further investigation.

The clinical effects of IL-6 and other cytokines are mediated partially by inappropriate up-regulation of nitric oxide [37]. In health, nitric oxide is a coronary vasodilator and myocardial protectant. However, nitric oxide at inappropriately high levels is a systemic vasodilator and direct myocardial depressant [38]. In addition, some experts believe that nitric oxide may mediate myocardial stunning and cell death through apoptosis, among other mechanisms [39].

Several small studies have tested the hypothesis that inhibiting nitric oxide production using the nitric oxide synthase inhibitor L-N(G)-monomethyl arginine (L-NMMA) has resulted in improved hemodynamic parameters and survival to hospital discharge [40,41]. However, the multicenter randomized trial testing this hypothesis has recently been stopped because of futility [42], leaving the nitric oxide–mediated inflammatory paradigm unproven, although a role for acute inflammation in the genesis of cardiogenic shock complicating MI remains compelling.

Other cardiac causes of shock

In all of the following causes of cardiogenic shock complicating acute MI, the primary problem is decreased forward cardiac output. However, the specific mechanism of decreased output is different in each case.

Right ventricular infarction

Patients who have right ventricular infarction have a distinct clinical picture with elevated right atrial pressures and low pulmonary capillary wedge pressures. After revascularization, optimal fluid resuscitation is the cornerstone of therapy for these patients to maintain right ventricular preload while not at the expense of left ventricular filling. Patients who have right ventricular MI are particularly sensitive to rhythm disturbances and depend on the atrial kick of sinus rhythm for ventricular filling. Inotropic therapy may be required to increase right ventricular performance.

Acute mitral regurgitation

Mitral regurgitation can occur with acute MI, resulting in dramatic pulmonary edema and hypotension. Although up to 15% of patients who have MI have an element of mitral regurgitation, acute mitral regurgitation caused by posterior papillary muscle rupture is a rare complication. It is usually associated with inferior and posterior MIs, but can also occur in the setting of anterior MI. Surgical repair is indicated to fix the mechanical problem, but strategies to decrease afterload and thereby the regurgitant fraction should be instituted.

Ventricular septal rupture and free wall rupture

Ventricular septal rupture and free wall rupture are both catastrophic events leading to cardiogenic shock. Medical stabilization is a temporizing measure until definitive therapy with primarily surgery can be instituted.

The capacity to have compound ischemic and mechanical factors contributing to cardiogenic shock constitutes the basis of practice guidelines that urge the use of expedited echocardiography coincident with emergency cardiac catheterization early in the course of shock. Diminished contractility, low cardiac output, mechanical ventilation, and intra-aortic balloon counterpulsation may all mask mechanical cardiac lesions.

Finally, recognition and rapid treatment of other causes of shock are essential to the management of these patients. Particularly important is volume status and treatment of hypovolemia. Also, sepsis can occur in patients who undergo prolonged ventilation and invasive procedures. Recognition and treatment of other reversible causes of shock is paramount in patients who have limited myocardial reserve.

Summary

Cardiogenic shock is a rapidly progressive, often fatal complication of MI. Rapid restoration of myocardial perfusion is the critical first step in preventing shock in acute MI and treating patients who have cardiogenic shock. The increasing mismatch between myocardial oxygen supply and demand in this syndrome and its consequences begins to explain the unrelenting nature of this condition as outlined above. Whether the inflammatory paradigm can be proven and mediated remains to be seen.

References

[1] Babaev A, Frederick PD, Pasta DJ, et al, NRMI Investigators. Trends in management and outcomes of patients with acute myocardial infarction complicated by cardiogenic shock. JAMA 2005;294(4):448–54.

[2] Hasdai D, Holmes DR Jr, Topol EJ, et al. Frequency and clinical outcome of cardiogenic shock during acute myocardial infarctionamong patients receiving reteplase or alteplase: results from GUSTO III. Eur Heart J 1999;20:128–35.

[3] Menon V, Hochman JS. Management of cardiogenic shock complicating acute myocardial infarction. Heart 2002;88:531–7.

[4] Hochman JS, Sleeper LA, Webb JG, et al. Early revascularization in acute myocardial infarction complicated by cardiogenic shock. SHOCK Investigators. Should we emergently revascularize occluded coronaries for cardiogenic shock. N Engl J Med 1999;341(9): 625–34.

[5] Ganz P, Braunwald E. Coronary blood flow and myocardial ischemia. In: Braunwald E, editor. Heart disease. A textbook of cardiovascular medicine. 5th edition. Philadelphia: WB Saunders; 1997. p. 1161–84.

[6] Bolli R. Why myocardial stunning is clinically important. Basic Res Cardiol 1998;93(3): 169–72.

[7] Camici PG, Rimoldi O. Myocardial hibernation vs repetitive stunning in patients. Cardiol Rev 1999;7(1):39–43.

[8] Kim SJ, Peppas A, Hong SK, et al. Persistent stunning induces myocardial hibernation and protection: flow/function and metabolic mechanisms. Circ Res 2003;92(11):1233–9.

[9] Heusch G, Schulz R, Rahimtoola SH. Myocardial hibernation: a delicate balance. Am J Physiol Heart Circ Physiol 2005;288(3):H984–99.

[10] Sonntag S, Sundberg S, Lehtonen LA, et al. The calcium sensitizer levosimendan improves the function of stunned myocardium after percutaneous transluminal coronary angioplasty in acute myocardial ischemia. J Am Coll Cardiol 2004;43(12):2177–82.

[11] Chen C, Li L, Chen LL, et al. Incremental doses of dobutamine induce a biphasic response in dysfunctional left ventricular regions subtending coronary stenoses. Circulation 1995;92(4): 756–66.

[12] Heusch G, Schulz R. Hibernating myocardium: a review. J Mol Cell Cardiol 1996;28(12): 2359–72.

[13] Bito V, Heinzel FR, Weidemann F, et al. Cellular mechanisms of contractile dysfunction in hibernating myocardium. Circ Res 2004;94(6):794–801.

[14] Schulz R, Rose J, Martin C, et al. Development of short-term myocardial hibernation. Its limitation by the severity of ischemia and inotropic stimulation. Circulation 1993;88(2): 684–95.

[15] Webb JG, Sleeper LA, Buller CE, et al. Implications of the timing of onset of cardiogenic shock after acute myocardial infarction: a report from the SHOCK Trial Registry. SHould we emergently revascularize occluded coronaries for cardiogenic shocK? J Am Coll Cardiol 2000;36(3 Suppl A):1084–90.

[16] Duvernoy CS, Bates ER. Management of cardiogenic shock attributable to acute myocardial infarction in the reperfusion era. J Intensive Care Med 2005;20(4):188–98.

[17] Hollenberg SM, Kavinsky CJ, Parrillo JE. Cardiogenic shock. Ann Intern Med 1999;131: 47–59.

[18] Page DL, Caulfield JB, Kastor JA, et al. Myocardial changes associated with cardiogenic shock. N Engl J Med 1971;285(3):133–7.

[19] Alonso DR, Scheidt S, Post M, et al. Pathophysiology of cardiogenic shock. Quantification of myocardial necrosis, clinical, pathologic and electrocardiographic correlations. Circulation 1973;48(3):588–96.

[20] Wong SC, Sanborn T, Sleeper LA, et al. Angiographic findings and clinical correlates in patients with cardiogenic shock complicating acute myocardial infarction: a report from the SHOCK Trial Registry. SHould we emergently revascularize occluded coronaries for cardiogenic shocK? J Am Coll Cardiol 2000;36(3 Suppl A):1077–83.

[21] Hasdai D, Topol EJ, Califf RM, et al. Cardiogenic shock complicating acute coronary syndromes. Lancet 2000;356:749–56.

[22] Hasdai D, Califf RM, Thompson TD, et al. Predictors of cardiogenic shock after thrombolytic therapy for acute myocardial infarction. J Am Coll Cardiol 2000;35:136–43.

[23] HOchman JS, Boland JS, Sleeper LA, et al. Current spectrum of cardiogenic shock and effect of early revascularization of mortality. Circulation 1995;91:873–81.

[24] Antman E, Anbe DT, Armstrong PW, et al. ACC/AHA guidelines for the management of patients with ST-Elevation myocardial infarction-executive summary: a report of the American College of Cardiology/American Heart Association Task Force on practice guidelines (writing committee to revise the 1999 guidelines for the management of patients with acute myocardial infarction). J Am Coll Cardiol 2004;44:671–719.

[25] Abbate A, Biondi-Zoccai GG, Bussani R, et al. Increased myocardial apoptosis in patients with unfavorable left ventricular remodeling and early symptomatic post-infarction heart failure. J Am Coll Cardiol 2003;41(5):753–60.

[26] Kostin S, Pool L, Elsasser A, et al. Myocytes die by multiple mechanisms in failing human hearts. Circ Res 2003;92:715–24.

[27] Chen C, Ma L, Linfert DR, et al. Myocardial cell death and apoptosis in hibernating myocardium. J Am Coll Cardiol 1997;30(5):1407–12.

[28] Moens AL, Claeys MJ, Timmermans JP, et al. Myocardial ischemia/reperfusion-injury, a clinical view on a complex pathophysiological process. Int J Cardiol 2005;100(2): 179–90.

[29] Michiels C. Physiological and pathological responses to hypoxia. Am J Pathol 2004;164: 1875–82.

[30] Giordano FJ. Oxygen, oxidative stress, hypoxia, and heart failure. J Clin Invest 2005;115: 500–8.

[31] Huang LE, Bunn HF. Hypoxia-inducible factor and its biomedical relevance. J Biol Chem 2003;278:19575–8.

[32] Picard MH, Davidoff R, Sleeper LA, et al. Echocardiographic predictors of survival and response to early revascularization in cardiogenic shock. Circulation 2003;107(2):279–84.

[33] Sleeper LA, Ramanathan K, Picard MH, et al. Functional status and quality of life after emergency revascularization for cardiogenic shock complicating acute myocardial infarction. J Am Coll Cardiol 2005;46(2):266–73.

[34] Kohsaka S, Menon V, Lowe AM, et al. Systemic inflammatory response syndrome after acute myocardial infarction complicated by cardiogenic shock. Arch Intern Med 2005; 165(14):1643–50.

[35] Geppert A, Dorninger A, Delle-Karth G, et al. Plasma concentrations of interleukin-6, organ failure, vasopressor support, and successful coronary revascularization in predicting 30-day mortality of patients with cardiogenic shock complicating acute myocardial infarction. Crit Care Med 2006;34(8):2035–42.

[36] Geppert A, Steiner A, Zorn G, et al. Multiple organ failure in patients with cardiogenic shock is associated with high plasma levels of interleukin-6. Crit Care Med 2002;30(9): 1987–94.

[37] Wildhirt SM, DUdek RR, Suzuki H, et al. Involvement of inducible nitric oxide synthase in the inflammatory process of myocardial infarction. Int J Cardiol 1995;50:253–61.

[38] Feng O, Lu X, Jones DL, et al. Increased inducible nitric oxide synthase expression contributes to myocardial dysfunction and higher mortality after myocardial infarction in mice. Circulation 2001;104:700-4.

[39] Li H, Forstermann U. Nitric oxide synthase in the pathogenesis of vascular disease. J Pathol 2000;190:244-54.

[40] Cotter G, Kaluski E, Blatt A, et al. L-NMMA (a nitric oxide synthase inhibitor) is effective in the treatment of cardiogenic shock. Circulation 2000;101:1358-61.

[41] Cotter G, Kaluski E, Milo O, et al. LINCS: L-NAME (a NO synthase inhibitor) in the treatment of refractory cardiogenic shock: a prospective randomized study. Eur Heart J 2003; 24(14):1287-95.

[42] TRIUMPH Investigators: Alexander JH, Reynolds HR, Stebbins AL, et al. Effect of tilarginine acetate in patients with acute myocardial infarction and cardiogenic shock: the TRIUMPH randomized controlled trial. JAMA 2007;297(15):1711-3.

ELSEVIER
SAUNDERS

Med Clin N Am 91 (2007) 713–727

THE MEDICAL
CLINICS
OF NORTH AMERICA

Cardiogenic Shock: Treatment

Zaza Iakobishvili, MD, PhD[a,b],
David Hasdai, MD[a,b],*

[a]Intensive Cardiac Care Unit, Department of Cardiology, Rabin Medical Center,
Beilinson Campus, 39 Jabotinsky Street, Petah Tikva, Israel 49100
[b]Tel Aviv University, P.O. Box 39040, Tel Aviv 69978, Israel

The treatment of cardiogenic shock patients consists of medical therapy, percutaneous revascularization procedures, cardiac surgery, and the implantation of devices. Because of the extreme complexity of their management, cardiogenic shock patients require reliable and precise hemodynamic monitoring. Invasive systemic blood pressure monitoring is highly recommended. In addition, many authorities advocate use of right heart catheterization or echocardiography for guiding therapeutic measures.

Right heart catheterization

The role of right heart catheterization in the management of cardiogenic shock patients remains controversial. On one hand, there are retrospective data on increased mortality hazard associated with this procedure [1]. On the other hand, data from the Global Use of Strategies to Open Occluded Coronary Arteries (GUSTO-I) trial [2] and the Should We Emergently Revascularize Occluded Coronaries in Cardiogenic Shock? (SHOCK) registry [3] suggest that it is not harmful, and possibly beneficial, in terms of outcome. The mortality rate was lower in patients who underwent right heart catheterization than in those who did not (45.2% versus 63.4%) in the GUSTO-I population. In the SHOCK registry, no increase was reported in the in-hospital mortality among patients undergoing right heart catheterization [3].

The current American and European guidelines recommend right heart catheterization for patients who have ST-elevation acute coronary

* Corresponding author. Intensive Cardiac Care Unit, Department of Cardiology, Rabin Medical Center, Beilinson Campus, 39 Jabotinsky Street, Petah Tikva, Israel 49100.
E-mail address: dhasdai@post.tau.ac.il (D. Hasdai).

0025-7125/07/$ - see front matter © 2007 Elsevier Inc. All rights reserved.
doi:10.1016/j.mcna.2007.02.007 *medical.theclinics.com*

syndromes (ACS), or who have progressive heart failure, cardiogenic shock, or mechanical complications, despite the paucity of evidence proving its efficacy [4,5]; however, the implementation of these guidelines is rather poor in current clinical practice. According to the Euro-Heart-ACS Survey, among 549 cardiogenic shock patients, right heart catheterization was performed only in 20.2% of cases [6]. It should be stressed that there are no data regarding the optimal hemodynamic values to be targeted in cardiogenic shock patients.

Echocardiography

Doppler echocardiography is an excellent bedside tool for hemodynamic assessment and for the evaluation of cardiac function, valvular status, and mechanical complications of ACS [7]. Its use has steadily increased over the years, and currently it is performed routinely among ACS patients in many institutions. Its use is also increasing among cardiogenic shock patients. In the SHOCK trial, 175 echocardiograms were performed within 24 hours of randomization [8]. In the Euro-Heart-ACS Survey, 68% of cardiogenic shock patients underwent an echocardiographic evaluation [7]. Perhaps this noninvasive, readily available method has supplanted right heart catheterization use in most situations.

Drug therapy

Inotropes

A mean arterial pressure of 60 mm Hg is generally necessary for tissue perfusion. Experience in patients who have septic shock has shown that further elevation of the mean blood pressure by norepinephrine did not further improve systemic perfusion, but did increase myocardial oxygen demands [9].

Large-scale controlled studies have not been performed to compare different combinations of inotropes in patients who have cardiogenic shock. Their efficacy can be influenced by the local tissue perfusion and metabolism that are progressively impaired in cardiogenic shock.

Dopamine and dobutamine are the most commonly used inotropic agents. They have different effects on hemodynamics, cardiac output, and systemic vascular resistance. Low-dose dopamine (0.5–2 µg/kg/minute) acts on the dopaminergic receptors, causing vasodilatation and theoretically preserving renal blood flow and natriuresis [10]; however, in a recent randomized placebo-controlled trial in intensive care patients, no nephroprotective benefit was reported from low-dose dopamine [11]. Dopamine's myocardial inotropic and chronotropic effects are mediated through myocardial β-1 adrenergic receptors, and are most evident with doses above

5 μg/kg/minute. The variable plasma-dopamine clearance in very sick patients can lead to unpredictable serum concentrations and consequently, variable clinical benefits [12].

Dobutamine has both α- and β-adrenergic agonistic activities. It increases myocardial contractility through β-adrenergic receptor stimulation, with only a minute peripheral vasodilatory effect. The drug is usually initiated at 2 μg/kg/minute and titrated upwards according to the patient's response, usually to a maximum of 20 μg/kg/minute. Dobutamine is often used together with low-dose dopamine for the inotropic effect of the former and the suggested renal vasodilator effect of the latter.

Norepinephrine is a potent α-adrenergic agonist with less marked β-1 adrenergic agonistic properties and a short half-life of 2 to 4 minutes. Vasoconstriction is dose-related, and the drug infusion is titrated upwards from an initial low dose of 0.02 to 0.04 μg/kg/minute to a dose that maintains adequate systemic blood pressure. Norepinephrine may be used in conjunction with dopamine and dobutamine; however, in the authors' practice the cardiac effects of these agents include worsening ischemia and serious arrhythmia, and the vasoconstriction induced by norepinephrine can lead to end-organ ischemia. Thus, we avoid prolonged "triple" or "double" inotropic treatment.

Milrinone, a second-generation phosphodiesterase inhibitor, can be used in cardiogenic shock patients. Milrinone prevents the breakdown of cyclic adenosine monophosphate (cAMP), the final common pathway for raising intracellular calcium, thus increasing inotropy. The significant vasodilatory effect and relatively long plasma half-life make milrinone difficult to use as monotherapy in patients who have cardiogenic shock. Milrinone can be used synergistically with other inotropic drugs to enhance myocardial contractility [13].

Levosimendan represents a new class of positive inotropic agents. Levosimendan causes conformational changes in cardiac troponin C during systole, leading to sensitization of the contractile apparatus to calcium ions [14,15]. In addition to its positive inotropic action, levosimendan possesses vasodilating properties that reduce cardiac preload and afterload. Vasodilation is attributed to the opening of adenosine triphosphate (ATP)-sensitive potassium channels in vascular smooth muscle and, in higher doses, to the inhibition of phosphodiesterase III. Moreover, coronary blood flow is enhanced and myocardial oxygen supply is increased [16,17].

At present, however, use of levosimendan is not recommended by the manufacturer for the sole treatment of cardiogenic shock, because of its vasodilatory properties. The combined use of levosimendan with other vasoactive drugs may be considered on an individual basis. Isolated case reports advocate the use of levosimendan as the sole inotrope in post-myocardial infarction cardiogenic shock patients [18].

Based on effects of vasopressin in septic shock [19], Jolly and colleagues [20] hypothesized that vasopressin would increase mean arterial pressure without altering pulmonary capillary wedge pressure or cardiac index. In the Toronto General Hospital database, they identified the patients who had refractory cardiogenic shock who were treated with vasopressin (median 3.6 U/min, 95% CI 2.5–4.7) or norepinephrine (median 19.5 μg/min, 95% CI 9.3–29.8), and invasive hemodynamic monitoring was established. Intravenous vasopressin therapy increased mean arterial pressure from 56 to 73 mm Hg at 1 hour ($P<.001$) and maintained it for 24 hours without changing pulmonary capillary wedge pressure, cardiac index, urine output, or other inotropic requirements. In a cohort of patients who developed refractory cardiogenic shock after myocardial infarction, vasopressin was associated with increased mean arterial pressure and no adverse effect on other hemodynamic parameters [20]. Randomized prospective trials are warranted to confirm the utility and safety of vasopressin in the setting of cardiogenic shock after myocardial infarction.

Diuretics and fluids

The patients in cardiogenic shock might need the optimization of left ventricular filling pressures, even in the presence of a priori elevated pulmonary capillary wedge pressure, to ensure maximal performance on Starling curve. In these difficult cases, right heart catheterization may be of value (see above). Commonly, readily available clinical parameters can be used for the estimation of filling pressure. For example, hourly monitored urinary output in conjunction with clear lung fields and absence of pulmonary congestion on chest radiograph may indicate a need for volume-replacement therapy, especially in the setting of right ventricular infarction, whereas progressive desaturation and pulmonary congestion obviate the need for diuretic therapy.

Thrombolysis

The outcome of cardiogenic shock is closely related to the patency of the culprit coronary arteries [21]. In some studies, thrombolytic therapy decreased the incidence of cardiogenic shock among patients who had ST-segment–elevation myocardial infarction [22,23]. According to GUSTO-I, tissue-plasminogen activator (tPA) is more efficacious than streptokinase in preventing shock. No difference was observed in GUSTO-III between newer thrombolytic agents and tPA in terms of prevention of cardiogenic shock [24].

The use of thrombolytic therapy for patients in cardiogenic shock has been disappointing, as noted in the Gruppo Italiano per lo Studio della Streptochinasi nell'Infarto Miocardico (GISSI)-I trial [25]. In the randomized SHOCK trial, thrombolytic therapy was an independent correlate of 12-month survival on univariate analysis (relative risk 0.5, $P = .008$), but not after adjustment for confounding factors (relative risk 0.72, $P = .15$)

[26]. The SHOCK registry data demonstrated that thrombolytic therapy in shock patients was associated with a lower mortality, but these results are biased, in that patients who did not receive thrombolytic therapy were at increased risk of dying independently of treatment received [27]. The lack of apparent benefit of thrombolytic agents in the treating cardiogenic shock may be the result of reduced lysis of thrombi in patients who have low perfusion pressures [28]. The use of intra-aortic balloon counterpulsation (IABP) may increase the efficacy of thrombolytic therapy in patients who have hypotension by increasing perfusion pressure.

Glycoprotein IIb/IIIa receptor antagonists

There is some evidence that cardiogenic shock outcomes are improved by the use of glycoprotein IIb/IIIa receptor antagonists. In the Platelet Glycoprotein IIb/IIIa in Unstable Angina: Receptor Suppression Using Integrilin Therapy (PURSUIT) trial, shock patients who received eptifibatide had a 50% reduction of 30-day mortality (58.5% versus 73.5% for placebo, OR 0.51, 95% CI 0.28, 0.94, $P = .03$) [29]. It is unclear if this effect can be explained by chance. Only 29% of enrolled patients in PURSUIT underwent angioplasty, so the observed reduction in mortality is unlikely to be related to coronary interventions. Platelet glycoprotein IIb/IIIa antagonists may have beneficial effects on the microvasculature. There may be severe abnormalities of microvascular tone in shock patients, which may further increase subendocardial ischemia. The available data favor administration of IIb/IIIa antagonists, particularly abciximab, in patients who have cardiogenic shock who are undergoing percutaneous intervention, unless the risk of bleeding is considered to be excessive. In the recently published trial [30], 40 patients who had ST-segment–elevation myocardial infarction and cardiogenic shock were treated with primary revascularization, abciximab, heparin, and aspirin. The reported mortality rate at 30 days was 42.5%. Abciximab seemed to improve outcomes of the younger population (<75 years) versus elderly (>75 years), with mortality rates of 24% versus 91%, respectively ($P < .001$) [30]. Stents and abciximab have been associated with improved acute angiographic and procedural success of percutaneous coronary intervention (PCI) for cardiogenic shock, leading to improved survival at short and mid-term [31] as well as at long-term—up to 2.5 years [32].

N-Monomethyl-L-Arginine

There is some evidence suggesting the role for inflammatory mediators in the pathogenesis of cardiogenic shock, as part of systemic inflammatory response syndrome [33]. These mediators include intrinsic nitric oxide synthase (iNOS) expression, which increases nitric oxide (NO) and peroxynitrite levels, resulting in further myocardial dysfunction and failure of an appropriate peripheral circulatory response. N-Monomethyl-L-Arginine

(L-NMMA), a NO inhibitor, was tested in 11 patients who had refractory cardiogenic shock after no improvement was achieved with maximal treatment—high-dose catecholamines, IABP, mechanical ventilation, and percutaneous revascularization. Urine output and blood pressure increased markedly, with a 72% 30-day survival rate [34]. The same group randomized 30 cardiogenic shock patients after revascularization of the culprit artery to supportive treatment or supportive treatment and L-NAME (L-NMMA prototype). One-month survival in the L-NAME group was 73% versus 33% in supportive treatment alone, with significant increase of mean arterial pressure and urinary output in the L-NAME group [35]. Based on the results of a multicenter, randomized clinical trial, SHOCK-II, the Food and Drug Administration (FDA) approved a prototype drug, tilarginine acetate injection (TAI), as an orphan drug for the treatment of cardiogenic shock. Tilarginine Acetate Injection (TAI) in a Randomized International Study in Unstable Acute Myocardial Infarction (AMI) Patients/Cardiogenic Shock—the TRIUMPH Study—was a Phase III international multicenter, prospective, randomized, double-blind, parallel arm, placebo-controlled investigation of the intravenous administration of TAI in patients who had cardiogenic shock complicating myocardial infarction. The TRIUMPH study population was 658 patients who had a diagnosis of cardiogenic shock complicating myocardial infarction, persistent shock for more than 1 hour after patency of the infarct-related artery was confirmed ($\leq 70\%$ stenosis with any thrombolysis in myocardial infarction [TIMI] flow grade), and systolic blood pressure measured at < 100 mm Hg. All 658 patients were to be randomized 1:1 to receive either TAI or placebo at approximately 120 centers worldwide. TAI or matching placebo was to be administered to patients as an intravenous (IV) bolus followed by a 5-hour infusion. The TAI dose was to be 1.0 mg/kg IV bolus, followed by 1.0 mg/kg/hr for 5 hrs. The primary end point was all-cause mortality at 30 days post-randomization [36]. This study was prematurely terminated by the investigators, however, indicating that the treatment was either ineffective or perhaps deleterious.

Complement blocking agents

The complement system is an important innate humoral modulator; it mediates defense mechanisms against infection, initiates and amplifies inflammation, bridges innate and adaptive immunity, induces apoptosis, and clears autoimmune and apoptotic material. Complement is also recognized as being an important contributor to ischemia-reperfusion injury [37]. Pexelizumab is a unique single-chain fragment of a humanized monoclonal antibody specifically directed against the complement protein C5 [38]. The administration of pexelizumab in patients who had an acute ST-segment–elevation myocardial infarction, managed with primary PCI, was associated with a substantial reduction in mortality and cardiogenic shock compared with placebo in the Complement Inhibition in Myocardial Infarction Treated with Angioplasty (COMMA) trial [39]. The benefits were achieved with no detectable effect on infarct size as measured by the area under the curve of creatine kinase MB isoenzyme (CK-MB) release, the trial's primary end point. This implied that nonconventional mechanisms could be operative and that further exploration was warranted. To evaluate further the role of complement system inhibition in acute ST-segment–elevation myocardial infarction undergoing primary angioplasty, a large phase three mortality trial with pexelizumab Assessment of Pexelizumab in Acute Myocardial Infarction (APEX-AMI) was conducted. The APEX-AMI study was stopped on March 2006 at its halfway point, at enrollment of about 5100 patients, after disappointing results of two major trials of this drug in coronary artery bypass surgery patients [40].

Metabolic agents

The rationale for the use of these agents derives from the field of reperfusion injury. The most studied drug to abolish the deleterious effects of reperfusion is adenosine, an endogenous purine nucleoside. In the Acute Myocardial Infarction Study of Adenosine (AMISTAD) trial [41], adenosine decreased infarct size in anterior wall myocardial infarction patients; however, there were nonsignificant increases in deaths (10% versus 6%), reinfarctions (7% versus 3%), heart failure (13% versus 8%), and cardiogenic shock (6% versus 4%) in the adenosine group. The trial was not powered for determining these subtle differences.

Sodium/hydrogen-exchange inhibitors

During ischemia, the falling pH activates anaerobic metabolism and sodium/hydrogen exchange, thus leading to intracellular sodium accumulation. This process eventually leads by sodium/calcium exchange to intracellular calcium accumulation and ultimately to cell death [42]. Two large trials—the Guard During Ischemia Against Necrosis (GUARDIAN) trial of 11,590 patients who had ACS [42] and the Evaluation of the Safety and Cardioprotective Effects of Eniporide in Acute Myocardial Infarction (ESCAMI) trial [43]—studied a new class of agents: sodium/hydrogen-exchange inhibitors. None of these trials demonstrated any benefit in terms of reduction in serious adverse outcomes.

Antioxidants

Recombinant human superoxide dismutase (h-SOD) failed to improve recovery of ventricular function after primary PCI [44]. In a very small placebo-controlled trial of 47 patients who had AMI, N-acetylcysteine was used adjunctively with reperfusion therapy, resulting in a smaller infarct sizes [45].

Glucose-insulin-potassium infusion

In a prospective study, glucose-insulin-potassium (GIK) was found to be beneficial, particularly in the subgroup of reperfused patients (relative risk of in-hospital mortality 0.34, $P = .008$). The frequency of cardiogenic shock was 4.6% in those who received GIK, compared with 7.6% in those who did not (relative risk 0.60, 95% CI 0.21–1.69, $P = NS$) [46]. In the Clinical Trial of Reviparin and Metabolic Modulation in Acute Myocardial Infarction Treatment Evaluation (CREATE) Estudios Cardiologicos Latinoamerica (ECLA) randomized controlled trial, high-dose GIK infusion had a neutral effect on mortality, cardiac arrest, and cardiogenic shock in patients who had acute ST-segment–elevation myocardial infarction [47].

Nonpharmacologic treatment of cardiogenic shock

Revascularization

Bypass surgery
  Early studies of coronary revascularization for cardiogenic chock focused on surgical revascularization. Several small surgical series reported relatively good outcomes in patients who had cardiogenic shock [48,49].
  According to SHOCK trial data, surgically revascularized patients benefited mostly—among 57 patients who underwent bypass surgery, 30-day mortality was 42.1%, versus 45.3% for those treated with PCI. The trial was not designed to compare between percutaneous and surgical revascularization strategies [50]. There are several surgical techniques designed to optimize outcomes for patients in cardiogenic shock: the use of warm blood cardioplegia enriched with glutamate and aspartate, grafting of large areas of viable myocardium first followed by treatment of infarct-related artery last, and preferential use of saphenous vein grafts for their high initial flow rates and because they can be rapidly harvested [51].

Coronary angioplasty
  Several retrospective analyses regarding coronary angioplasty in cardiogenic shock are available [52–55]. In the GUSTO-I trial, an aggressive revascularization strategy was associated with reduced 30-day mortality (odds ratio, 0.43 (CI, 0.34–0.54), $P = .0001$) [56].
  These retrospective analyses of patients who did and did not undergo revascularization for shock suffer from selection bias regarding the use of mechanical revascularization—the sickest patients usually were treated conservatively.
  Two prospective randomized trials evaluated the role of revascularization among patients who had cardiogenic shock. The SMASH trial (Swiss Multicenter trial of Angioplasty for Shock) involved 55 patients who had AMI complicated by cardiogenic shock. They were randomized to undergo revascularization (surgical or percutaneous) versus medical therapy alone [57].

SMASH was stopped prematurely because of low enrollment and because of physician perception that revascularization was beneficial based on retrospective analyses of registries. In this small, undersized cohort, a 9% absolute reduction in 30-day mortality was seen among patients treated with revascularization (69% versus 78%, $P = .68$ log rank test), which did not achieve statistical significance.

In the second randomized study, the SHOCK trial, patients who developed cardiogenic shock within the first 36 hours of AMI (either ST-segment elevation, or new left bundle-branch block) were eligible for enrollment; patients who had mechanical causes for shock or predominantly right-ventricular infarction were excluded [26,50]. In the SHOCK trial, an aggressive, invasive approach (angioplasty or coronary artery bypass surgery— emergency revascularization [ERV], generally with IABP) was compared with medical treatment—initial medical stabilization (IMS), including thrombolytic therapy and IABP. Randomization was required within 12 hours of shock onset. Most patients randomized to the ERV (n = 152) underwent coronary angiography (97%), and 87% underwent revascularization (surgical or percutaneous). The primary end point of the study was 30-day mortality. In the ERV arm, the mortality was 46.7%, as compared with 56.0% in the conservative arm ($P = .11$). The mortality difference at 6 months achieved statistical significance, and was lower in the ERV group (50.3% versus 63.1%, $P = .027$) [51]. The survival curves continued to diverge at 12 months of follow-up [26]. In a prespecified subgroup analysis, the benefit of ERV were seen only in patients younger than 75 years of age, in whom the 30-day mortality was 56.8% for the conservative arm versus 41.4% for the ERV arm, relative risk 0.73 (95% CI 0.56–0.95)); however, 30-day survival among medically treated patients older than 75 years tended to be better than that of older patients in the ERV arm (53.1% versus 75.0%, relative risk 1.41 (95% CI of 0.95 to 2.11), $P = $ NS).

The 13% absolute reduction in mortality at 6 months associated with the aggressive revascularization strategy (50.3% versus 63.1%t, $P = .027$) was both statistically and clinically significant. On the basis of the SHOCK trial, the American College of Cardiology/American Heart Association (ACC/AHA) guidelines for the treatment of patients who have myocardial infarction have included early revascularization for shock as a Class I indication, particularly for those less than 75 years of age [4].

Of note, while analyzing the subgroup of elderly patients in SHOCK registry, Dzavik and colleagues [58] found that those who underwent early revascularization had lower in-hospital mortality rates—48% versus 81% ($P = .0003$)—and after exclusion of 65 early deaths and covariate adjustment, the relative risk was 0.76 (0.59, 0.99; $P = .045$) in patients aged <75 years and 0.46 (0.28, 0.75; $P = .002$) in patients aged 75 years or older.

Despite the guidelines' recommendations, good clinical judgment has to be applied while treating elderly patients who have myocardial infarction complicated by cardiogenic shock. In a prospective registry of consecutive

PCI interventions in northern New England [59] the mortality rate for elderly shock patients undergoing PCI was 46%, which is significantly lower than previously reported in randomized clinical trials.

In a recent analysis of percutaneous revascularization from the SHOCK trial, Webb and colleagues [60] examined the clinical, angiographic, and procedural characteristics determining survival after percutaneous revascularization for cardiogenic shock. Restoration of coronary blood flow appeared to be a major predictor of survival in cardiogenic shock. Coronary revascularization benefits shock patients beyond the accepted 12-hour post-infarction window. Severe mitral regurgitation in shock patients after percutaneous revascularization was associated with 67% 1-year mortality—thus surgery should be considered in shock patients who have severe mitral insufficiency or multivessel disease not amenable to relatively complete percutaneous revascularization. In another analysis [61] of the same data set, left ventricular function and culprit vessel patency were independent correlates of 1-year survival in revascularized patients.

In the Global Registry of Acute Coronary Events (GRACE) study, percutaneous revascularization with coronary stenting was the most powerful predictor of hospital survival among shock patients (odds ratio 3.99, 95% CI 2.41–6.62) [62].

There are very limited data on revascularization for non–ST-segment-elevation shock. In the SHOCK registry, the authors found a nonsignificant survival benefit for patients who had non–ST-segment elevation who underwent revascularization, after adjustment for patient age and several treatment characteristics [63].

The growing body of evidence suggests that rapid revascularization reduces mortality in patients who have myocardial infarction complicated by cardiogenic shock, be it percutaneous or surgical. Thus, it is perplexing that in the Euro Heart Survey of ACS, it was found that fewer than one half of cardiogenic shock patients received any revascularization [64].

Intra-aortic balloon counterpulsation

IABP increases diastolic coronary artery perfusion and decreases systemic afterload without increasing myocardial oxygen demand. Few data are available to support its use in improving outcomes of patients who have shock.

Patients treated with IABP in conjunction with thrombolytic therapy had the lowest in-hospital mortality rate (47%) in the SHOCK registry. Patients who had ST-elevation myocardial infarction who did not receive IABP or thrombolytic therapy had the worst baseline risk status [27]. The SHOCK registry data suggest that initial stabilization of cardiogenic shock patients using an IABP may be associated with a 20% absolute risk reduction in mortality. Similarly, retrospective analysis from the United States National Registry of Myocardial Infarction [65] has shown a 6% absolute reduction in hospital mortality associated with IABP use among cardiogenic shock patients.

In the Thrombolysis and Counterpulsation to Improve Cardiogenic Shock Survival (TACTICS) trial, the only randomized trial examining the role of IABP deployment (within 3 hours of thrombolysis), enrollment was terminated after random assignment of 57 patients, though in the subset of 31 patients who had "classic" shock, mortality at 6 months was 39% in the patients randomly assigned to receive IABP, whereas it was 80% in those randomly assigned to thrombolysis alone ($P < .05$) [66].

IABP was recommended in the SHOCK Trial protocol and used in 87% of patients, for a median duration of approximately 3 days. Overall, IABP usage was not an independent predictor of mortality at 12 months; however, in patients who had systemic hypoperfusion and whose hemodynamics and end-organ perfusion were improved by IABP, the mortality rates were lower at 12 months in both the initial medical stabilization and the ERV treatment groups (both $P < .01$). The combination of IABP and thrombolytic therapy did not significantly increase the incidence of bleeding requiring transfusion, although patients who also underwent revascularization were at higher risk of bleeding [67]. Peripheral vascular disease and physicians' unfamiliarity with bedside IABP insertion may preclude using this useful therapeutic tool for initial stabilization and transportation to a facility with catheterization and percutaneous or surgical revascularization capabilities.

IABP use is strongly advised in current guidelines for the treatment of cardiogenic shock patients [4,5]. Despite this, a perplexingly low rate of use of IABP in cardiogenic shock patients was found in The Euro Heart Survey of ACS [64].

According to accumulated data and accepted guidelines, all patients having cardiogenic shock without contraindications should receive IABP for at least 3 days or longer if clinically indicated, for recovery from myocardial stunning.

Other procedures

There are several additional possible approaches to support the patients who have cardiogenic shock. Left ventricular assist devices were described in a few retrospective single-center based studies as a promising modality in the post-myocardial infarction setting [68,69]. Anecdotal case reports and case series were published during the last year confirming the emerging role of urgent cardiac resynchronization therapy (CRT) in inotrope-dependent patients [70–72]. Urgent cardiac transplantation should be considered in cardiogenic shock patients. At the present time all of the above treatment modalities should be considered on an individual basis.

Summary

Cardiogenic shock remains a grim complication of acute myocardial infarction. Alertness of managing physicians to the possibility of its occurrence and timely establishment of aggressive reperfusion therapy, along with various pharmacologic and mechanical means, make it possible to achieve significant progress in the treatment of this complicated subset of patients.

References

[1] Connors AFJ, Speroff T, Dawson NV, et al. The effectiveness of right heart catheterization in the initial care of critically ill patients. SUPPORT investigators. JAMA 1996;276:889–97.

[2] Hasdai D, Holmes DR Jr, Califf RM, et al. Cardiogenic shock complicating acute myocardial infarction: predictors of death. Am Heart J 1999;138:21–31.

[3] Menon V, Sleeper LA, Fincke R, et al. Outcomes with pulmonary artery catheterization in cardiogenic shock [abstract]. J Am Coll Cardiol 1998;31(Suppl A):397A.

[4] Antman EM, Anbe DT, Armstrong PW, et al. ACC/AHA guidelines for the management of patients with ST-elevation myocardial infarction: executive summary: a report of the ACC/AHA Task Force on Practice Guidelines (Committee to Revise the 1999 Guidelines on the Management of Patients with Acute Myocardial Infarction). J Am Coll Cardiol 2004;44:671–719.

[5] Van de Werf F, Ardissino D, Betriu A, et al. Management of acute myocardial infarction in patients presenting with ST-segment elevation. The Task Force on the Management of Aacute Myocardial Infarction of the European Society of Cardiology. Eur Heart J 2003;24:28–66.

[6] Porter A, Iakobishvili Z, Haim M, et al. Balloon-floating right heart catheter monitoring for acute coronary syndromes complicated by heart failure—discordance between guidelines and reality. Cardiology 2005;104:186–90.

[7] Hasdai D, Lev EI, Behar S, et al. Acute coronary syndromes in patients with pre-existing moderate to severe valvular disease of the heart: lessons from the Euro-Heart Survey of Acute Coronary Syndromes. Eur Heart J 2003;24:623–9.

[8] Picard MH, Davidoff R, Sleeper LA, et al. Echocardiographic predictors of survival and response to early revascularization in cardiogenic shock. Circulation 2003;107:279–84.

[9] LeDoux D, Astiz ME, Carpati CM, et al. Effects of perfusion pressure on tissue perfusion in septic shock. Crit Care Med 2000;28:2729–32.

[10] Denton MD, Chertow GM, Brady HR. "Renal-dose" dopamine for the treatment of acute renal failure: scientific rationale, experimental studies and clinical trials. Kidney Int 1996;50:4–14.

[11] Australian and New Zealand Intensive Care Society (ANZICS) Clinical Trials Group. Low-dose dopamine in patients with early renal dysfunction: a placebo-controlled randomised trial. Lancet 2000;356:2139–43.

[12] Juste RN, Moran L, Hooper J, et al. Dopamine clearance in critically ill patients. Intensive Care Med 1998;24:1217–20.

[13] Colucci WS, Denniss AR, Leatherman GF, et al. Intracoronary infusion of dobutamine to patients with and without severe congestive heart failure: dose-response relationships, correlation with circulating catecholamines, and effect of phosphodiesterase inhibition. J Clin Invest 1988;81:1103–10.

[14] Haikala H, Kaheinen P, Levijoki J, et al. The role of cAMP- and cGMP-dependent protein kinases in the cardiac actions of the new calcium sensitizer, levosimendan. Cardiovasc Res 1997;34:536–46.

[15] Figgitt DP, Gillies PS, Goa KL. Levosimendan. Drugs 2001;61:613–27.

[16] Lilleberg J, Nieminen MS, Akkila J, et al. Effects of a new calcium sensitizer, levosimendan, on haemodynamics, coronary blood flow and myocardial substrate utilization early after coronary artery bypass grafting. Eur Heart J 1998;19:660–8.

[17] Cleland JG, McGowan J. Levosimendan: a new era for inodilator therapy for heart failure? Curr Opin Cardiol 2002;17:257–65.

[18] Ellger BM, Zahn PK, Van Aken HK, et al. Levosimendan: a promising treatment for myocardial stunning? Anaesthesia 2006;61:61–3.

[19] Holmes CL, Walley KR, Chittock DR, et al. The effects of vasopressin on hemodynamics and renal function in severe septic shock: a case series. Intensive Care Med 2001;27:1416–21.

[20] Jolly S, Newton G, Horlock E, et al. Effect of vasopressin on hemodynamics in patients with refractory cardiogenic shock complicating acute myocardial infarction. Am J Cardiol 2005; 96:1617–20.

[21] Bengtson JR, Kaplan AJ, Pieper KS, et al. Prognosis in cardiogenic shock after acute myocardial infarction in the interventional era. J Am Coll Cardiol 1992;20:1482–9.

[22] AIMS Trial Study Group. Effect of intravenous APSAC on mortality after acute myocardial infarction: preliminary report of a placebo-controlled clinical trial. Lancet 1988;8585: 545–9.

[23] Wilcox RG, von der Lippe G, Olsson CG, et al. Trial of tissue plasminogen activator for mortality reduction in acute myocardial infarction: Anglo-Scandinavian Study of Early Thrombolysis (ASSET). Lancet 1988;8585:525–30.

[24] Hasdai D, Holmes DR Jr, Topol EJ, et al. Frequency and clinical outcome of cardiogenic shock during acute myocardial infarction among patients receiving reteplase or alteplase: results from GUSTO III. Eur Heart J 1999;20:128–35.

[25] Effectiveness of intravenous thrombolytic treatment in acute myocardial infarction. Gruppo Italiano per lo Studio della Streptochinasi nell'Infarto Miocardico (GISSI). Lancet 1986; 8478:397–402.

[26] Hochman JS, Sleeper LA, White HD, et al. One-year survival following early revascularization for cardiogenic shock. JAMA 2001;285:190–2.

[27] Sanborn TA, Sleeper LA, Bates ER, et al. Impact of thrombolysis, intra-aortic balloon pump counterpulsation, and their combination in cardiogenic shock complicating acute myocardial infarction: a report from the SHOCK trial registry. J Am Coll Cardiol 2000;36: 1123–9.

[28] Prewitt RM, Gu S, Schick U, et al. Intraaortic balloon counterpulsation enhances coronary thrombolysis induced by intravenous administration of a thrombolytic agent. J Am Coll Cardiol 1994;23:794–8.

[29] Hasdai D, Harrington RA, Hochman JS, et al. Platelet glycoprotein IIb/IIIa blockade and outcome of cardiogenic shock complicating acute coronary syndromes without persistent ST-segment elevation. J Am Coll Cardiol 2000;36:685–92.

[30] Zeymer U, Tebbe U, Weber M, et al, on behalf of ALKK Study Group. Prospective evaluation of early abciximab and primary percutaneous intervention for patients with ST elevation myocardial infarction complicated by cardiogenic shock: results of the REO-SHOCK trial. J Invasive Cardiol 2003;15(7):385–9.

[31] Antoniucci D, Valenti R, Migliorini A, et al. Abciximab therapy improves survival in patients with acute myocardial infarction complicated by early cardiogenic shock undergoing coronary artery stent implantation. Am J Cardiol 2002;90(4):353–7.

[32] Chan AW, Chew DP, Bhatt DL, et al. Long-term mortality benefit with the combination of stents and abciximab for cardiogenic shock complicating acute myocardial infarction. Am J Cardiol 2002;89(2):132–6.

[33] Hochman JS. Cardiogenic shock complicating acute myocardial infarction: expanding the paradigm. Circulation 2003;107:2998–3002.

[34] Cotter G, Kaluski E, Blatt A, et al. L-NMMA (a nitric oxide synthase inhibitor) is effective in the treatment of cardiogenic shock. Circulation 2000;101:1358–61.

[35] Cotter G, Kaluski E, Milo O, et al. LINCS: L-NAME (a NO synthase inhibitor) in the treatment of refractory cardiogenic shock: a prospective randomized study. Eur Heart J 2003;24: 1287–95.

[36] Waknine Y. FDA approvals: orphan drugs troxatyl, tilarginine acetate, aerosolized gene therapy. Available at: http://www.medscape.com/viewarticle/507286. Accessed June 24, 2005.

[37] Vakeva AP, Agah A, Rollins SA, et al. Myocardial infarction and apoptosis after myocardial ischemia and reperfusion: role of the terminal complement components and inhibition by anti-C5 therapy. Circulation 1998;97:2259–67.

[38] Fitch JC, Rollins S, Matis L, et al. Pharmacology and biological efficacy of a recombinant, humanized, single-chain antibody C5 complement inhibitor in patients undergoing coronary artery bypass graft surgery with cardiopulmonary bypass. Circulation 1999;100:2499–506.

[39] Granger CB, Mahaffey KW, Weaver WD, et al. Pexelizumab. An anti-C5 complement antibody, as adjunctive therapy to primary percutaneous coronary intervention in acute myocardial infarction: the COMplement inhibition in Myocardial infarction treated with Angioplasty (COMMA) trial. Circulation 2003;108:1184–91.

[40] Hughes S. Apex AMI pexelizumab trial to be stopped early. Available at: www.theheart.org/article/640883.do. Accessed February 3, 2006.

[41] Mahaffey KW, Puma JA, Barbagelata A, et al. Adenosine as an adjunct to thrombolytic therapy for acute myocardial infarction: results of a multicenter, randomized, placebo-controlled trial: the Acute Myocardial Infarction Study of Adenosine (AMISTAD) trial. J Am Coll Cardiol 1999;34:1711–20.

[42] Théroux P, Chaitman BR, Danchin N, et al. Inhibition of the sodium-hydrogen exchanger with cariporide to prevent myocardial infarction in high-risk ischemic situations: main results of the GUARDIAN trial. Circulation 2000;102:3032–8.

[43] Zeymer U, Suryapranata H, Monassier JP, et al. The Na^+/H^+ exchange inhibitor eniporide as an adjunct to early reperfusion therapy for acute myocardial infarction. Results of the Evaluation of the Safety and Cardioprotective Effects of Eniporide in Acute Myocardial Infarction (ESCAMI) trial. J Am Coll Cardiol 2001;38:1644–50.

[44] Flaherty JT, Pitt B, Gruber JW, et al. Recombinant human superoxide dismutase (h-SOD) fails to improve recovery of ventricular function in patients undergoing coronary angioplasty forAMI. Circulation 1994;89:1982–91.

[45] Zhang Y, Patel AA, Juergens C, et al. N-Acetylcysteine improves myocardial salvage after reperfusion therapy in humans [abstract]. Circulation 1999;100(Suppl I):I-371.

[46] Diaz R, Paolasso EA, Piegas LS, et al. Metabolic modulation of acute myocardial infarction. The ECLA (Estudios Cardiologicos Latinoamerica) Collaborative Group. Circulation 1998;98:2227–34.

[47] Mehta SR, Yusuf S, Diaz R, et al. CREATE-ECLA Trial Group investigators. Effect of glucose-insulin-potassium infusion on mortality in patients with acute ST-segment elevation myocardial infarction: the CREATE-ECLA randomized controlled trial. JAMA 2005;293(4):437–46.

[48] Dunkman WB, Leinbach RC, Buckley MJ, et al. Clinical and hemodynamic results of intra-aortic balloon pumping and surgery for cardiogenic shock. Circulation 1972;46:465–77.

[49] Subramanian VA, Roberts AJ, Zema MJ, et al. Cardiogenic shock following acute myocardial infarction; late functional results after emergency cardiac surgery. N Y State J Med 1980;80(6):947–52.

[50] Hochman JS, Sleeper LA, Webb JG, et al. Early revascularization in acute myocardial infarction complicated by cardiogenic shock. SHOCK Investigators. Should we emergently revascularize occluded coronaries for cardiogenic shock. N Engl J Med 1999;341:625–34.

[51] Duvernoy CS, Bates ER. Management of cardiogenic shock attributable to acute myocardial infarction in the reperfusion era. J Intensive Care Med 2005;20:188–98.

[52] Lee L, Bates ER, Pitt B, et al. Percutaneous transluminal coronary angioplasty improves survival in acute myocardial infarction complicated by cardiogenic shock. Circulation 1988;78:1345–51.

[53] Lee L, Erbel R, Brown TM, et al. Multicenter registry of angioplasty therapy of cardiogenic shock: initial and long term survival. J Am Coll Cardiol 1991;17:599–603.

[54] Verna E, Repetto S, Boscarini M, et al. Emergency coronary angioplasty in patients with severe left ventricular dysfunction or cardiogenic shock after acute myocardial infarction. Eur Heart J 1989;10:58–66.

[55] Disler L, Haitas B, Benjamin J, et al. Cardiogenic shock in evolving myocardial infarction: treatment by angioplasty and streptokinase. Heart Lung 1987;16:649–52.

[56] Berger PB, Holmes DR Jr, Stebbins AL, et al. Impact of an aggressive invasive catheterization and revascularization strategy on mortality in patients with cardiogenic shock in the Global Utilization of Streptokinase and Tissue Plasminogen Aactivator for Occluded Coronary Arteries (GUSTO-I) trial. An observational study. Circulation 1997;96:122–7.

[57] Urban P, Stauffer JC, Bleed D, et al. A randomized evaluation of early revascularization to treat shock complicating acute myocardial infarction: the (Swiss) Multicenter Trial of Angioplasty for Shock—(S)MASH. Eur Heart J 1999;96:1030–8.

[58] Dzavik V, Sleeper LA, Cocke TP, et al. Early revascularization is associated with improved survival in elderly patients with acute myocardial infarction complicated by cardiogenic shock: a report from the SHOCK trial registry. Eur Heart J 2003;24:828–37.

[59] Dauerman HL, Ryan TJ Jr, Piper WD, et al. Outcomes of percutaneous coronary intervention among elderly patients in cardiogenic shock: a multicenter, decade-long experience. J Invasive Cardiol 2003;15:380–4.

[60] Webb JG, Lowe AM, Sanborn TA, et al. Percutaneous coronary intervention for cardiogenic shock in the SHOCK trial. J Am Coll Cardiol 2003;42:1380–6.

[61] Sanborn T, Sleeper L, Webb J, et al. Correlates of one-year survival inpatients with cardiogenic shock complicating acute myocardial infarction: angiographic findings from the SHOCK trial. J Am Coll Cardiol 2003;42:1373–9.

[62] Dauerman HL, Goldberg RJ, White K, et al. Revascularization, stenting, and outcomes of patients with acute myocardial infarction complicated by cardiogenic shock. Am J Cardiol 2002;90:838–42.

[63] Jacobs AK, French JK, Col J, et al. Cardiogenic shock with non–ST-segment elevation myocardial infarction: a report from the SHOCK trial registry. J Am Coll Cardiol 2000;36(3 Suppl A):1091–6.

[64] Iakobishvili Z, Behar S, Boyko V, et al. Does current treatment of cardiogenic shock complicating the acute coronary syndromes comply with guidelines? Am Heart J 2005;149(1): 98–103.

[65] Rogers WJ, Canto JG, Lambrew CT, et al. Temporal trends in the treatment of over 1.5 million patients with myocardial infarction in the US from 1990 through 1999:the national registry of myocardial infarction 1, 2 and 3. J Am Coll Cardiol 2000;36:2056–66.

[66] Ohman ME, Nannas J, Stomel RJ. Thrombolysis and Counterpulsation to Improve Cardiogenic Shock Survival (TACTICS): results of a prospective randomized trial [abstract]. Circulation 2000;102(Suppl II):600.

[67] French JK, Miller D, Palmieri S, et al. Cardiogenic shock treated with thrombolytic therapy and intra-aortic balloon counter pulsation: a report from the SHOCK trial [abstract]. Circulation 1999;100:(Suppl I):I-370.

[68] Leshnower BG, Gleason TG, O'Hara ML, et al. Safety and efficacy of left ventricular assist device support in postmyocardial infarction cardiogenic shock. Ann Thorac Surg 2006; 81(4):1365–70.

[69] Tayara W, Starling RC, Yamani MH, et al. Improved survival after acute myocardial infarction complicated by cardiogenic shock with circulatory support and transplantation: comparing aggressive intervention with conservative treatment. J Heart Lung Transplant 2006; 25(5):504–9.

[70] James KB, Militello M, Gus B, et al. Biventricular pacing for heart failure patients on inotropic support, a review of 38 consecutive cases. Tex Heart Inst J 2006;33(1):19–22.

[71] Konstantino Y, Iakobishvili Z, Arad O, et al. Urgent cardiac resynchronization therapy in patients with decompensated chronic heart failure receiving inotropic therapy. A case series. Cardiology 2006;106(1):59–62.

[72] Cowburn PJ, Patel H, Jolliffe RE, et al. Cardiac resynchronization therapy: an option for inotrope-supported patients with end-stage heart failure? Eur J Heart Fail 2005;7(2): 215–7.

ELSEVIER
SAUNDERS

THE MEDICAL
CLINICS
OF NORTH AMERICA

Med Clin N Am 91 (2007) 729–749

New Trials and Therapies for Acute Myocardial Infarction

Richard J. Gumina, MD, PhD

*Division of Cardiovascular Medicine, The Ohio State University,
Columbus, OH 43210, USA*

Acute coronary syndromes (ACSs), which include the clinical entities of unstable angina (UA), non–ST-segment elevation myocardial infarction (NSTEMI), and ST-segment elevation myocardial infarction (STEMI), account for more than 1.5 million hospital admissions annually in the United States alone. Approximately 1 million of these admissions are classified as UA/NSTEMI and approximately 500,000 are STEMI [1]. Because of the overwhelming number of studies on ACSs over the past several years, this article focuses on new trials and therapies for treating patients diagnosed with STEMI.

The adage "time is myocardium" is central to the treatment of STEMI [2]. Percutaneous coronary intervention (PCI) has been shown to be superior to thrombolytic therapy in several studies [3]. However, because coronary catheterization laboratories are not available in all communities, several studies have evaluated the optimal reperfusion strategy for patients who present to hospitals without invasive facilities. Specifically, the Danish Trial in Acute Myocardial Infarction (DANAMI-2) and the Primary Angioplasty in Acute Myocardial Infarction Patients from German Community Hospitals Transported to Percutaneous Transluminal Coronary Angioplasty Units versus Emergency Thrombolysis (PRAGUE-2) showed a reduction in the incidence of major adverse cardiac events (MACE) at 30 days in the invasive strategy groups. These studies highlight the superiority of PCI over on-site fibrinolytic therapy despite the additional time-to-treatment incurred during patient transfer. A recent meta-analysis comparing primary PCI with in-hospital fibrinolytic therapy supports this finding, showing that PCI was associated with a significantly lower 30-day mortality rate regardless of the treatment delay. The time to PCI in both studies was short (97 minutes in PRAGUE-2 and 114 minutes in DANAMI-2).

E-mail address: Richard.Gumina@osumc.edu

0025-7125/07/$ - see front matter © 2007 Published by Elsevier Inc.
doi:10.1016/j.mcna.2007.04.003   *medical.theclinics.com*

Several reports have shown the adverse impact of longer time-to-treatment, finding that infarct size and 1-year mortality were worse in patients who experienced treatment delay [4–6]. The American College of Cardiology/American Heart Association (ACC/AHA) Guidelines for the Management of Patients with ST-Elevation Myocardial Infarction, updated in 2004, reflect these issues in their recommendations [1]. Because of the inherent delay associated with patient transfers, several recent studies have evaluated whether combined pharmacologic and mechanical reperfusion strategies (facilitated PCI) in patients who have STEMI improves clinical outcomes.

Percutaneous coronary intervention after thrombolytic therapy in ST-segment elevation myocardial infarction

The timing of PCI after administration of fibrinolytic therapy can be classified as immediate (ie, as soon as possible after thrombolysis, or *facilitated PCI*), rescue (ie, performed only for failed fibrinolysis), or deferred (ie, greater than 24 hours after fibrinolysis) [7].

Rescue percutaneous coronary infarction

Approximately 20% of patients treated with thrombolytic therapy experience incomplete reperfusion or reocclusion of the culprit artery. Therefore, the Rescue Angioplasty versus Conservative Treatment or Repeat Thrombolysis (REACT) trial recently evaluated the role of rescue angioplasty, randomizing 427 patients who showed no ST-segment resolution 90 minutes after thrombolytic therapy to one of three treatment arms: (1) rescue PCI, (2) repeat thrombolysis using tissue-type plasminogen activator or reteplase, or (3) conservative care [8]. The primary end point of combined death, reinfarction, stroke, or severe heart failure within 6 months was significantly reduced in the rescue PCI arm compared with the repeat thrombolytic arm and conservative care (15.5% versus 31.0% versus 29.8%, respectively; $P < .01$). Additionally, less ischemia-driven revascularization was required in the rescue PCI arm. These data also suggest that rescue PCI is associated with a reduction in adverse clinical outcomes in patients who undergo failed thrombolysis.

Facilitated percutaneous coronary intervention

Immediate PCI after thrombolytic administration is often referred to as *facilitated PCI*. Several early clinical trials showed poorer clinical outcomes in patients who underwent fibrinolytic therapy followed by immediate angioplasty [9–12]. However, in the modern era of antiplatelet agents, more recent trials have revisited this hypothesis and expanded the concept of facilitated PCI to encompass the planned use of immediate PCI after administration of a pharmacologic regimen, including thrombolytic therapy, glycoprotein (GP) IIb/IIIa antagonist therapy, and combination therapy, to obtain patency of the culprit artery. Several recent clinical trials have evaluated facilitated PCI.

In the Combined Angioplasty and Pharmacological Intervention versus Thrombolytics Alone in Acute Myocardial Infarction (CAPITAL AMI) study, tenecteplase plus immediate angioplasty (median door-to-balloon time, 95 minutes) was found to be superior to tenecteplase alone in 170 patients who had high-risk STEMI [13]. MACEs were significantly reduced at 30 days (9.3% versus 21.7%; $P = .03$) and 6 months (11.6% versus 24.4%; $P = .04$) in the tenecteplase–facilitated PCI group, because of reductions in recurrent unstable ischemia and reinfarction. No increase in the incidence of major bleeding was observed.

The Bavarian Reperfusion Alternatives Evaluation (BRAVE) trial randomized 253 patients who had STEMI to undergo facilitated PCI with half-dose reteplase plus abciximab versus abciximab alone [14]. Despite the delay in PCI (74% of patients required transfer for PCI), the primary end point of infarct size measured with technetium Tc 99m sestamibi was similar between the groups (13.0% versus 11.5%; $P = .81$). However, major bleeding was higher in the facilitated PCI group (5.6% versus 1.6%; $P = .16$). Furthermore, this study did not include a placebo group that underwent PCI only, making interpretation difficult.

The Assessment of the Safety and Efficacy of a New Treatment Strategy with Percutaneous Coronary Intervention (ASSENT-4 PCI), the largest of the facilitated PCI trials, was designed to determine if primary PCI was superior to facilitated PCI [15]. This trial planned to randomized 4000 patients who experienced STEMI less than 6 hours from symptom onset to undergo treatment with weight-adjusted tenecteplase with unfractionated heparin (UFH) (facilitated PCI arm) or UFH alone (PCI arm) before PCI. The Data Monitoring and Safety Board stopped the trial at 1667 patients because of higher in hospital mortality (6% versus 3%; $P = .0105$). The primary end point of the 90-day composite of death, congestive heart failure, or cardiogenic shock was significantly higher in the facilitated PCI arm than the primary PCI arm (19% versus 13%; $P = .0045$).

Additionally, a meta-analysis of 17 randomized trials comparing facilitated and primary PCI in 4504 patients who had acute ST-elevation myocardial infarction showed that, despite a greater than twofold increase in preprocedural thrombosis in myocardial infarction (TIMI)-3 flow (facilitated PCI, 37% versus primary PCI, 15%), facilitated PCI resulted in increased mortality and greater rates of reinfarction, urgent repeat revascularization, major bleeding, hemorrhagic stroke, and total stroke [16]. Death, recurrent ischemia, and major hemorrhagic complications were increased with preintervention thrombolytic therapy with or without GP IIb/IIIa inhibitors, whereas use of an upfront GP IIb/IIIa inhibitor was not harmful but also not beneficial.

The ongoing Facilitated Intervention with Enhanced Reperfusion Speed to Stop Events (FINESSE) is a double-blind, placebo-controlled, trial randomizing 3000 patients to one of three arms comparing the efficacy and safety of (1) facilitated PCI with reduced-dose reteplase plus abciximab bolus doses given in the emergency department, (2) facilitated PCI with an abciximab bolus injection administered in the emergency department, and (3) primary PCI with abciximab given in the cardiac catheterization laboratory immediately before the procedure [17]. The primary end point is a composite of death, heart failure, ventricular function, or shock at 90 days, with a substudy comparing the effect of UFH and low molecular weight heparin (LMWH).

The use of abciximab as an adjunct to reperfusion in STEMI has been studied in registries and randomized clinical trials. De Luca and colleagues [18] performed a meta-analysis of 11 trials including 27,115 patients treated with primary PCI and fibrinolysis. The authors found that abciximab administration was associated with a significant reduction in both 30-day and 6- to 12-month mortality in patients undergoing primary angioplasty (30-day mortality was 2.4% with abciximab versus 3.4% for control [$P = .047$] and the respective 6- to 12-month mortality was 4.4% versus 6.2% [$P = .01$]). The administration of abciximab was also associated with a reduction in reinfarction despite whether the trial included primary PCI or fibrinolysis. Although abciximab did not cause increased intracranial hemorrhage, it was associated with a higher risk for major bleeding when given with fibrinolysis.

Summary

Although facilitated PCI has theoretical benefit, given the data from ASSENT-4 PCI and a meta-analysis of 17 studies of facilitated PCI, the routine use of fibrinolytic therapy before PCI cannot be recommended outside of clinical trials. Whether facilitated PCI is a viable option in patients transferred from remote areas, where a significant delay occurs before arrival at PCI-capable hospital, is uncertain.

Antiplatelet therapy with percutaneous coronary intervention/thrombolytics

Glycoprotein IIb/IIIa antagonists in ST-segment elevation myocardial infarction

Although the benefit of potent antiplatelet therapy in conjunction with a fibrinolytic agent is not yet established, several trials have confirmed the benefit of GP IIb/IIIa antagonists, specifically abciximab, used in conjunction with primary PCI [19–23]. These trials showed that abciximab was associated with a significant reduction in death, myocardial infarction, and urgent revascularization at 30 days, and long-term benefit [18].

In these previous studies, GP IIb/IIIa antagonists were primarily administered at PCI. The Ongoing Tirofiban in Myocardial Infarction Evaluation (ON-TIME) trial randomized 507 patients who had STEMI requiring transfer for PCI to undergo prehospital administration of tirofiban (facilitated) versus primary PCI [24]. No difference in post-PCI perfusion was seen, as assessed using final TIMI flow grade, blush score, or corrected TIMI frame counts. However, a trend toward increased MACE in the facilitated group was seen at 30 days (8.6% versus 4.4%; $P = .06$), but no difference in death or recurrent myocardial infarction at 1 year.

In the BRAVE trial, combination therapy with reteplase and abciximab had higher rates of major bleeding (5.6% versus 1.6%; $P = .16$) with comparable infarct size [14].

The Time to Integrelin Therapy in Acute Myocardial Infarction (TITAN)-TIMI-34 study was a smaller trial of 343 patients comparing early administration of the GP IIb/IIIa inhibitor eptifibatide in the emergency department versus its later administration in the cardiac catheterization laboratory, with the primary end point of corrected TIMI frame count. Early administration of eptifibatide led to faster coronary flow as assessed using corrected TIMI frame count (77.5 versus 84.3 frames; $P = .049$) and a higher frequency of TIMI grade 3 flow (24.3% versus 14.2%; $P = .026$) [25].

Meta-analysis of 17 randomized trials comparing facilitated and primary angioplasty showed an increase in mortality and greater rates of reinfarction, urgent repeat revascularization, major bleeding, hemorrhagic stroke, and total stroke [16]. In the GP IIb/IIIa–facilitated studies, no difference was seen in 30-day mortality, but also no increase in adverse clinical outcomes occurred in patients treated with GP IIb/IIIa antagonists. Two ongoing trials are addressing the use of GP IIb/IIIa antagonists in facilitated regimens.

The Combined Abciximab Reteplase Stent Study in Acute Myocardial Infarction (CARESS) in 1800 patients who have STEMI is comparing the primary end point of the combined incidence of death, myocardial infarction, or refractory ischemia at 30 days in patients presenting to hospitals without PCI capabilities who are treated with abciximab and half-dose reteplase, with rescue PCI in the case of reperfusion failure, versus referral for facilitated PCI after early administration of abciximab and a half dose of reteplase [26].

GRACIA-3: A Randomized Trial to Evaluate the Role of Paclitaxel Eluting Stent and Tirofiban to Improve the Results of Facilitated PCI in the Treatment of Acute ST-Segment Elevation Myocardial Infarction will determine the efficacy of a paclitaxel-eluting stent compared with conventional bare stent in terms of restenosis [27]. A total of 436 patients will be initially treated with tenecteplase and enoxaparin (facilitated PCI). Tirofiban will start 120 minutes after tenecteplase administration in patients randomized to tirofiban therapy. Patients will proceed to PCI with randomization to either a paclitaxel-eluting stent or bare metal stent.

Summary

In patients undergoing primary PCI for STEMI, the early administration of a GP IIb/IIIa antagonist seems to provide better infarct-related artery patency.

Oral antiplatelet agents in ST-segment elevation myocardial infarction

Although the antiplatelet agent clopidogrel added to aspirin provides clinical benefit in patients undergoing stent implantation and those who have ACSs without ST-segment elevation, the role of clopidogrel therapy in patients who have STEMI was unclear. Two recent clinical trials evaluated the efficacy of early clopidogrel administration on clinical outcomes in patients who had STEMI.

The Clopidogrel and Metoprolol in Myocardial Infarction Trial (COMMIT) was a two-by-two trial designed to evaluate the efficacy of metoprolol and clopidogrel in 45,852 patients who presented within 24 hours of symptoms and were found to have either new left bundle branch block (6%), ST-segment elevation (87%), or ST-segment depression within 24 hours of suspected acute myocardial infarction symptom onset [28]. Of the randomized patients, 54% were treated with thrombolytic agents (predominantly urokinase) before or after entry in the study. The results showed that the group receiving aspirin (162 mg daily) plus clopidogrel (75 mg daily) experienced a significant reduction in death, reinfarction, or stroke compared with the group given aspirin plus placebo (9.2% clopidogrel versus 10.1% placebo; $P = .002$). The effects on death, reinfarction, and stroke were independent of other treatments, which is important because only 54% of patients underwent primary reperfusion therapy in the form of thrombolytic therapy. In addition, a reduction in any death occurred (7.5% versus 8.1%; $P = .03$) and no significant excess bleeding risk was noted with clopidogrel (0.58% versus 0.55%; $P = .59$).

The Clopidogrel as Adjunctive Reperfusion Therapy–Thrombolysis in Myocardial Infarction (CLARITY TIMI) 28 trial randomized 3491 patients to treatment with clopidogrel (300-mg loading dose, then 75 mg once daily) or placebo within 12 hours after the onset of an STEMI [29]. The primary efficacy end point, a composite of an occluded infarct-related artery (defined by a TIMI flow grade of 0 or 1) on angiography or death or recurrent myocardial infarction before angiography, was significantly lower in the clopidogrel-treated group (placebo, 21.7% versus clopidogrel, 15%; $P < .001$). At 30 days, the composite end point of death from cardiovascular causes, recurrent myocardial infarction, or recurrent ischemia leading to the need for urgent revascularization was significantly lower in the clopidogrel-treated group (placebo, 14.1% versus clopidogrel, 11.6%; $P = .03$). No significant differences were seen in rates of major bleeding (placebo, 1.1% versus clopidogrel, 1.3%; $P = .64$) and intracranial hemorrhage (0.7% versus 0.5%; $P = .38$).

The PCI-CLARITY study prospectively analyzed 1863 patients from the CLARITY–TIMI 28 study who underwent PCI as a result of findings from the mandated angiography [30]. Pretreatment with clopidogrel significantly reduced the combined end point of cardiovascular death, myocardial infarction, or stroke after PCI (3.6% versus 6.2%; $P = .008$), without an increase in bleeding (pretreatment, 2.0% versus non-pretreatment, 1.9%; $P > .99$). This difference was observed despite a loading dose of clopidogrel administered in the catheterization laboratory for patients treated with placebo, and the use of GP IIb/IIIa inhibitors at the operator's discretion.

Summary

In patients presenting with STEMI, the addition of clopidogrel (75 mg daily) to aspirin markedly improves clinical outcomes regardless of administration of thrombolytic therapy. In patients undergoing aspirin and thrombolytic therapy for STEMI, administration of clopidogrel improves culprit artery patency and reduces mortality.

Optimal anticoagulation in ST-segment elevation myocardial infarction

UFH has been used for more than 40 years in the treatment of STEMI. With the advent of low molecular weight heparins (LMWHs), direct thrombin inhibitors, and compounds with anti-Factor Xa activity, several recent studies have focused on the optimal anticoagulation therapy with either thrombolytic therapy or primary PCI for treating STEMI.

Low molecular weight heparin in ST-segment elevation myocardial infarction

In the Clinical Trial of Reviparin and Metabolic Modulation in Acute Myocardial Infarction Treatment Evaluation (CREATE), 15,570 patients who had STEMI were randomized to receive, before or within 15 minutes of thrombolytic therapy, the LMWH reviparin or placebo for 7 days [31]. A benefit to treatment with reviparin was seen with a lower primary composite end point of death, reinfarction, or stroke at 7 days (control, 11.0% versus reviparin, 9.6%, $P = .005$) that persisted at 30 days (13.6% versus 11.3%; $P = .001$). However, reviparin therapy resulted in increased life-threatening bleeding at 7 days (control, 0.1% versus reviparin, 0.2%; $P = .07$).

The Enoxaparin and Thrombolysis Reperfusion for Acute Myocardial Infarction Treatment—Thrombolysis in Myocardial Infarction 25 (ExTRACT-TIMI-25) study randomized 20,506 patients undergoing thrombolytic therapy for treatment of a STEMI to receive either enoxaparin for 7 days or UFH for at least 48 hours [32]. The primary end point of death or nonfatal recurrent myocardial infarction at 30 days was significantly lower in the group treated with enoxaparin (9.9% versus 12.0%; $P < .001$). This benefit persisted in patients who underwent subsequent PCI. However, although no difference was seen in mortality (UFH, 7.5% versus enoxaparin, 6.9%; $P = .11$), bleeding complications in the enoxaparin-treated group were significantly higher (2.1% versus 1.4%; $P < .001$), which was consistent with findings from previous studies.

Direct thrombin inhibitors in ST-segment elevation myocardial infarction

One previously published large-scale study, the Hirulog Early Reperfusion Occlusion 2 (HERO-2) trial, evaluated 17,073 patients who had acute myocardial infarction who were treated with streptokinase and then randomized to receive UFH or the direct thrombin inhibitor bivalirudin [33]. Although no difference was seen in the primary end point of 30-day mortality (bivalirudin, 10.8% versus UFH, 10.9%; $P = .85$), the bivalirudin group showed increased rates of mild and moderate bleeding and a trend toward increased intracranial hemorrhage. The Harmonizing Outcomes with Revascularization and Stents (HORIZONS AMI) trial, an ongoing comparison of UFH with a GP IIb/IIIa inhibitor versus bivalirudin at primary PCI for STEMI, will help define the role of direct thrombin inhibitors in the treatment of STEMI [34]. Currently, direct thrombin inhibitors have a role only in patients who have heparin-induced thrombocytopenia.

Factor Xa inhibitors in ST-segment elevation myocardial infarction

The MICHELANGELO Organization to Assess Strategies in Acute Ischemic Syndromes (OASIS)-6 trial studied the effect of fondaparinux on mortality and reinfarction in patients who experienced acute STEMI, comparing fondaparinux, a Factor Xa inhibitor, with UFH in 12,092 patients who experienced STEMI [35]. Fondaparinux administration was associated with a reduced incidence of the primary end point of death and reinfarction at 30 days compared with control treatment (UFH, 11.2% versus fondaparinux, 9.7%; $P = .008$), with no increase in bleeding complications. Patients treated with thrombin-specific thrombolytic agents showed a reduction in 30-day mortality or myocardial infarction. However, subgroup analysis showed no benefit of fondaparinux treatment in patients undergoing primary PCI. Furthermore, an increased risk for catheter thrombosis was seen that was prevented by coadministration of heparin.

Summary

Enoxaparin administration with thrombolysis is associated with improved clinical outcomes but higher bleeding complications. The role of direct thrombin inhibitors in STEMI remains undefined. Fondaparinux seems to provide clinical benefit in patients treated with thrombolytics or conservative therapy without excess bleeding; an increase in catheter thrombosis is seen in patients who undergo PCI.

Optimal stents in primary percutaneous coronary intervention for ST-segment elevation myocardial infarction

Although prior studies have clearly shown the superiority of catheter-based reperfusion over fibrinolytic therapy [3], whether drug-eluting stents are beneficial or harmful in the treatment of STEMI has not been determined.

Paclitaxel-eluting stents in ST-segment elevation myocardial infarction

The Paclitaxel-Eluting Stent versus Conventional Stent for STEMI (PASSION) trial evaluated the 1-year occurrence of the composite of cardiovascular death, recurrent myocardial infarction, or target lesion revascularization in 619 patients presenting within 6 hours of symptom onset with STEMI [36]. Patients were randomized to receive either the paclitaxel-eluting stent (TAXUS, Boston Scientific, Natick, Massachusetts) or a conventional bare-metal stent (Express Stent, Boston Scientific). At 1 year, the primary end point was not statistically different between the groups (paclitaxel-eluting stent, 8.8% versus bare metal stent, 12.8%; $P = .09$). The ongoing HORIZONS AMI [34] and GRACIA-3 [27] trials will compare the paclitaxel-eluting stent to bare-metal stents in patients who have STEMI.

Sirolimus-eluting stents in ST-segment elevation myocardial infarction

The Trial to Assess the Use of Cypher Stent in Acute Myocardial Infarction Treated with Balloon Angioplasty (TYPHOON) was a multicenter prospective randomized open-label study of 712 patients presenting within 12 hours of symptom onset with STEMI [37]. Patients were randomized to treatment with either a sirolimus-eluting stent (CYPHER stent, Cordis Corporation) or a bare-metal stent. A prespecified subgroup of 200 patients underwent angiographic follow-up at 8 months. The primary end point of target vessel failure at 1 year, defined as target vessel revascularization, cardiac death, or recurrent myocardial infarction, was significantly higher in the bare-metal than the sirolimus-eluting stent group (14.3% versus 7.3%; $P = .004$). This difference was driven primarily by a lower incidence of target lesion revascularization in the sirolimus-eluting stent group. The angiographic follow-up cohort showed significantly lower in-stent late loss and binary restenosis in the sirolimus-eluting stent group. These results were duplicated in the smaller Sirolimus Stent vs Bare Stent in Acute Myocardial Infarction (SESAMI) trial that randomized 320 patients presenting with STEMI who were to undergo either primary PCI or rescue PCI to receive either a sirolimus-eluting stent (CYPHER stent) or a bare-metal stent [38]. The primary end point of angiographic binary restenosis occurred less often in the sirolimus-eluting stent group (9.3% versus 21.3%; $P = .032$).

Summary

No difference in acute or subacute stent thrombosis was observed. Using drug-eluting stents in PCI to treat STEMI seems to have no adverse effects. A reduction in restenosis is seen with the use of sirolimus-eluting stents for PCI in patients who have a STEMI.

Adjunctive therapy for myocardial protection in ST-segment elevation myocardial infarction

Despite the rapid and effective delivery of reperfusion therapy for patients who have a STEMI, a substantial number still develop large infarcts, resulting in reduced left ventricular function and increased mortality. Therefore, adjunctive therapies designed to reduce ischemic injury or protect against reperfusion injury have been studied extensively. Based on preclinical models showing myocardial salvage, recent clinical trials have evaluated many promising pharmacologic agents and nonpharmacologic strategies.

Thrombectomy/distal protection device to protect the myocardium in ST-segment elevation myocardial infarction

Several devices have been designed to protect the microvasculature from distal embolization of debris released during PCI. Because of the thrombus burden and debris released into the distal microvascular bed during primary PCI in STEMI, several studies have examined whether reduction of distal embolization during primary PCI for STEMI improves perfusion and clinical outcomes. The Enhanced Myocardial Efficacy and Removal by Aspiration of Liberated Debris (EMERALD) trial used the GuardWire balloon occlusion and aspiration system (Medtronic, Santa Rosa, California) during the angioplasty procedure [39]. Although 73% of cases treated with the protection device retrieved visible debris, no improvement occurred in TIMI flow grade, myocardial perfusion, or infarct size, and no reduction in clinical events was observed (10.0% versus 11.0%; $P = .66$).

In the X-Sizer in Acute Myocardial Infarction for Negligible Embolization and Optimal ST Resolution (X AMINE ST) trial, adjunctive thrombectomy with the X-Sizer device (ev3, White Bear Lake, Minnesota) resulted in improved ST-segment resolution [40]. In the Protection Devices in PCI-Treatment of Myocardial Infarction for Salvage of Endangered Myocardium (PROMISE) trial, the FilterWire-EX (Boston Scientific) was used to limit distal embolization, but failed to improve maximal adenosine-induced Doppler flow velocity in the infarct-related artery post-PCI, or infarct size according to MRI [41].

The AngioJet in Acute Myocardial Infarction (AiMI) trial randomized more than 480 patients to undergo primary PCI with or without rheolytic thrombectomy using the AngioJet device (Possis Medical Inc., Minneapolis, Minnesota) followed by PCI with stenting and use of a GP IIb/IIIa inhibitor versus no pretreatment with the AngioJet device [42]. The primary end point of infarct size according to single-photon emission computed tomographic (SPECT) imaging was higher in the thrombectomy group (12.5% versus 9.8%; $P = .03$), particularly in patients presenting with inferior infarcts, and a significantly higher incidence of MACE occurred at 30 days (6.7% versus 1.7%, $P < .01$), which was driven primarily by a difference in mortality. The AngioJET Rheolytic Thrombectomy Before Direct Infarct Artery Stenting in Patients Undergoing Primary PCI for Acute Myocardial Infarction (JETSTENT) study is evaluating treatment with AngioJet RT immediately before direct infarct artery stenting versus direct stenting alone in patients who have STEMI and angiographically visible thrombus presenting within 6 hours of symptom onset for primary PCI [43].

Summary

Recent studies do not support the routine use of thrombectomy or distal protection devices during PCI for STEMI. Whether the use of these devices is efficacious in select patients who have a large thrombus burden remains to be investigated.

Metabolic/ionic protection

Hyperoxemia in ST-segment elevation myocardial infarction

The Acute Myocardial Infarction with Hyperoxemic Therapy (AMI-HOT) trial investigated the use of hyperoxemic reperfusion with aqueous oxygen during STEMI [44]. After stent implantation, patients in the aqueous oxygen group underwent a 90-minute intracoronary infusion of blood supersaturated with oxygen. One important difference in study design, compared with previous reperfusion trials, was that patients were eligible for enrollment up to 24 hours from symptom onset. Hyperoxemic reperfusion was safe and well tolerated; however, no significant improvement was seen in the primary study end points (ST-segment resolution, regional wall motion according to serial echocardiography, and SPECT infarct size). Examination of a prespecified subset of patients who had anterior STEMI treated within 6 hours of symptom onset suggested benefit of therapy. The AMIHOT II trial is a randomized noninferiority trial designed to evaluate the effect of hyperoxemia on infarct size and 30-day MACE in patients who have anterior STEMI treated within 6 hours of symptom onset [45].

Hypothermia in ST-segment elevation myocardial infarction

The use of hypothermia to limit infarct size and preserve myocardium has been evaluated in several trials. The most recent, the Intravascular Cooling Adjunctive to Percutaneous Coronary Intervention for Acute Myocardial Infarction (ICE-IT) study, randomized patients who had STEMI to undergo hypothermia through cooling with an endovascular cooling catheter for 6 hours (Innercool Inc., San Diego, California) [46]. The trial was discontinued due to no difference in the primary end point of final infarct size in the hypothermia group. Post-hoc analysis showed that patients who had anterior myocardial infarction who underwent sufficient cooling before reperfusion seemed to experience a reduction in infarct size. This finding is consistent with data from the Cooling as an Adjunctive Therapy to Percutaneous Intervention in Patients with Acute Myocardial Infarction (COOL MI) trial. The recently initiated COOL-MI-2 trial will specifically evaluate infarct size and improvement in left ventricular ejection fraction in 225 patients who experience anterior STEMI less than 6 hours before presentation [47].

Glucose–insulin–potassium in ST-segment elevation myocardial infarction

Several studies have suggested a benefit from glucose–insulin–potassium (GIK) therapy in controlling metabolism in patients who have a STEMI. The Effect of Glucose–Insulin–Potassium Infusion on Mortality in Patients with Acute ST-Segment Elevation Myocardial Infarction (CREATE-ECLA) trial randomized 20,201 patients who had a STEMI presenting within 12 hours from symptom onset to receive either a high-dose GIK infusion for 24 hours or usual care [48]. In this study, fewer than 2000 patients were treated with primary PCI. No difference was seen in the primary end point of all-cause mortality at 30 days (control, 9.7% versus GIK, 10.0%; $P = .45$) or any secondary outcome measures, including cardiac arrest, cardiogenic shock, or reinfarction. Similarly, in the randomized, open label Glucose-Insulin-Potassium Study in Patients with ST Elevation Myocardial Infarction without Signs of Heart Failure (GIPS)-II trial, 889 patients who had a STEMI with no signs of heart failure underwent reperfusion therapy (primary PCI, 88%, thrombolytics, 7%) and either high-dose GIK or control. The study was terminated early after an interim analysis showed no reduction in infarct size or mortality [49]. Thus, based on these two large-scale studies, the routine use of GIK in the treatment of patients who have STEMI cannot be recommended.

Sodium/calcium exchange inhibition in ST-segment elevation myocardial infarction

The use of pharmacologic agents to alter the metabolic milieu and reduce calcium overload has been the focus of several studies. The Caldaret in ST-Elevation Myocardial Infarction (CASTEMI) trial treated 387 patients who had a STEMI with two doses (a low dose of 57.5 mg and a high dose of 172.5 mg) of intravenous MCC-135 (caldaret, a sodium/calcium exchanger inhibitor) [50]. Although no difference was seen in the primary end point (infarct size at day 7), a benefit was seen in patients in the high-dose group who experienced anterior myocardial infarction. The Evaluation of MCC-135 for Left Ventricular Salvage in Acute MI (EVOLVE) study is a phase 2a, multicenter, randomized, double-blind, placebo-controlled trial that will evaluate safety and efficacy of MCC-135 in STEMI [51].

Nicorandil in ST-segment elevation myocardial infarction

Nicorandil, a potassium channel opener and nitric oxide donor, has been shown in preclinical studies to provide significant cardioprotection [52,53]. Several small clinical studies have also suggested benefit in the treatment of STEMI. Most recently, a larger single-center trial of 368 patients showed that an intravenous bolus of nicorandil (12 mg) markedly reduced death and heart failure and improved TIMI flow, TIMI frame count, and ST-segment resolution compared with placebo [54]. The Japan-Working Groups of Acute Myocardial Infarction for the Reduction of Necrotic Damage by a K-ATP Channel Opener (J-WIND-KATP) is a 26-center prospective, randomized, multicenter study designed to evaluate whether nicorandil reduces myocardial infarct size and improves regional wall motion when used as an adjunctive therapy in patients treated for STEMI [55].

Adenosine in ST-segment elevation myocardial infarction

Administration of adenosine reduces myocardial infarct size and improves coronary flow reserve in several preclinical studies. In the Acute Myocardial Infarction Study of Adenosine (AMISTAD) trial, a trend toward reduction in infarct size was observed in patients who experienced anterior STEMI [56]. In the AMISTAD-II trial, which investigated whether intravenous adenosine administered before reperfusion would reduce infarct size or improve clinical outcomes, patients undergoing thrombolytic therapy or primary PCI were randomized to undergo a 3-hour infusion of adenosine (50 or 70 μg/kg/min) or placebo [57]. No difference was seen in the primary end point (new congestive heart failure, first rehospitalization for congestive heart failure, or death within 6 months) between the placebo and the pooled adenosine dose groups (17.9% versus 16.3%; $P = .43$). Although the pooled adenosine group trended toward a smaller median infarct size than the placebo group (17% versus 27%; $P = .074$), a dose–response relationship in median infarct size was observed (high dose, 11% versus placebo, 27%; $P = .023$, and low dose, 23% versus placebo, 27%; $P = .41$). Whether high-dose adenosine is efficacious requires a large-scale clinical trial.

Postconditioning in ST-segment elevation myocardial infarction

Postconditioning is a cardioprotective phenomenon that is induced by a sequence of reversible, brief episodes of ischemia–reperfusion performed immediately after a prolonged ischemic insult [58–60]. Protection afforded by postconditioning seems as potent as that provided by ischemic preconditioning [59]. Based on promising preclinical work, a randomized study of postconditioning was conducted in 30 patients undergoing primary PCI for STEMI [61]. After reperfusion through direct stenting, control subjects underwent no further intervention, whereas postconditioning with four episodes of 1-minute inflation and 1-minute deflation of the angioplasty balloon was performed within 1 minute of reflow. The primary end point of infarct size, assessed through measuring the area under the curve for total creatine kinase release over 72 hours, was significantly reduced in the postconditioning group compared with the control group ($208,984 \pm 26,576$ versus $326,095 \pm 48,779$ arbitrary units; $P < .05$). Blush grade, a marker of myocardial reperfusion, was also significantly increased in the patients who underwent postconditioning compared with controls (2.44 ± 0.17 versus 1.95 ± 0.27; $P < .05$).

Pexelizumab in ST-segment elevation myocardial infarction

Preclinical data have suggested that modulation of the complement system provides significant cardioprotection. In the Complement Inhibition in Myocardial Infarction Treated with Angioplasty (COMMA) study [62], pexelizumab, a novel humanized monoclonal antibody fragment that binds specifically to C5 complement and prevents its cleavage and terminal complement activation, showed no significant effect on the primary end point of infarct size, but a reduction in 90-day mortality occurred compared with placebo (1.8% versus 5.9%; $P = .014$) [63]. The Assessment of Pexelizumab in Acute Myocardial Infarction (APEX AMI), a multicenter, randomized, double-blind, parallel-group, placebo-controlled study of pexelizumab in patients who have acute myocardial infarction undergoing primary PCI trial [64], randomized 5745 patients undergoing primary PCI for STEMI to receive placebo versus pexelizumab bolus and infusion for 24 hours. The primary efficacy analysis of all-cause mortality at day 30 was lower than expected in this trial and no difference in 30-day mortality was observed (placebo: 4.06% versus pexelizumab: 3.92%; $P = .78$).

Metoprolol in ST-segment elevation myocardial infarction

Although prior studies have emphasized the prognostic importance of β-blocker therapy in patients treated with PCI for STEMI, showing an association with a reduction in mortality, the metoprolol arm of the COMMIT trial suggested the possibility of harm from the use of β-blockers in STEMI [65]. This trial randomized 45,852 patients within 24 hours of suspected acute myocardial infarction to receive metoprolol (up to 15 mg intravenous then 200 mg oral daily) or matching placebo. The coprimary outcomes of the composite of death, reinfarction, or cardiac arrest (metoprolol, 9.4% versus placebo, 9.9%; $P = .1$) or death from any cause during the scheduled treatment period (7.7% versus 7.8%; $P = .69$) were not significantly reduced by metoprolol therapy. Although metoprolol therapy was associated with fewer patients experiencing reinfarction (metoprolol, 2.0% versus placebo, 2.5%; $P = .001$) or ventricular fibrillation (2.5% versus 3.0%; $P = .001$), significantly more patients developed cardiogenic shock (5.0% versus 3.9%; $P < .0001$), predominantly during the first 24 hours of admission. The results from COMMIT have raised questions regarding the use of β-blockers (intravenous then oral dosing) in the early stages of STEMI. Notably, patients with Killip Class II/III were included in COMMIT.

As outlined in the ACC/AHA guidelines [1], relative contraindications to the use of β-blockers in STEMI include heart rate less than 60 bpm, systolic blood pressure less than 100 mm Hg, moderate or severe left ventricular failure, shock, PR interval on the EKG more than 0.24 seconds, second- or third-degree heart block, and active asthma/reactive airways disease.

Summary

Although no evaluated mechanisms have shown superior clinical efficacy in reducing myocardial damage and improving clinical outcomes, several therapies have suggested efficacy in patients who have anterior STEMI. The routine use of GIK provides no benefit in the treatment of patients who have STEMI, whereas the use of β-blocker therapy in patients who have STEMI reduces the risks for reinfarction and ventricular fibrillation, but increases the risk for cardiogenic shock, especially during the first day. As outlined in the ACC/AHA guidelines, clinical judgment should be used when considering β-blockers for patients who have STEMI.

Optimizing therapy for cardiogenic shock in ST-segment elevation myocardial infarction

Despite advances in primary reperfusion and adjunctive therapy, the prognosis for patients who have STEMI who develop cardiogenic shock remains poor even with early reperfusion. Several new percutaneous hemodynamic support devices have been developed. One is the TandemHeart percutaneous assist device (Cardiac Assist Inc., Pittsburgh, Pennsylvania), which can provide hemodynamic support up to 4.0 L/min [66]. Two randomized studies have reported a superiority of the TandemHeart assist device in providing hemodynamic support and improving clinical parameters and possibly outcomes when compared with intra-aortic balloon counterpulsation in patients who have cardiogenic shock complicating STEMI [67,68].

Levosimendan, a calcium-sensitizing agent, improves hemodynamic parameters and has shown safety and efficacy in patients who have acute decompensated heart failure [69] and left ventricular failure caused by an acute myocardial infarction. A randomized, placebo-controlled, double-blind study, the Randomized Study on Safety and Effectiveness of Levosimendan in Patients with Left Ventricular Failure After an Acute Myocardial Infarct (RUSSLAN), evaluated the safety and efficacy of levosimendan in 504 patients who had left ventricular failure complicating acute myocardial infarction [70]. Mortality was lower with levosimendan compared with placebo at 14 days (11.7% versus 19.6%; $P = .031$). Two additional smaller studies have also suggested improved hemodynamics in patients who have cardiogenic shock from STEMI [71,72]. The Safety and Efficacy of Levosimendan in Patients With Acute Myocardial Infarction Complicated by Symptomatic Left Ventricular Failure study will, in a double-blind, placebo-controlled fashion, examine whether a 24-hour infusion with levosimendan improves regional contractility measured with echocardiography improves brain natriuretic protein levels, reduces the levels of proinflammatory cytokines, and improves symptoms in 60 patients who have PCI-treated acute STEMI complicated with decompensated heart failure.

Summary

Decompensated heart failure remains a major cause of mortality in patients who have STEMI. Therapy with percutaneous ventricular assist devices and calcium-sensitizing agents seem promising in early studies.

Cell-based cardiac repair after ST-segment elevation myocardial infarction

Cell therapy for treatment of myocardial infarction has received enormous attention because of the potential for stem cells, bone marrow cells, and skeletal myoblasts to enhance myocardial recovery after STEMI. Numerous studies have been reported with the evolution to recent randomized control studies. A detailed discussion of these is beyond the scope of this article, and the reader is referred to the article by Gulati and Simari elsewhere in this issue.

Summary

Over the past several years, numerous studies on treatment for STEMI have focused on prompt reperfusion therapy for achieving culprit artery patency and microvascular reperfusion, with the goal of reducing myocardial infarct size and left ventricular dysfunction. In patients who have STEMI treated with primary PCI, early administration of GP IIb/IIIa inhibitors improves patency rates, and in patients treated with thrombolytic therapy, administration of clopidogrel provides a significant morality advantage. In contrast, the most recent trial of facilitated PCI, which administered thrombolytics before PCI, showed increased adverse clinical outcomes [15]. Ongoing trials will provide the definitive answer to this treatment modality. Although routine use of distal protection/thrombectomy devices is not supported in several studies, their use in patients who have angiographically evident large thrombus burden remains to be determined. Promising initial results with cardioprotective agents, such as nicorandil and adenosine, and postconditioning warrant further investigation. In the treatment of cardiogenic shock, the TandemHeart and other assist devices may allow bridging to recovery of cardiac function, transplant, or destination therapy in appropriate patients. Cell-based therapies have now progressed into large-scale clinical trials that will address clinical efficacy. Trials evaluating the treatment for patients who have STEMI continues to progress rapidly. Currently, prompt early reperfusion is clearly the most efficacious therapy; whether additional therapy can impact myocardial infarct size and clinical outcomes remains to be shown.

References

[1] Antman EM, Anbe DT, Armstrong PW, et al. ACC/AHA guidelines for the management of patients with ST-elevation myocardial infarction. J Am Coll Cardiol 2004;44:671–719.

[2] Gibson CM. Time is myocardium and time is outcomes. Circulation 2001;104:2632–4.

[3] Keeley EC, Boura JA, Grines CL. Primary angioplasty versus intravenous thrombolytic therapy for acute myocardial infarction: a quantitative review of 23 randomised trials. Lancet 2003;361:13–20.

[4] De Luca G, Ernst N, Suryapranata H, et al. Relation of interhospital delay and mortality in patients with ST-segment elevation myocardial infarction transferred for primary coronary angioplasty. Am J Cardiol 2005;95:1361–3.

[5] De Luca G, Suryapranata H, Ottervanger JP, et al. Time delay to treatment and mortality in primary angioplasty for acute myocardial infarction: every minute of delay counts. Circulation 2004;109:1223–5.

[6] De Luca G, van't Hof AWJ, de Boer M-J, et al. Time-to-treatment significantly affects the extent of ST-segment resolution and myocardial blush in patients with acute myocardial infarction treated by primary angioplasty. Eur Heart J 2004;25:1009–13.

[7] Cantor C. Rationale and lexicon of primary angioplasty. Totawa (NJ): Humana Press; 2002: 1–7.

[8] Gershlick AH, Stephens-Lloyd A, Hughes S, et al. Rescue angioplasty after failed thrombolytic therapy for acute myocardial infarction. N Engl J Med 2005;353:2758–68.

[9] Immediate vs delayed catheterization and angioplasty following thrombolytic therapy for acute myocardial infarction. TIMI II A results. The TIMI Research Group. JAMA 1988; 260:2849–58.

[10] SWIFT trial of delayed elective intervention v conservative treatment after thrombolysis with anistreplase in acute myocardial infarction. SWIFT (Should We Intervene Following Thrombolysis?) Trial Study Group. BMJ 1991;302:555–60.

[11] Simoons ML, Arnold AE, Betriu A, et al. Thrombolysis with tissue plasminogen activator in acute myocardial infarction: no additional benefit from immediate percutaneous coronary angioplasty. Lancet 1988;1:197–203.

[12] Topol EJ, Califf RM, George BS, et al. A randomized trial of immediate versus delayed elective angioplasty after intravenous tissue plasminogen activator in acute myocardial infarction. N Engl J Med 1987;317:581–8.

[13] Le May MR, Wells GA, Labinaz M, et al. Combined angioplasty and pharmacological intervention versus thrombolysis alone in acute myocardial infarction (CAPITAL AMI study). J Am Coll Cardiol 2005;46:417–24.

[14] Kastrati A, Mehilli J, Schlotterbeck K, et al. Early administration of reteplase plus abciximab vs abciximab alone in patients with acute myocardial infarction referred for percutaneous coronary intervention: a randomized controlled trial. JAMA 2004;291:947–54.

[15] Assessment of the Safety and Efficacy of a New Treatment Strategy with Percutaneous Coronary Intervention (ASSENT-4 PCI) Investigators. Primary versus tenecteplase-facilitated percutaneous coronary intervention in patients with ST-segment elevation acute myocardial infarction (ASSENT-4 PCI): randomised trial. Lancet 2006;367:569–78.

[16] Keeley EC, Boura JA, Grines CL. Comparison of primary and facilitated percutaneous coronary interventions for ST-elevation myocardial infarction: quantitative review of randomised trials. Lancet 2006;367:579–88.

[17] Ellis SG, Armstrong P, Betriu A, et al. Facilitated percutaneous coronary intervention versus primary percutaneous coronary intervention: design and rationale of the Facilitated Intervention with Enhanced Reperfusion Speed to Stop Events (FINESSE) trial. Am Heart J 2004;147:e16.

[18] De Luca G, Suryapranata H, Stone GW, et al. Abciximab as adjunctive therapy to reperfusion in acute ST-segment elevation myocardial infarction: a meta-analysis of randomized trials. JAMA 2005;293:1759–65.

[19] Antoniucci D, Migliorini A, Parodi G, et al. Abciximab-supported infarct artery stent implantation for acute myocardial infarction and long-term survival: a prospective, multicenter, randomized trial comparing infarct artery stenting plus abciximab with stenting alone. Circulation 2004;109:1704–6.

[20] Brener SJ, Barr LA, Burchenal JE, et al. Randomized, placebo-controlled trial of platelet glycoprotein IIb/IIIa blockade with primary angioplasty for acute myocardial infarction. ReoPro and Primary PTCA Organization and Randomized Trial (RAPPORT) Investigators. Circulation 1998;98:734–41.

[21] Montalescot G, Barragan P, Wittenberg O, et al. Platelet glycoprotein IIb/IIIa inhibition with coronary stenting for acute myocardial infarction. N Engl J Med 2001;344:1895–903.

[22] Neumann FJ, Kastrati A, Schmitt C, et al. Effect of glycoprotein IIb/IIIa receptor blockade with abciximab on clinical and angiographic restenosis rate after the placement of coronary stents following acute myocardial infarction. J Am Coll Cardiol 2000;35:915–21.

[23] Tcheng JE, Kandzari DE, Grines CL, et al. Benefits and risks of abciximab use in primary angioplasty for acute myocardial infarction: the Controlled Abciximab and Device Investigation to Lower Late Angioplasty Complications (CADILLAC) trial. Circulation 2003;108:1316–23.

[24] van't Hof AW, Ernst N, de Boer MJ, et al. Facilitation of primary coronary angioplasty by early start of a glycoprotein 2b/3a inhibitor: results of the ongoing tirofiban in myocardial infarction evaluation (On-TIME) trial. Eur Heart J 2004;25:837–46.

[25] Gibson C. Time to Integrilin Therapy in Acute Myocardial Infarction (TITAN-TIMI 34) Presented at the AHA Scientific Sessions 2005. Dallas (TX), November 13–15, 2005.

[26] Di Mario C, Bolognese L, Maillard L, et al. Combined Abciximab REteplase Stent Study in acute myocardial infarction (CARESS in AMI). Am Heart J 2004;148:378–85.

[27] ClinicalTrials.gov. Available at: http://clinicaltrials.gov/show/NCT00306228.

[28] Chen ZM, Jiang LX, Chen YP, et al. Addition of clopidogrel to aspirin in 45,852 patients with acute myocardial infarction: randomised placebo-controlled trial. Lancet 2005;366: 1607–21.

[29] Sabatine MS, Cannon CP, Gibson CM, et al. Addition of clopidogrel to aspirin and fibrinolytic therapy for myocardial infarction with ST-segment elevation. N Engl J Med 2005;352: 1179–89.

[30] Sabatine MS, Cannon CP, Gibson CM, et al. Effect of clopidogrel pretreatment before percutaneous coronary intervention in patients with ST-elevation myocardial infarction treated with fibrinolytics: the PCI-CLARITY study. JAMA 2005;294:1224–32.

[31] Yusuf S, Mehta SR, Xie C, et al. Effects of reviparin, a low-molecular-weight heparin, on mortality, reinfarction, and strokes in patients with acute myocardial infarction presenting with ST-segment elevation. JAMA 2005;293:427–35.

[32] Antman EM, Morrow DA, McCabe CH, et al. Enoxaparin versus unfractionated heparin with fibrinolysis for ST-elevation myocardial infarction. N Engl J Med 2006;354:1477–88.

[33] White H. Thrombin-specific anticoagulation with bivalirudin versus heparin in patients receiving fibrinolytic therapy for acute myocardial infarction: the HERO-2 randomised trial. Lancet 2001;358:1855–63.

[34] ClincalTrials.gov. Available at: http://clinicaltrials.gov/show/NCT00433966.

[35] Yusuf S, Mehta SR, Chrolavicius S, et al. Effects of fondaparinux on mortality and reinfarction in patients with acute ST-segment elevation myocardial infarction: the OASIS-6 randomized trial. JAMA 2006;295:1519–30.

[36] Laarman GJ, Suttorp MJ, Dirksen MT, et al. Paclitaxel-eluting versus uncoated stents in primary percutaneous coronary intervention. N Engl J Med 2006;355:1105–13.

[37] Spaulding C, Henry P, Teiger E, et al. Sirolimus-eluting versus uncoated stents in acute myocardial infarction. N Engl J Med 2006;355:1093–104.

[38] Menichelli M, Parma A, Pucci E, et al. Randomized trial of Sirolimus-Eluting Stent Versus Bare-Metal Stent in Acute Myocardial Infarction (SESAMI). J Am Coll Cardiol 2007;49: 1924–30.

[39] Stone GW, Webb J, Cox DA, et al. Distal microcirculatory protection during percutaneous coronary intervention in acute ST-segment elevation myocardial infarction: a randomized controlled trial. JAMA 2005;293:1063–72.

[40] Lefevre T, Garcia E, Reimers B, et al. X-sizer for thrombectomy in acute myocardial infarction improves ST-segment resolution: results of the X-sizer in AMI for negligible embolization and optimal ST resolution (X AMINE ST) trial. J Am Coll Cardiol 2005;46: 246–52.

[41] Gick M, Jander N, Bestehorn HP, et al. Randomized evaluation of the effects of filter-based distal protection on myocardial perfusion and infarct size after primary percutaneous catheter intervention in myocardial infarction with and without ST-segment elevation. Circulation 2005;112:1462–9.

[42] Ali A, Cox D, Dib N, et al. Rheolytic thrombectomy with percutaneous coronary intervention for infarct size reduction in acute myocardial infarction: 30-day results from a multicenter randomized study. J Am Coll Cardiol 2006;48:244–52.

[43] Antoniucci D. Rheolytic thrombectomy in acute myocardial infarction: the Florence experience and objectives of the multicenter randomized JETSTENT trial. J Invasive Cardiol 2006;18:32c–4c.

[44] O'Neill W. Acute Myocardial Infarction With Hyperoxemic Therapy (AMIHOT): a prospective, randomized, multicenter trial. Presented at the Annual Scientific Session of the American College of Cardiology. New Orleans (Louisiana), March 2004.

[45] ClincalTrials.gov. Available at: http://clinicaltrials.gov/show/NCT00175058.

[46] Grines C. Intravascular cooling adjunctive to percutaneous coronary intervention for acute myocardial infarction. Presented at the Transcatheter Cardiovascular Therapeutics 2004, Washington, DC, September 2004.

[47] ClincalTrials.gov. Available at: http://clinicaltrials.gov/show/NCT00248196.

[48] Mehta SR, Yusuf S, Diaz R, et al. Effect of glucose-insulin-potassium infusion on mortality in patients with acute ST-segment elevation myocardial infarction: the CREATE-ECLA randomized controlled trial. JAMA 2005;293:437–46.

[49] Timmer JR, Svilaas T, Ottervanger JP, et al. Glucose-insulin-potassium infusion in patients with acute myocardial infarction without signs of heart failure: the Glucose-Insulin-Potassium Study (GIPS)-II. J Am Coll Cardiol 2006;47:1730–1.

[50] Bar FW, Tzivoni D, Dirksen MT, et al. Results of the first clinical study of adjunctive CAldaret (MCC-135) in patients undergoing primary percutaneous coronary intervention for ST-elevation myocardial infarction: the randomized multicentre CASTEMI study. Eur Heart J 2006;27:2516–23.

[51] Jang IK, Pettigrew V, Picard MH, et al. A randomized, double-blind, placebo-controlled study of the safety and efficacy of intravenous MCC-135 as an adjunct to primary percutaneous coronary intervention in patients with acute myocardial infarction: rationale and design of the evaluation of MCC-135 for left ventricular salvage in acute MI (EVOLVE) study. J Thromb Thrombolysis 2005;20:147–53.

[52] Gross GJ, Auchampach JA, Maruyama M, et al. Cardioprotective effects of nicorandil. J Cardiovasc Pharmacol 1992;20(Suppl 3):S22–8.

[53] Lamping KA, Christensen CW, Pelc LR, et al. Effects of nicorandil and nifedipine on protection of ischemic myocardium. J Cardiovasc Pharmacol 1984;6:536–42.

[54] Ishii H, Ichimiya S, Kanashiro M, et al. Impact of a single intravenous administration of nicorandil before reperfusion in patients with ST-segment-elevation myocardial infarction. Circulation 2005;112:1284–8.

[55] Minamino T, Jiyoong K, Asakura M, et al. Rationale and design of a large-scale trial using nicorandil as an adjunct to percutaneous coronary intervention for ST-segment elevation acute myocardial infarction: Japan-Working groups of acute myocardial infarction for the reduction of Necrotic Damage by a K-ATP channel opener (J-WIND-KATP). Circ J 2004;68:101–6.

[56] Mahaffey KW, Puma JA, Barbagelata NA, et al. Adenosine as an adjunct to thrombolytic therapy for acute myocardial infarction: results of a multicenter, randomized, placebo-controlled trial: the Acute Myocardial Infarction STudy of ADenosine (AMISTAD) trial. J Am Coll Cardiol 1999;34:1711–20.

[57] Ross AM, Gibbons RJ, Stone GW, et al. A randomized, double-blinded, placebo-controlled multicenter trial of adenosine as an adjunct to reperfusion in the treatment of acute myocardial infarction (AMISTAD-II). J Am Coll Cardiol 2005;45:1775–80.

[58] Philipp S, Yang XM, Cui L, et al. Postconditioning protects rabbit hearts through a protein kinase C-adenosine A2b receptor cascade. Cardiovasc Res 2006;70:308–14.

[59] Zhao ZQ, Corvera JS, Halkos ME, et al. Inhibition of myocardial injury by ischemic postconditioning during reperfusion: comparison with ischemic preconditioning. Am J Physiol Heart Circ Physiol 2003;285:H579–88.

[60] Zhao ZQ, Vinten-Johansen J. Postconditioning: reduction of reperfusion-induced injury. Cardiovasc Res 2006;70:200–11.

[61] Staat P, Rioufol G, Piot C, et al. Postconditioning the human heart. Circulation 2005;112:2143–8.

[62] Granger CB, Mahaffey KW, Weaver WD, et al. Pexelizumab, an anti-C5 complement antibody, as adjunctive therapy to primary percutaneous coronary intervention in acute myocardial infarction: the COMplement inhibition in Myocardial infarction treated with Angioplasty (COMMA) trial. Circulation 2003;108:1184–90.

[63] Fitch JC, Rollins S, Matis L, et al. Pharmacology and biological efficacy of a recombinant, humanized, single-chain antibody C5 complement inhibitor in patients undergoing coronary artery bypass graft surgery with cardiopulmonary bypass. Circulation 1999;100:2499–506.

[64] APEX AMI Investigators: Armstrong PW, Granger CB, Adams PX, et al. Pexelizumab for acute ST-elevation myocardial infarction in patients undergoing primary percutaneous coronary intervention: a randomized controlled trial. JAMA 2007;297:43–51.

[65] Chen ZM, Pan HC, Chen YP, et al. Early intravenous then oral metoprolol in 45,852 patients with acute myocardial infarction: randomised placebo-controlled trial. Lancet 2005;366: 1622–32.

[66] Vranckx P, Foley DP, de Feijter PJ, et al. Clinical introduction of the Tandemheart, a percutaneous left ventricular assist device, for circulatory support during high-risk percutaneous coronary intervention. Int J Cardiovasc Intervent 2003;5:35–9.

[67] Burkhoff D, Cohen H, Brunckhorst C, et al. A randomized multicenter clinical study to evaluate the safety and efficacy of the tandemHeart percutaneous ventricular assist device versus conventional therapy with intraaortic balloon pumping for treatment of cardiogenic shock. Am Heart J 2006;152:469, e1–8.

[68] Thiele H, Sick P, Boudriot E, et al. Randomized comparison of intra-aortic balloon support with a percutaneous left ventricular assist device in patients with revascularized acute myocardial infarction complicated by cardiogenic shock. Eur Heart J 2005;26:1276–83.

[69] Follath F, Cleland JGF, Just H, et al. Efficacy and safety of intravenous levosimendan compared with dobutamine in severe low-output heart failure (the LIDO study): a randomised double-blind trial. Lancet 2002;360:196–202.

[70] Moiseyev VS, Poder P, Andrejevs N, et al. Safety and efficacy of a novel calcium sensitizer, levosimendan, in patients with left ventricular failure due to an acute myocardial infarction. A randomized, placebo-controlled, double-blind study (RUSSLAN). Eur Heart J 2002;23: 1422–32.

[71] García-González M, Domínguez-Rodríguez A, Ferrer-Hita J. Utility of levosimendan, a new calcium sensitizing agent, in the treatment of cardiogenic shock due to myocardial stunning in patients with ST elevation myocardial infarction: a series of cases. J Clin Pharmacol 2005;45:704–8.

[72] Sonntag S, Sundberg S, Lehtonen LA, et al. The calcium sensitizer levosimendan improves the function of stunned myocardium after percutaneous transluminal coronary angioplasty in acute myocardial ischemia. J Am Coll Cardiol 2004;43:2177–82.

ELSEVIER
SAUNDERS

THE MEDICAL
CLINICS
OF NORTH AMERICA

Med Clin N Am 91 (2007) 751–768

Outcome and Quality of Care of Patients who have Acute Myocardial Infarction

Wissam A. Jaber, MD*,
David R. Holmes, Jr., MD, FACC, FSCAI

*Division of Cardiovascular Diseases, Mayo Clinic, 200 First Street SW,
Rochester, MN 55905, USA*

Because coronary artery disease (CAD) is the number one killer in developed countries, with lifetime prevalence of up to 50% in American men [1], a substantial volume of the medical literature has been dedicated to studying the outcome of this dreadful disease. Multiple life-saving therapies after acute myocardial infarction (AMI) have emerged in the last few decades, backed up by a large number of well conducted studies [2,3], but despite the publication of management guidelines adopting these therapies, appropriate implementation of the guidelines is still less than optimal. Recently, large efforts have been focused on finding means to improve the quality of care (QC) after AMI in an attempt to improve its outcome [4]. This has been accompanied by a gradual shift by the national payers and policy makers toward linking quality performance and outcome to hospital reimbursement and accreditation [5].

This article illustrates the outcome after AMI as related to QC, describes the underuse of evidence-based therapies, and discusses reasons and factors associated with poor adherence to guidelines. It also gives an overview of current quality improvement projects, and some available means to measure and optimize the QC for patients who have AMI.

Outcome after acute myocardial infarction

Despite an aging population, the last 2 decades have witnessed a significant decrease in mortality after AMI [6–11]. In one population, between 1985 and 1995 mortality from CAD fell by 31% for men and 41% for

---

* Corresponding author.
E-mail address: jaber.wissam@mayo.edu (W.A. Jaber).

women [8]. By 1995, the 28-day case fatality among hospitalized AMI patients was 7% to 10% [8]. A separate study in multiple communities in the United States between 1987 and 1994 measured an overall adjusted 28-day mortality of 10.6% for women and 9.0% for men. The in-hospital mortality fell by 4.1% per year in men and 9.8% per year in women [10]. In an analysis of data of over 1.5 million patients who had AMI enrolled in the National Registry of Myocardial Infarction (NRMI) 1, 2, and 3 between 1990 and 1999, the median duration of hospital stay after AMI decreased from 8.3 to 4.3 days, and hospital mortality dropped from 11.2% to 9.4% [12]. Similar trends were found around the world [6,7]. Most of the observed decrease in mortality can be attributed to increased use of appropriate therapy, including primary percutaneous coronary intervention (PCI) for ST segment-elevation myocardial infarction (STEMI), aspirin, angiotensin-converting enzyme (ACE) inhibitors, and beta blockers, in addition to improvement in risk factor modification through secondary prevention.

Morbidity after AMI remains substantial. Recurrent myocardial infarction occurs in up to 33% of patients, heart failure develops in up to 30%, and stroke in 9% to 13% [13]. Events tend to occur more commonly in women, but this is probably because of the higher age of women presenting with AMI as compared with men [11].

Outcome following AMI varies significantly with the characteristics of the patient at presentation. Poor prognostic indicators include older age, larger AMI, prior AMI, heart failure, anterior AMI, hypotension, tachycardia, baseline risk factors for CAD, elevated cardiac biomarkers, elevated serum creatinine, and ST segment deviation on the electrocardiogram [14–20]. Multiple risk scores have been derived to predict the mortality risk based on these clinical indicators.

Mortality also depends on the type of myocardial infarction. In-hospital mortality has been around 2% in most clinical trials of non-ST segment-elevation myocardial infarction (NSTEMI) [21,22], and 3% to 5% in STEMI [23,24]. In registries, as opposed to clinical trials, in-hospital mortality rates are higher, being around 5% to 7% for NSTEMI and 7% to 9% for STEMI [25–29]. The high likelihood of receiving optimal medical care and the exclusion of high-risk patients in most trials contribute to the lower mortality rate in patients enrolled in clinical trials when compared with registries [30].

In contrast to the short-term outcome, long-term mortality is higher after NSTEMI than after STEMI. In the GUSTO-IIb trial, 1-year mortality was 11.1% in NSTEMI and 9.6% in STEMI [31]; the 2-year mortality was 20% for NSTEMI and 11% for STEMI in a community-based observational study [32]. The likely explanation for this discrepancy is that patients who have STEMI have larger infarcts, and thus worse immediate outcome, whereas NSTEMI patients often have a higher risk profile, higher incidence of multivessel disease, a greater likelihood of residual ischemia, and thus worse long-term outcome [31,33,34]. This underlines the importance of secondary medical prevention to improve survival in AMI patients.

Quality of care after acute myocardial infarction

Survival after AMI has been improving; CAD, however, remains the leading cause of death in the United States. Despite the publication and dissemination of guidelines on the management of patients who have AMI by the American College of Cardiology (ACC) and the American Heart Association (AHA) [2,3,35], the implementation of appropriate treatment is still not optimal [16,36–46].

How well do we perform?

Frequent studies assessing adherence to guidelines have yielded disappointing results. An analysis of over 64,000 NSTEMI patients enrolled in the CRUSADE (Can Rapid Risk Stratification of Unstable Angina Patients Suppress Adverse Outcomes With Early Implementation of the ACC/AHA Guidelines) National Quality Improvement Initiative showed a large variation among hospitals in the percentage of adherence to the ACC/AHA Class I recommendations in the treatment of NSTEMI [47]. The adherence score of each individual hospital ranged from as low as 40% to as high as 85%. Strikingly, outcome differed significantly between the hospitals based on their level of adherence: every decrease in 10% in adherence to guidelines corresponded to a 10% increase in mortality at that hospital.

Multiple other studies have documented the underuse of evidence-based therapies in patients who have AMI [16,37–45]. In the NRMI-4, among all patients who had acute NSTEMI who were eligible for glycoprotein (GP) IIb/IIIa inhibitors, only 25% received that therapy, despite the fact that it is a Class I indication in the ACC/AHA guidelines [2]. The poor performance is not only limited to the United States. European studies have shown similarly low numbers, with wide variation between hospitals [48].

Table 1 shows recently reported rates of adherence to multiple quality indicators, as measured in some registries and databases. Although some measures have shown significantly better implementation with time, the numbers remain disappointing.

Performance does not only lie in the use of medical therapy, but also in the speed and efficiency of administering timely treatment. In STEMI, the shorter the time from hospital arrival to reperfusion therapy (fibrinolysis or primary PCI), the lower the mortality [49,50]. The ACC/AHA have recommended a time to fibrinolysis of less than 30 minutes and time to PCI of less than 90 minutes [3,35]. The current numbers, however, are far from meeting the guidelines. Analysis of the NRMI-3 and -4 showed that in 1999, only 46% of STEMI patients receiving fibrinolytic therapy were treated within 30 minutes, and only 35% of patients treated with primary PCI were treated within 90 minutes [51]. Over the next 3 years, these proportions increased by only 1% and 2%, respectively [51]. In 2005, Medicare data indicated that more than one third of patients who have

Table 1
Rates of adherence to quality indicators as reported in selected observational studies depicting care and outcome in patients with AMI

Quality indicator	Study [reference], years conducted, type of AMI and adherence percentages				
	Medicare data [41], 1998–99, STEMI	GAP [91], 1998–99, STEMI	CRUSADE [47], 2000–02, NSTEMI	NRMI 3 [12,45], 1999, all AMI	National average [52], 2005, all AMI
Aspirin on admission	84%	81%	90%	85%	91%
Beta blocker on admission	64%	65%	37%	54%	85%
Aspirin at discharge	85%	84%	89%	80%	88%
Beta blocker at discharge	72%	89%	80%	62%	87%
ACE inhibitor for LVEF <40%	71%	80%	59%	40%	80%
Smoking cessation counseling	40%	53%	57%	38%	77%
Lipid lowering treatment	—	68%	73%	32%	—
In-hospital mortality	—	13.6%	4.9%	9.8%	—

Abbreviation: LVEF, left ventricular ejection fraction.

STEMI undergoing primary PCI are treated after 120 minutes of presentation [52].

Where do we perform poorly?

For reasons not fully understood, certain high-risk patients presenting with AMI tend to be undertreated with evidence-based therapy when compared with lower-risk patients. These include the elderly, diabetics, women, African Americans, patients who have renal insufficiency, and heart failure patients [39,53–55]. Because adherence to guidelines improves outcome, and because high-risk patients have a higher mortality [14–16,19,20], these patients should receive therapy that most closely matches the guidelines. The opposite, however, happens in practice.

Analysis of the CRUSADE data [56] and a separate analysis from Canada [57] showed that patients over the age of 75 presenting with AMI received significantly less aspirin, beta blockers, and statins at discharge, and are less likely to have their lipids tested. GP IIb/IIIa inhibitors in the CRUSADE data were also much less commonly used in the elderly. Partly because they represent an older population, Medicare and Veterans Affairs AMI patients witness an underuse of angiography when this procedure is actually indicated [58]. Similar disparities exist for African Americans when compared with whites [39,59–61], and for women when compared with men. Although they have a greater incidence of death, recurrent AMI, and heart failure after AMI, women are treated in accordance to the ACC/AHA guidelines less often than are men. They are specifically less likely to receive angiography, percutaneous coronary intervention, bypass surgery, and GP IIb/IIIa inhibitors [59,62,63].

Diabetes [64], heart failure, and mildly increased troponin levels [65] are all well-established poor prognostic indicators that are paradoxically associated with a lower adherence to the management guidelines. Similarly, although patients who have NSTEMI have equal or higher long-term mortality when compared with STEMI patients [31,32] and thus deserve equal or better secondary preventive measures, they are actually less likely than STEMI patients to receive aspirin, beta-blockers, ACE inhibitors, lipid-lowering agents, smoking cessation counseling, and cardiac rehabilitation referral [66].

Barriers to implementing guidelines

Multiple factors have been linked to poor adherence to treatment guidelines. Non-teaching or for-profit hospitals tend to score lower than academic or not-for-profit hospitals [67,68]. This translates into a survival advantage for teaching over non-teaching hospitals, which is attenuated but not eliminated by controlling for baseline patient characteristics [67]. It appears that hospital therapy tradition and structure of care play roles in the different outcome among hospitals [48]. In fact, in a study of

Medicare patients who had AMI treated in 1994 and 1995, admission to a hospital ranked high on the "America's Best Hospitals" list published annually by the *US News & World Report* [69] was associated with a lower 30-day mortality, linked to a higher rate of use of aspirin and beta blockers by these hospitals [70].

It is interesting that most studies looking at outcome by treating physician found that the outcome of AMI patients is better when the care is assumed by a cardiologist [39,71–73]. Although specialists may be treating patients with less comorbid conditions, attempts to adjust for baseline patient characteristics did not eliminate the difference in in-hospital or one year mortality [71,73]. It is the better implementation of recommended medical therapy and the higher use of reperfusion therapy by cardiologists that could account for most of the observed difference in outcome [71–73]. Although this finding calls for better implementation of the guidelines by all treating physicians, it does not justify a universal call on all AMI patients to be cared for by cardiologists only [73,74].

The factors that may prevent a physician from applying the guidelines are complex and poorly understood [36]. The physician may simply be unaware of the presence of the guidelines, or may be unfamiliar with their contents. Even when aware of them, some may disagree with the guidelines, believe that they are overwhelming and confusing, have poor outcome expectancy, or find it hard to change practices they are already used to [75].

Measurement of quality of care

With the existence of enough data to suggest that better adherence to guidelines and better care after AMI improves outcome, there has been a significant recent growth in importance accorded to measurement, reporting, and improvement of quality of health care.

Definition of quality of care

QC has been defined by the Institute of Medicine (IOM) as "the degree to which health services for individuals and populations increase the likelihood of desired health outcomes and are consistent with current professional knowledge" [76]. In a specific health care setting, QC is determined on three levels: structure, process, and outcome [77]. Structure refers to the setting in which a patient who has AMI is being treated, including the organization of an institution, the abundance and experience of the health care professionals, the emergency department triage system, the availability of specialized treatment and equipment in the treating center, and quality improvement infrastructure [78]. Process involves the application of diagnostic and therapeutic measures by the practitioner, in addition to the appropriateness and timing of these measures. Outcome is exemplified by mortality, morbidity, cost, and patient satisfaction.

Quantifying quality of care

The ability to measure QC is a prerequisite to the improvement of this care. As described by the AMI Working Group of the first ACC/AHA Scientific Forum on Quality of Care and Outcomes Research in Cardiovascular Disease and Stroke [74], performance measurements must be meaningful to the patient's outcome, must be reliably and accurately measured, can account for patient variability, can be adaptable to changes with care standards over time, and must be feasible.

Measuring structure can be hard to do, costly, and may not be necessarily directly related to outcome [74]. On the other hand, outcome may be more linked to the patient's baseline characteristics than to the process or structure of care, and cause of mortality may be hard to ascertain. Because some processes of care have been shown to be closely related to outcome (eg, use of aspirin, beta blockers, lipid management, time to reperfusion, counseling for smoking cessation) [47,49,79–85], failure to implement these processes translates into a worse care. Thus, the adherence to such measures by an institution can be used to quantify the QC at that specific institution [4]. The availability of these data, with feedback to the treating physician accompanied by a comparison to the national or regional performance, can stimulate better adherence to the guidelines, and, as a result, better QC.

Performance measures

As part of a nationwide effort to improve QC after AMI, the ACC and AHA have issued clinical performance measures for adults who have STEMI and NSTEMI [86]. These are mostly based on the Class I and Class III recommendations of the ACC/AHA guidelines for the management of AMI patients [2,3,35], and include eleven measures, shown in Box 1.

The ACC and AHA are not alone in their endeavor. The IOM has started an ongoing effort designed to evaluate and advance the QC in the United States [76]. As part of this effort, the IOM has recently issued a set of quality measures that can be used to assess the QC [87]. Among other general measures, those related to CAD include prescribing a drug therapy to lower LDL cholesterol, beta blocker prescription at discharge after AMI, and persistent beta-blocker treatment 6 months after discharge.

In 2002, the Joint Commission on Accreditation of Healthcare Organizations (JCAHO) implemented similar standardized measures of performance for AMI, heart failure, and pneumonia [88]. For AMI, these measures resemble the ones adopted by the ACC/AHA working group [86], in addition to one clinical outcome: death in the hospital after AMI. Accredited hospitals under this program are required to collect and report to JCAHO their own data on performance measures, while receiving comparative feedback reports on a quarterly basis.

Box 1. ACC/AHA AMI performance measures

Aspirin at arrival
Aspirin at discharge
Beta blocker at arrival (within 24 hours)
Beta blocker at discharge
Low-density lipoprotein (LDL) cholesterol assessment
Lipid lowering therapy at discharge (for patients who have
  LDL > 100 mg/dL)
ACE inhibitor or angiotensin receptor blockers (ARB) for left
  ventricular (LV) dysfunction at discharge
Median time from arrival to fibrinolytic therapy ≤ 30 min in
  STEMI/new left-bundle branch block (LBBB) patients
Median time from arrival to PCI ≤ 90 min in STEMI/new LBBB
  patients
Reperfusion therapy for STEMI patients
Adult smoking cessation advice/counseling for patients who have
  a history of smoking cigarettes

Adapted from Krumholz HM, Anderson JL, Brooks NH, et al. ACC/AHA clinical
performance measures for adults with ST-elevation and non–ST-elevation myocardial infarction: a report of the American College of Cardiology/American Heart
Association Task Force on Performance Measures (Writing Committee to Develop
Performance Measures on ST-Elevation and Non-ST-Elevation Myocardial Infarction). J Am Coll Cardiol 2006;47:236–65.

There is a strong current trend to use such performance indicators to determine hospital reimbursement [5]. It is believed that payment and public
reporting initiatives may help to stimulate the use of guidelines, and thus improve outcome [89].

Improving quality of care

Quality initiative projects

Devising means to measure quality and identifying areas of poor performance is the first step toward improving QC. The next step would be to implement programs designed to improve adherence to the quality measures.

One successful program was the Guidelines Applied in Practice (GAP)
project, conceived at the University of Michigan and sponsored by the
ACC. The GAP project was a multifaceted intervention designed to improve the adherence to the guidelines for STEMI management in Southeast-
ern Michigan. The crucial elements of the program were the identification
of strong local physician and nurse opinion leaders, the routine use of standard AMI admission orders and patient discharge instruction form and

contract, chart stickers, pocket guides, and hospital performance charts [90]. Implementation of the project between the years 1998 and 2000 led to a significant increase in the adherence to key treatments in participating hospitals, as shown in Fig. 1 [91,92]. The effect was most prominent in the populations that were most undertreated (Medicare beneficiaries, elderly, women, black). The use of GAP tools correlated with a 21% to 26 % decrease in adjusted mortality, both in-hospital and at 1 year [81]. An additional improvement in quality was obtained when the project was repeated, now with more emphasis on standard AMI admission orders and discharge tools [92]. The GAP tool kits can be found at the official ACC website, http://.acc.org/qualityandscience/gap/mi/ami_gap.htm.

Likewise, the AHA sponsored a separate program called "Get With the Guidelines" in New England in the year 2000. The program, focusing on discharge planning of patients who have AMI, consisted of a Web-based data collection system for individual hospitals to monitor their progress, and for treating physicians to receive reminders on acute care and secondary prevention [93]. This resulted in a substantial increase in adherence to treatment guidelines in smoking cessation counseling, lipid treatment, LDL measurement, and cardiac rehabilitation referral.

The Center for Medicare and Medicaid Services (CMS), through its Cooperative Cardiovascular Project, used peer review organizations to collect data on quality indicators of Medicare patients treated for AMI, and then provided feedback to the practitioners to encourage quality improvement activities [94]. Under this program, there was a 20% absolute increase in the rate of beta blocker administration at discharge, with significant but less prominent increase in ACE inhibitor and aspirin use, and a decrease in the time to reperfusion [95].

Multiple other initiatives, mostly focusing on data feedback systems, have been successful in improving the rate of adherence to guidelines. Examples are the Partnership for Change collaborative [96], the Cardiac Hospitalization Atherosclerosis Management Program [97], and the JCAHO's incorporation of performance measures in its hospital accreditation program [88]. CRUSADE, a national quality improvement initiative, was designed by the Duke Clinical Research Institute to improve the QC in high-risk NSTEMI patients [98]. CRUSADE involves a dynamic registry that measures the use of acute treatment modalities, and provides feedback to the treating physicians on their adherence scores to the NSTEMI treatment guidelines with comparison to national norms, accompanied by educational material. This registry has also allowed obtaining a better insight into current care for NSTEMI patients and identifying necessary areas for improvement [39,47].

The effort by the IOM to improve the QC is more extensive, and is not only limited to treatment of AMI. The approach is multifaceted, and includes redesigning care delivery, coordinating government roles, quality measurement and reporting, reforming health profession education, and encouraging the implementation of information technology [76,87].

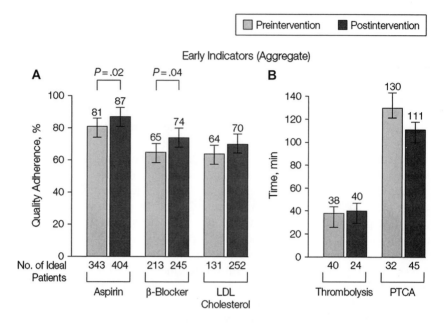

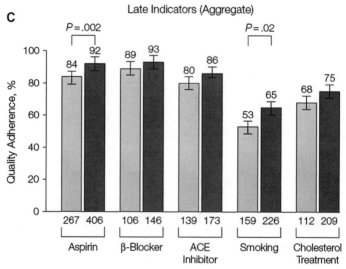

Fig. 1. Overall Effects of the Guidelines Applied in Practice (GAP) intervention on early (*A, B*) and late (*C*) quality indicators. (*From* Mehta RH, Montoye CK, Gallogly M, et al. Improving quality of care for acute myocardial infarction: The Guidelines Applied in Practice (GAP) initiative. JAMA 2002;287:1273; with permission. Copyright © 2002, American Medical Association. All rights reserved.)

Recently, multiple public agencies such as the CMS and JCAHO collaborated with private consumer groups to form the Hospital Quality Alliance (HQA). Under the HQA, hospitals from all over the United States report to the CMS data on their performance in key measures for AMI, heart failure, and pneumonia care [68]. For AMI, the measures are identical to the ones recommended by the ACC/AHA and shown in Box 1, excluding lipid assessment and management. Information on the program is available at www.cms.hhs.gov/HospitalQualityInits. An important element of the HQA was the creation in April 2005 of a Web site that publicly reports and compares the QC in the US hospitals, www.hospitalcompare.hhs.gov. Along the same line, there are other groups that publicly rate hospitals, such as the Leapfrog group (www.leapfroggroup.org). These measures are believed to encourage hospitals to implement their own quality improvement initiatives and force them to better adhere to the guidelines.

How can we be successful in implementing quality improvement?

As the authors have discussed so far, despite prior efforts to improve care and disseminate AMI treatment guidelines, full adherence to guidelines is not yet achieved. It is through active, multifaceted quality improvement projects that care can be improved further. Some practicing groups have been more successful than others at implementing these projects and at improving their care. A few key factors have been identified as crucial to such a success. These include local opinion leaders, feedback on performance, multidisciplinary interventions, public reporting, use of standard admission and discharge forms, and incorporation of ongoing quality improvement projects in the structure of care [91,99–103].

Bradley and colleagues [104] conducted a qualitative study to isolate the characteristics that enabled the top 11 hospitals in the NRMI registry to improve their door-to-balloon time in STEMI patients treated with primary PCI between the years 1999 and 2002. The factors that mostly characterized those hospitals included a clear shared goal for improvement, strong administrative support, flexible and innovative protocols, clinical opinion leaders, multidisciplinary collaboration, and data feedback systems.

Limitations of quality measures

The current indicators of QC are not perfect. Although they measure adherence to the most obvious evidence-based treatment strategies, they do not account for other, less easily measurable aspects of care [74]. For example, overuse (eg, performing a cardiac catheterization when not indicated), misuse (eg, ongoing use of ACE inhibitors despite potassium levels reaching dangerous levels, inappropriate medication doses, and so forth), and misdiagnosis can be hard to ascertain. Because not all hospitals use electronic records, reviewing medical charts of individual patients to assess appropriateness of treatment can be cumbersome and costly. This is likely to change with the advances of electronic records. Simply measuring outcome may not be the solution to these problems. Patient outcome may reflect more their baseline characteristics than the QC delivered. Moreover, the usual outcome reported is in-hospital mortality, whereas many of the processes performed during hospitalization for AMI also affect long-term outcome [81].

As more and more efforts are invested in this field, more improvement measures and initiatives can be devised [74]. Care for AMI starts with the recognition of the symptoms by the patient and the mobilization of the emergency response systems. Better organization of the ambulance system [80] and access to early electrocardiograms [105] decrease the time to treatment. Care is also likely to improve with better organization and incorporation of protocols for early triage and risk assessment for AMI in the emergency departments [50,106,107]. Long-term patient follow up with ongoing implementation of secondary preventive measures is not less important than acute management of AMI. Quantification of the process of transferring care from the inpatient to the outpatient setting may also prove to be a necessary measure of quality [74].

Summary

Treatment of AMI has evolved significantly over the last years, accompanied by a decrease in mortality. Outcome can be further improved by a better adherence to the evidence-based therapies as recommended by the ACC/AHA guidelines [2,3]. Performance measures for the treatment of AMI have been published [86], and individual hospital adherence scores are publicly reported. Interest has grown in implementing quality improvement projects, both at the local and national level. Some of these projects have identified a few key elements that help close the gap between guidelines and practice: integration of dynamic, ongoing quality improvement initiatives into clinical practice; adoption of a multifaceted approach guided by opinion leaders; and use of simple discharge tools.

With current quality measures relying on the process of care, more research is needed to identify means to assess and improve the structure of care, and to integrate into the performance measures baseline risk-adjusted patient outcome, including not only mortality, but also morbidity, cost, and patient satisfaction [74]. Studies are also needed to compare different quality improvement initiatives and identify the most successful elements.

References

[1] Lloyd-Jones DM, Larson MG, Beiser A, et al. Lifetime risk of developing coronary heart disease. Lancet 1999;353:89–92.

[2] Braunwald E, Antman EM, Beasley JW, et al. ACC/AHA guideline update for the management of patients with unstable angina and non–ST-segment elevation myocardial infarction—2002: summary article: a report of the American College of Cardiology/American Heart Association Task Force on Practice Guidelines (Committee on the Management of Patients With Unstable Angina). Circulation 2002;106:1893–900.

[3] Antman EM, Anbe DT, Armstrong PW, et al. ACC/AHA guidelines for the management of patients with ST-elevation myocardial infarction—executive summary: a report of the American College of Cardiology/American Heart Association Task Force on Practice Guidelines (Writing Committee to Revise the 1999 Guidelines for the Management of Patients With Acute Myocardial Infarction). Circulation 2004;110:588–636.

[4] Spertus JA, Eagle KA, Krumholz HM, et al. American College of Cardiology and American Heart Association methodology for the selection and creation of performance measures for quantifying the quality of cardiovascular care. Circulation 2005;111: 1703–12.

[5] Epstein AM, Lee TH, Hamel MB. Paying physicians for high-quality care. N Engl J Med 2004;350:406–10.

[6] Capewell S, Beaglehole R, Seddon M, et al. Explanation for the decline in coronary heart disease mortality rates in Auckland, New Zealand, between 1982 and 1993. Circulation 2000;102:1511–6.

[7] Capewell S, Morrison CE, McMurray JJ. Contribution of modern cardiovascular treatment and risk factor changes to the decline in coronary heart disease mortality in Scotland between 1975 and 1994. Heart 1999;81:380–6.

[8] McGovern PG, Jacobs DR Jr, Shahar E, et al. Trends in acute coronary heart disease mortality, morbidity, and medical care from 1985 through 1997: the Minnesota Heart Survey. Circulation 2001;104:19–24.

[9] McGovern PG, Pankow JS, Shahar E, et al. Recent trends in acute coronary heart disease—mortality, morbidity, medical care, and risk factors. The Minnesota Heart Survey investigators. N Engl J Med 1996;334:884–90.

[10] Rosamond WD, Chambless LE, Folsom AR, et al. Trends in the incidence of myocardial infarction and in mortality due to coronary heart disease, 1987 to 1994. N Engl J Med 1998; 339:861–7.

[11] Guidry UC, Evans JC, Larson MG, et al. Temporal trends in event rates after Q-wave myocardial infarction: the Framingham Heart Study. Circulation 1999;100:2054–9.

[12] Rogers WJ, Canto JG, Lambrew CT, et al. Temporal trends in the treatment of over 1.5 million patients with myocardial infarction in the US from 1990 through 1999: the National Registry of Myocardial Infarction 1, 2 and 3. J Am Coll Cardiol 2000;36: 2056–63.

[13] Thom T, Kannel WB, Silbershatz S, et al. Incidence, prevalence, and mortality of cardiovascular diseases in the United States. In: Alexander R, Schlant RC, Fuster V, et al, editors. Hurst's the heart. 9th edition. New York: McGraw Hill; 1998. p. 3.

[14] Granger CB, Goldberg RJ, Dabbous O, et al. Predictors of hospital mortality in the global registry of acute coronary events. Arch Intern Med 2003;163:2345–53.

[15] Becker RC, Burns M, Gore JM, et al. Early assessment and in-hospital management of patients with acute myocardial infarction at increased risk for adverse outcomes: a nationwide perspective of current clinical practice. The National Registry of Myocardial Infarction (NRMI-2) participants. Am Heart J 1998;135:786–96.

[16] Califf RM, Pieper KS, Lee KL, et al. Prediction of 1-year survival after thrombolysis for acute myocardial infarction in the global utilization of streptokinase and TPA for occluded coronary arteries trial. Circulation 2000;101:2231–8.

[17] Morrow DA, Antman EM, Charlesworth A, et al. TIMI risk score for ST-elevation myocardial infarction: a convenient, bedside, clinical score for risk assessment at presentation: an Intravenous nPA for Treatment of Iinfarcting Myocardium Early II trial substudy. Circulation 2000;102:2031–7.

[18] Eagle KA, Lim MJ, Dabbous OH, et al. A validated prediction model for all forms of acute coronary syndrome: estimating the risk of 6-month postdischarge death in an international registry. JAMA 2004;291:2727–33.

[19] Antman EM, Cohen M, Bernink PJ, et al. The TIMI risk score for unstable angina/non-ST elevation MI: a method for prognostication and therapeutic decision making. JAMA 2000; 284:835–42.

[20] Boersma E, Pieper KS, Steyerberg EW, et al. Predictors of outcome in patients with acute coronary syndromes without persistent ST-segment elevation. Results from an international trial of 9461 patients. The PURSUIT Investigators. Circulation 2000;101:2557–67.

[21] F Ragmin, Fast Revascularisation during instability in coronary artery disease investigators. Invasive compared with non-invasive treatment in unstable coronary-artery disease: FRISC II prospective randomised multicentre study. Lancet 1999;354:708–15.

[22] Cannon CP, Weintraub WS, Demopoulos LA, et al. Comparison of early invasive and conservative strategies in patients with unstable coronary syndromes treated with the glycoprotein IIb/IIIa inhibitor tirofiban. N Engl J Med 2001;344:1879–87.

[23] Stone GW, Grines CL, Cox DA, et al. Comparison of angioplasty with stenting, with or without abciximab, in acute myocardial infarction. N Engl J Med 2002;346: 957–66.

[24] Cannon CP, Gibson CM, Lambrew CT, et al. Relationship of symptom-onset-to-balloon time and door-to-balloon time with mortality in patients undergoing angioplasty for acute myocardial infarction. JAMA 2000;283:2941–7.

[25] Steg PG, Goldberg RJ, Gore JM, et al. Baseline characteristics, management practices, and in-hospital outcomes of patients hospitalized with acute coronary syndromes in the Global Registry of Acute Coronary Events (GRACE). Am J Cardiol 2002;90:358–63.

[26] Hasdai D, Behar S, Wallentin L, et al. A prospective survey of the characteristics, treatments and outcomes of patients with acute coronary syndromes in Europe and the Mediterranean basin; the Euro Heart Survey of Acute Coronary Syndromes (Euro Heart Survey ACS). Eur Heart J 2002;23:1190–201.

[27] Savonitto S, Ardissino D, Granger CB, et al. Prognostic value of the admission electrocardiogram in acute coronary syndromes. JAMA 1999;281:707–13.

[28] Bahit MC, Cannon CP, Antman EM, et al. Direct comparison of characteristics, treatment, and outcomes of patients enrolled versus patients not enrolled in a clinical trial at centers participating in the TIMI 9 Trial and TIMI 9 Registry. Am Heart J 2003;145: 109–17.

[29] Roe MT, Ohman EM, Pollack CV Jr, et al. Changing the model of care for patients with acute coronary syndromes. Am Heart J 2003;146:605–12.

[30] Kandzari DE, Roe MT, Chen AY, et al. Influence of clinical trial enrollment on the quality of care and outcomes for patients with non-ST-segment elevation acute coronary syndromes. Am Heart J 2005;149:474–81.

[31] Armstrong PW, Fu Y, Chang WC, et al. Acute coronary syndromes in the GUSTO-IIb trial: prognostic insights and impact of recurrent ischemia. The GUSTO-IIb Investigators. Circulation 1998;98:1860–8.

[32] Furman MI, Dauerman HL, Goldberg RJ, et al. Twenty-two year (1975 to 1997) trends in the incidence, in-hospital and long-term case fatality rates from initial Q-wave and non-Q-wave myocardial infarction: a multi-hospital, community-wide perspective. J Am Coll Cardiol 2001;37:1571–80.

[33] Behar S, Haim M, Hod H, et al. Long-term prognosis of patients after a Q wave compared with a non-Q wave first acute myocardial infarction. Data from the SPRINT Registry. Eur Heart J 1996;17:1532–7.

[34] Haim M, Behar S, Boyko V, et al. The prognosis of a first Q-wave versus non-Q-wave myocardial infarction in the reperfusion era. Am J Med 2000;108:381–6.

[35] Smith SC Jr, Feldman TE, Hirshfeld JW Jr, et al. ACC/AHA/SCAI 2005 guideline update for percutaneous coronary intervention—summary article: a report of the American

College of Cardiology/American Heart Association Task Force on Practice Guidelines (ACC/AHA/SCAI Writing Committee to Update the 2001 Guidelines for Percutaneous Coronary Intervention). J Am Coll Cardiol 2006;47:216–35.

[36] Bassand J-P, Priori S, Tendera M. Evidence-based vs. 'impressionist' medicine: how best to implement guidelines. Eur Heart J 2005;26:1155–8.

[37] Hemingway H, Crook AM, Feder G, et al. Underuse of coronary revascularization procedures in patients considered appropriate candidates for revascularization. N Engl J Med 2001;344:645–54.

[38] Califf RM, DeLong ER, Ostbye T, et al. Underuse of aspirin in a referral population with documented coronary artery disease. Am J Cardiol 2002;89:653–61.

[39] Bhatt DL, Roe MT, Peterson ED, et al. Utilization of early invasive management strategies for high-risk patients with non-ST-segment elevation acute coronary syndromes: results from the CRUSADE quality improvement initiative. JAMA 2004;292:2096–104.

[40] Mehta RH, Ruane TJ, McCargar PA, et al. The treatment of elderly diabetic patients with acute myocardial infarction: insight from Michigan's cooperative cardiovascular project. Arch Intern Med 2000;160:1301–6.

[41] Jencks SF, Cuerdon T, Burwen DR, et al. Quality of medical care delivered to Medicare beneficiaries: a profile at state and national levels. JAMA 2000;284:1670–6.

[42] Schiele F, Meneveau N, Seronde MF, et al. Compliance with guidelines and 1-year mortality in patients with acute myocardial infarction: a prospective study. Eur Heart J 2005;26: 873–80.

[43] Gurwitz JH, Goldberg RJ, Chen Z, et al. Beta-blocker therapy in acute myocardial infarction: evidence for underutilization in the elderly. Am J Med 1992;93:605–10.

[44] McLaughlin TJ, Soumerai SB, Willison DJ, et al. Adherence to national guidelines for drug treatment of suspected acute myocardial infarction: evidence for undertreatment in women and the elderly. Arch Intern Med 1996;156:799–805.

[45] Fonarow GC, French WJ, Parsons LS, et al. Use of lipid-lowering medications at discharge in patients with acute myocardial infarction: data from the National Registry of Myocardial Infarction 3. Circulation 2001;103:38–44.

[46] Ellerbeck EF, Jencks SF, Radford MJ, et al. Quality of care for Medicare patients with acute myocardial infarction. A four-state pilot study from the Cooperative Cardiovascular Project. JAMA 1995;273:1509–14.

[47] Peterson ED, Roe MT, Mulgund J, et al. Association between hospital process performance and outcomes among patients with acute coronary syndromes. JAMA 2006;295: 1912–20.

[48] Stenestrand U, Lindback J, Wallentin L. Hospital therapy traditions influence long-term survival in patients with acute myocardial infarction. Am Heart J 2005;149:82–90.

[49] McNamara RL, Wang Y, Herrin J, et al. Effect of door-to-balloon time on mortality in patients with ST-segment elevation myocardial infarction. J Am Coll Cardiol 2006;47:2180–6.

[50] Gersh BJ, Stone GW, White HD, et al. Pharmacological facilitation of primary percutaneous coronary intervention for acute myocardial infarction: is the slope of the curve the shape of the future? JAMA 2005;293:979–86.

[51] McNamara RL, Herrin J, Bradley EH, et al. Hospital improvement in time to reperfusion in patients with acute myocardial infarction, 1999 to 2002. J Am Coll Cardiol 2006;47: 45–51.

[52] U.S. Department of Health & Human Services. Available at: www.hospitalcompare.hhs.gov, Accessed July 13, 2006.

[53] Ohman EM, Roe MT, Smith SC Jr, et al. Care of non-ST-segment elevation patients: insights from the CRUSADE national quality improvement initiative. Am Heart J 2004; 148:S34–9.

[54] Roe MT, Peterson ED, Newby LK, et al. The influence of risk status on guideline adherence for patients with non–ST-segment elevation acute coronary syndromes. Am Heart J 2006; 151:1205–13.

[55] Brogan GX Jr, Peterson ED, Mulgund J, et al. Treatment disparities in the care of patients with and without diabetes presenting with non–ST-segment elevation acute coronary syndromes. Diabetes Care 2006;29:9–14.

[56] Alexander KP, Roe MT, Chen AY, et al. Evolution in cardiovascular care for elderly patients with non–ST-segment elevation acute coronary syndromes: results from the CRUSADE National Quality Improvement Initiative. J Am Coll Cardiol 2005;46:1479–87.

[57] Tran CT, Laupacis A, Mamdani MM, et al. Effect of age on the use of evidence-based therapies for acute myocardial infarction. Am Heart J 2004;148:834–41.

[58] Petersen LA, Normand SL, Leape LL, et al. Regionalization and the underuse of angiography in the Veterans Affairs Health Care System as compared with a fee-for-service system. N Engl J Med 2003;348:2209–17.

[59] Schulman KA, Berlin JA, Harless W, et al. The effect of race and sex on physicians' recommendations for cardiac catheterization. N Engl J Med 1999;340:618–26.

[60] Anand SS, Xie CC, Mehta S, et al. Differences in the management and prognosis of women and men who suffer from acute coronary syndromes. J Am Coll Cardiol 2005;46:1845–51.

[61] Sonel AF, Good CB, Mulgund J, et al. Racial variations in treatment and outcomes of black and white patients with high-risk non–ST-elevation acute coronary syndromes: insights from CRUSADE (Can Rapid Risk Stratification of Unstable Angina Patients Suppress Adverse Outcomes With Early Implementation of the ACC/AHA Guidelines?) 10.1161/01.CIR.0000157732.03358.64. Circulation 2005;111:1225–32.

[62] Jani SM, Montoye C, Mehta R, et al. Sex differences in the application of evidence-based therapies for the treatment of acute myocardial infarction: the American College of Cardiology's guidelines applied in practice projects in Michigan. Arch Intern Med 2006;166: 1164–70.

[63] Blomkalns AL, Chen AY, Hochman JS, et al. Gender disparities in the diagnosis and treatment of non–ST-segment elevation acute coronary syndromes: large-scale observations from the CRUSADE (Can Rapid Risk Stratification of Unstable Angina Patients Suppress Adverse Outcomes With Early Implementation of the American College of Cardiology/ American Heart Association Guidelines) national quality improvement initiative. J Am Coll Cardiol 2005;45:832–7.

[64] Vikman S, Niemela K, Ilva T, et al. Underuse of evidence-based treatment modalities in diabetic patients with non-ST elevation acute coronary syndrome. A prospective nation wide study on acute coronary syndrome (FINACS). Diabetes Res Clin Pract 2003;61:39–48.

[65] Roe MT, Peterson ED, Li Y, et al. Relationship between risk stratification by cardiac troponin level and adherence to guidelines for non–ST-segment elevation acute coronary syndromes. Arch Intern Med 2005;165:1870–6.

[66] Roe MT, Parsons LS, Pollack CV Jr, et al. Quality of care by classification of myocardial infarction: treatment patterns for ST-segment elevation vs non-ST-segment elevation myocardial infarction. Arch Intern Med 2005;165:1630–6.

[67] Allison JJ, Kiefe CI, Weissman NW, et al. Relationship of hospital teaching status with quality of care and mortality for Medicare patients with acute MI. JAMA 2000;284: 1256–62.

[68] Jha AK, Li Z, Orav EJ, et al. Care in U.S. hospitals—the hospital quality alliance program. N Engl J Med 2005;353:265–74.

[69] U.S. News & World Report. Available at: www.usnews.com/usnews/health/best-hospitals/ tophosp.htm, Accessed July 13, 2006.

[70] Chen J, Radford MJ, Wang Y, et al. Do "America's best hospitals" perform better for acute myocardial infarction? 10.1056/NEJM199901283400407. N Engl J Med 1999;340:286–92.

[71] Chen J, Radford MJ, Wang Y, et al. Care and outcomes of elderly patients with acute myocardial infarction by physician specialty: the effects of comorbidity and functional limitations. Am J Med 2000;108:460–9.

[72] Gottwik M, Zahn R, Schiele R, et al. Differences in treatment and outcome of patients with acute myocardial infarction admitted to hospitals with compared to without departments

of cardiology; results from the pooled data of the Maximal Individual Therapy in Acute Myocardial Infarction (MITRA 1+2) Registries and the Myocardial Infarction Registry (MIR). Eur Heart J 2001;22:1794–801.

[73] Jollis JG, DeLong ER, Peterson ED, et al. Outcome of acute myocardial infarction according to the specialty of the admitting physician. N Engl J Med 1996;335:1880–7.

[74] Spertus JA, Radford MJ, Every NR, et al. Challenges and opportunities in quantifying the quality of care for acute myocardial infarction: summary from the acute myocardial infarction working group of the American Heart Association/American College of Cardiology First Scientific Forum on Quality of Care and Outcomes Research in Cardiovascular Disease and Stroke. J Am Coll Cardiol 2003;41:1653–63.

[75] Cabana MD, Rand CS, Powe NR, et al. Why don't physicians follow clinical practice guidelines?: a framework for improvement. JAMA 1999;282:1458–65.

[76] Institute of Medicine of the National Academies. Available at: http://www.iom.edu/?id=19174, Accessed July 13, 2006.

[77] Donabedian A. The quality of care. How can it be assessed? JAMA 1988;260:1743–8.

[78] Nolan TW. Understanding medical systems. Ann Intern Med 1998;128:293–8.

[79] Stenestrand U, Wallentin L. Early revascularisation and 1-year survival in 14-day survivors of acute myocardial infarction: a prospective cohort study. Lancet 2002;359:1805–11.

[80] Kalla K, Christ G, Karnik R, et al. Implementation of guidelines improves the standard of care: the Viennese registry on reperfusion strategies in ST-elevation myocardial infarction (Vienna STEMI registry). Circulation 2006;113:2398–405.

[81] Eagle KA, Montoye CK, Riba AL, et al. Guideline-based standardized care is associated with substantially lower mortality in Medicare patients with acute myocardial infarction: the American College of Cardiology's Guidelines Applied in Practice (GAP) projects in Michigan. J Am Coll Cardiol 2005;46:1242–8.

[82] Jaber WA, Lennon RJ, Mathew V, et al. Application of evidence-based medical therapy is associated with improved outcomes after percutaneous coronary intervention and is a valid quality indicator. J Am Coll Cardiol 2005;46:1473–8.

[83] Kernis SJ, Harjai KJ, Stone GW, et al. Does beta-blocker therapy improve clinical outcomes of acute myocardial infarction after successful primary angioplasty? J Am Coll Cardiol 2004;43:1773–9.

[84] Newby LK, Rutsch WR, Califf RM, et al. Time from symptom onset to treatment and outcomes after thrombolytic therapy. GUSTO-1 Investigators. J Am Coll Cardiol 1996;27:1646–55.

[85] De Luca G, Suryapranata H, Zijlstra F, et al. Symptom-onset-to-balloon time and mortality in patients with acute myocardial infarction treated by primary angioplasty. J Am Coll Cardiol 2003;42:991–7.

[86] Krumholz HM, Anderson JL, Brooks NH, et al. ACC/AHA clinical performance measures for adults with ST-elevation and non–ST-elevation myocardial infarction: a report of the American College of Cardiology/American Heart Association Task Force on Performance Measures (Writing Committee to Develop Performance Measures on ST-Elevation and Non–ST-Elevation Myocardial Infarction). J Am Coll Cardiol 2006;47:236–65.

[87] Committee on Redesigning Health Insurance Performance Measures, and Payment Performance Improvement Programs. Performance measurement: accelerating improvement. Washington, DC: National Academies Press; 2006.

[88] Williams SC, Schmaltz SP, Morton DJ, et al. Quality of care in U.S. hospitals as reflected by standardized measures, 2002–2004. N Engl J Med 2005;353:255–64.

[89] Galvin R, Milstein A. Large employers' new strategies in health care. N Engl J Med 2002;347:939–42.

[90] Eagle KA, Gallogly M, Mehta RH, et al. Taking the national guideline for care of acute myocardial infarction to the bedside: developing the Guidelines Applied in Practice (GAP) initiative in Southeast Michigan. Jt Comm J Qual Improv 2002;28:5–19.

[91] Mehta RH, Montoye CK, Gallogly M, et al. Improving quality of care for acute myocardial infarction: the Guidelines Applied in Practice (GAP) initiative. JAMA 2002;287:1269–76.

[92] Mehta RH, Montoye CK, Faul J, et al. Enhancing quality of care for acute myocardial infarction: shifting the focus of improvement from key indicators to process of care and tool use: the American College of Cardiology Acute Myocardial Infarction Guidelines Applied in Practice Project in Michigan: Flint and Saginaw expansion. J Am Coll Cardiol 2004;43: 2166–73.

[93] LaBresh KA, Ellrodt AG, Gliklich R, et al. Get with the guidelines for cardiovascular secondary prevention: pilot results. Arch Intern Med 2004;164:203–9.

[94] Marciniak TA, Ellerbeck EF, Radford MJ, et al. Improving the quality of care for Medicare patients with acute myocardial infarction: results from the cooperative cardiovascular project. JAMA 1998;279:1351–7.

[95] Burwen DR, Galusha DH, Lewis JM, et al. National and state trends in quality of care for acute myocardial infarction between 1994–1995 and 1998–1999: the Medicare health care quality improvement program. Arch Intern Med 2003;163:1430–9.

[96] Zhang H, Alexander JA, Luttrell J, et al. Data feedback and clinical process improvement in acute myocardial infarction. Am Heart J 2005;149:856–61.

[97] Fonarow GC, Gawlinski A, Moughrabi S, et al. Improved treatment of coronary heart disease by implementation of a Cardiac Hospitalization Atherosclerosis Management Program (CHAMP). Am J Cardiol 2001;87:819–22.

[98] Hoekstra JW, Pollack CV Jr, Roe MT, et al. Improving the care of patients with non–ST-elevation acute coronary syndromes in the emergency department: the CRUSADE Initiative 10.1197/aemj.9.11.1146. Acad Emerg Med 2002;9:1146–55.

[99] Soumerai SB, McLaughlin TJ, Gurwitz JH, et al. Effect of local medical opinion leaders on quality of care for acute myocardial infarction: a randomized controlled trial. JAMA 1998; 279:1358–63.

[100] Davis DA, Thomson MA, Oxman AD, et al. Changing physician performance. A systematic review of the effect of continuing medical education strategies. JAMA 1995;274:700–5.

[101] Grol R. Improving the quality of medical care: building bridges among professional pride, payer profit, and patient satisfaction. JAMA 2001;286:2578–85.

[102] Roe MT. Success stories: how hospitals are improving care. Am Heart J 2004;148:S52–5.

[103] Bradley EH, Holmboe ES, Mattera JA, et al. A qualitative study of increasing beta-blocker use after myocardial infarction: why do some hospitals succeed? JAMA 2001;285:2604–11.

[104] Bradley EH, Curry LA, Webster TR, et al. Achieving rapid door-to-balloon times: how top hospitals improve complex clinical systems. Circulation 2006;113:1079–85.

[105] Kudenchuk PJ, Maynard C, Cobb LA, et al. Utility of the prehospital electrocardiogram in diagnosing acute coronary syndromes: the Myocardial Infarction Triage and Intervention (MITI) Project. J Am Coll Cardiol 1998;32:17–27.

[106] Farkouh ME, Smars PA, Reeder GS, et al. A clinical trial of a chest-pain observation unit for patients with unstable angina. Chest Pain Evaluation in the Emergency Room (CHEER) investigators. N Engl J Med 1998;339:1882–8.

[107] Gomez MA, Anderson JL, Karagounis LA, et al. An emergency department-based protocol for rapidly ruling out myocardial ischemia reduces hospital time and expense: results of a randomized study (ROMIO). J Am Coll Cardiol 1996;28:25–33.

ELSEVIER
SAUNDERS

Med Clin N Am 91 (2007) 769–785

THE MEDICAL
CLINICS
OF NORTH AMERICA

Cell Therapy for Acute Myocardial Infarction

Rajiv Gulati, MD, PhD, Robert D. Simari, MD*

*Division of Cardiovascular Diseases and Internal Medicine, Mayo Clinic College of Medicine,
200 First Street SW, Rochester, MN 55905, USA*

In the United States, myocardial infarction occurs in approximately 1 million patients annually, with a mortality of approximately 25% over 3 years. A considerable proportion of these patients will develop chronic congestive heart failure, which carries a mortality of approximately 20% per year in those who have symptoms [1]. Advances in mechanical and pharmacologic therapies have reduced early and late mortality after acute myocardial infarction. However, a significant proportion of survivors will have reduced cardiac reserve relating predominantly to an early and extensive loss of functioning cardiac myocytes.

The compelling clinical need for a means to reduce this loss, together with supportive preclinical data and intuitive appeal, has underpinned an increasing interest over the past 10 years in the concept of myocyte replacement therapy, or cell-based cardiac repair. Evidence suggesting that postnatal bone marrow and circulating blood may harbor myocardial and vascular progenitor cells was the basis for preclinical studies of adult progenitor cell therapy for acute myocardial infarction. Promising reports in murine studies prompted a rapid initiation of clinical trials using local myocardial delivery of autologous cells as adjunctive therapies for acute and chronic left ventricular dysfunction. Although clinical cell transplantation trials originally began with the explicit goal of myocardial regeneration, the emphasis has shifted recently to attempted modulation of myocardial remodeling through other processes, such as mechanical strengthening of scar tissue and promotion of myocardial tissue survival through cellular paracrine effects.

* Corresponding author.
E-mail address: simari.robert@mayo.edu (R.D. Simari).

0025-7125/07/$ - see front matter © 2007 Elsevier Inc. All rights reserved.
doi:10.1016/j.mcna.2007.03.003   *medical.theclinics.com*

Can adult cells regenerate myocardium?

The traditional paradigm of the heart as a terminally differentiated organ maintains that the total number of cardiomyocytes reaches a maximum of approximately 5 billion soon after birth and progressively diminishes thereafter. This paradigm has been challenged by studies suggesting a capability for myocyte turnover in mammalian hearts [2,3]. Moreover, several high-profile studies have suggested that a source of regenerative myocytes (in addition to vascular cells, hepatocytes, and neurons) might include bone marrow and circulating precursors [4–15].

One of the earliest studies purporting an unexpected plasticity of adult cells was reported by Orlic and colleagues [11] who sorted lineage-negative (Lin-), c-kit positive stem cells from the bone marrow of transgenic mice expressing green fluorescent protein. After induction of myocardial infarction through coronary ligation, Lin- c-kit+ cells were injected into the infarct border zone. Newly formed (green-fluorescing) myocardium reportedly occupied 68% of the infarcted portion of the ventricle 9 days after bone marrow cell injection. Analysis of this developing tissue reportedly showed proliferating myocytes and vascular structures, prompting the authors to suggest that autologous bone marrow may be able to generate de novo myocardium. Using fluorescence in situ hybridization for the Y chromosome, the same group identified recipient myocytes within postmortem hearts of patients who underwent transplantation [16]. Both studies provided a platform from which numerous clinical trials of bone marrow cell myocardial administration have been launched [17–20].

The findings of the initial studies, however, have been challenged recently. Murry and colleagues [21] studied a transgenic mouse line in which a cardiac-specific -myosin heavy chain promoter drives expression of a LacZ reporter to monitor cardiomyogenic transdifferentiation events after induction of infarction. No bone marrow cell–derived myocytes were identified. Differences are likely to have arisen from increasingly recognized difficulties in tracking the fate of transplanted cells within the heart. Orlic and colleagues [11] relied on detecting myocyte and stem cell markers using fluorescently tagged antibodies. Murry and colleagues [21], however, created intrinsic genetic markers that can be recognized without antibody staining. Because of its high density of muscle-specific contractile proteins, myocardium possesses high intrinsic background fluorescence and can also display nonspecific antibody–muscle protein binding, potentially leading to the misinterpretation of fluorescent signal and consequent (incorrect) conclusion that there was evidence of transdifferentiation. Moreover, because of difficulties in detecting cell borders with confocal microscopy, Y chromosome–containing nuclei are likely to have been (mis)identified as cardiomyocytes when they, in fact, belonged to overlying inflammatory leukocytes [22].

Cell fusion may also account for some reports of transdifferentiation. This issue was raised when murine bone marrow cells were shown to spontaneously fuse with embryonic stem cells in culture. In probing for tissue-specific protein expression, bone marrow cells would thus give the (misleading) appearance of having adopted the phenotype of their fused partners [23,24]. Subsequent studies suggested fusion events might account for some reports of apparent transdifferentiation of transplanted bone marrow into myocytes, hepatocytes, and Purkinje fibers [25–30].

Recent studies have proposed the existence of cardiac stem cell populations within the myocardium, residing in protected niches. Hierlihy and colleagues [31] first described an endogenous resident cardiac stem cell in mice in 2002 and some experts currently propose that these are undifferentiated cells that express the stem cell antigens c-kit, MDR1, and Sca-1 in variable combinations [32]. These resident cells have been characterized in mice, rats, dogs, and humans, but their ability to differentiate into viable functioning myocardium remains to be clarified [32].

Concerns about technical aspects of tissue-specific protein identification and cell fusion processes have tempered initial enthusiasm regarding adult stem cell plasticity. Although consensus has not been reached, the most convincing body of evidence suggests that adult stem regenerative events are rare in organs such as the heart, liver, and brain. In contrast, stem cell events may be much more frequent in the vasculature through precursor contribution to capillary angiogenesis and large vessel neointimal formation. Technical issues outlined above have not been specifically limiting for the vasculature. Endothelial cells and smooth muscle cells are readily identifiable morphologically and spatially within arterial cross sections, even before protein expression is used to confirm phenotype. Moreover, a recent chimeric study that specifically sought for fusion events was unable to identify more than two sex chromosomes in more than 4000 endothelial cells examined, consistent with an absence of cell fusion in this model [33]. Likewise, Caplice and colleagues [34] and Simper and colleagues [35] performed ploidy analysis of human tissue obtained from transplant recipients and did not identify any evidence of nuclear fusion in the vasculature.

Thus, although the initial studies by Quaini and colleagues [16] and Orlic and colleagues [36] suggested significant potential for adult bone marrow to regenerate myocardium, more detailed studies using intrinsic genetic markers suggest this may not be the case [21]. However, specific bone marrow populations, such as mesenchymal stem cells and resident myocardial populations, may be capable of myositic differentiation. Although this differentiation is clearly not sufficient in a physiologic sense, the possibility remains that such or similar cell fractions may be isolatable and expandable for use in a therapeutic setting.

Preclinical studies of exogenous cell transplantation

The most appropriate cell type for restoration of damaged myocardial tissue has not yet been defined (Fig. 1). Variable degrees of improvement

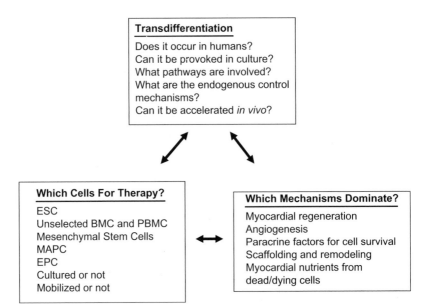

Transdifferentiation

Does it occur in humans?
Can it be provoked in culture?
What pathways are involved?
What are the endogenous control
mechanisms?
Can it be accelerated *in vivo*?

Which Cells For Therapy?

ESC
Unselected BMC and PBMC
Mesenchymal Stem Cells
MAPC
EPC
Cultured or not
Mobilized or not

Which Mechanisms Dominate?

Myocardial regeneration
Angiogenesis
Paracrine factors for cell survival
Scaffolding and remodeling
Myocardial nutrients from
dead/dying cells

Fig. 1. Issues that must be addressed at a cellular, organ, and animal level. Clinical cell therapy trials for myocardial infarction were initiated with the understanding that adult bone marrow contains cells capable of differentiation into de novo cardiac myocytes, although recent evidence has called this into question. Whether some or any adult cells are capable of this transdifferentiation is unclear. Moreover, the mechanisms through which cell therapy produces benefit in preclinical models is still not well understood.

in cardiac function in preclinical models have been observed with transplantation of embryonic stem cells, skeletal myoblasts, bone marrow cells, and resident cardiac progenitors. The possible mechanisms involved in improving cardiac function include mechanical effects on ventricular remodeling, promotion of angiogenesis, and the provision of bona fide regenerating myocytes. The ability of this surprisingly wide range of nonmyogenic cell types to improve ventricular function supports the notion that the benefit of cell transplantation may result from mechanisms distinct from regeneration. Moreover, despite approximately 6000-fold differences in numbers of cells delivered across a broad range of studies, the scale of improvement in myocardial function seems somewhat similar in each case [37]. In this regard, therapeutic effects of cell delivery may be partially indirect, relating to paracrine effects of delivered cells on threatened native myocardial and vascular tissue in the setting of acute injury.

Theoretically, various cell populations, including stem and progenitor cells, could be used to promote cardiac repair. Each cell type offers potential advantages and limitations in addition to practicability in the setting of acute disease. Only a few comparative studies exist of the protective and regenerative capacity of distinct cell populations [38–40]. Features of specific cell populations in terms of clinical suitability are discussed as follows.

Embryonic stem cells

Embryonic stem cells (ESCs), derived from the inner cell mass of preimplantation mouse and human embryos, reliably generate cardiac myocytes in vitro [41]. ESC-derived cardiomyocytes express cardiac molecular markers (such as sarcomeric myosin heavy chain and troponin I) and beat, leaving little doubt about their cardiac-specific phenotype. The ability of ESC-derived cardiomyocytes to electromechanically couple and electrophysiologically specialize adds to their versatility, offering great promise for regenerative therapy after acute myocardial infarction. However, translational efforts have been hampered by the formation of teratomas (a tumor containing cells derived from all three embryonic germ layers) in preclinical models of ESC transplantation [41]. Although a strategy to predifferentiate ESCs to committed myocytes without tumorigenic potential might circumvent this concern [42], translation to human studies remain limited by ethical concerns and immunologic incompatibility. Ethical concerns are also a limitation in the use of fetal or neonatal cardiomyocytes which, when implanted into the postinfarcted heart, can form electrical connections with native cardiomyocytes [2]. ESC-derived cardiomyocytes from humans, unlike mice, possess a high-proliferative capacity [43], providing a unique human model system to analyze mechanisms that control cardiomyocyte proliferation and differentiation. Insights gained from studies might perhaps offer therapeutic potential distinct from cellular transplantation.

Skeletal myoblasts

Skeletal myoblasts represent an autologous source of cells that show a contractile phenotype. Implantation of autologous skeletal myoblasts at the site of myocardial injury was shown to result in new myofiber formation [44,45] and produce significant improvements in left-ventricular function [45]. The mechanism underlying this benefit remains unclear, but seems neither to be related to transdifferentiation of skeletal myoblasts into cardiomyocytes nor electrical integration of engrafted myoblasts with native myocytes [46]. Although clinical trials using skeletal myoblast transfer have been performed, these have all been in the setting of chronic myocardial dysfunction. Because several weeks of culture expansion are required, a skeletal myoblast transfer approach does not seem feasible as a therapy for acute myocardial injury.

Bone marrow–derived cells

Adult bone marrow is heterogeneous. Hematopoietic stem cells, mesenchymal stem cells (MSCs), and potentially endothelial progenitor cells (EPCs) and multipotent adult progenitor cells are vastly outnumbered by committed hematopoietic progenitors and differentiated progeny, which comprise more than 99.9%. Kamihata and colleagues [47] performed an early preclinical study showing the therapeutic potential of an unselected bone marrow cell preparation. In a porcine model, these investigators injected bone marrow mononuclear cells into the infarct zone and peri-infarct region after induction of myocardial infarction through coronary artery ligation. Cell injection was associated with an improvement in myocardial perfusion through contrast echocardiography, increased numbers of capillaries and collaterals through angiography, improved ejection fraction, and reduction in infarct size compared with controls. Although many of the newly formed capillary endothelial cells seemed to be derived from injected cells, the fibroblasts in the scar did not, suggesting that the injected cells favored angiogenic rather than fibrotic differentiation.

Many investigators have since adopted this pragmatic approach of delivering unfractionated bone marrow mononuclear cells, given the potential efficacy of individual subpopulations and the prospect of synergistic effects obtained from transplanting a heterogeneous population [48–50]. Moreover, ease of harvest and lack of requirement for ex vivo manipulation offer further practical advantages of unselected bone marrow cells in the clinical setting of acute myocardial infarction.

Preclinical studies initially suggested that hematopoietic subsets were capable of regenerating multiple myocardial elements after acute infarction. Jackson and colleagues [10] transplanted an enriched, side-population subset of bone marrow hematopoietic cells ($CD34^-$/low, c-Kit^+, Sca-1^+) into lethally irradiated mice rendered acutely ischemic through transient coronary ligation. Results suggested that delivered cells, or their progeny, were able to generate de novo myocytes and endothelium. Similarly, Orlic and colleagues [11] selected populations enriched for lineage-negative (lin−) c-kit+ cells and presented evidence to suggest transdifferentiation of delivered cells into myocytes. A corresponding improvement in myocardial and hemodynamic parameters was seen after only 9 days. The same group suggested that mobilization of lin− c-kit+ cells with granulocyte colony-stimulating factor (GCSF) and stem cell factor before and after myocardial infarction in mice resulted in growth of new cardiomyocytes in the infarct zone, improved ventricular function, and substantial improvement in survival [36]. In contrast, Murry and colleagues [21] and Balsam and colleagues [51] reported that lin− c-kit+ cells did not differentiate into cardiomyocytes and suggested that earlier reports could be explained by limitations in identifying delivered cells. However, although bone marrow cells transplanted into ischemic myocardium adopted hematopoietic fates rather than transdifferentiating into myocardium in the latter of these studies, cell administration still prevented left ventricular (LV) dilatation and dysfunction associated with postinfarction remodeling.

Cells with phenotypic and functional characteristics similar to endothelium can be generated from adult bone marrow and circulating blood [52,53]. These cells, often collectively termed *endothelial progenitor cells*, may consist of monocyte-dominant and diverse true precursor populations

[54]. Kocher and colleagues [55] intravenously injected human marrow–derived CD34+ EPCs after experimentally induced myocardial infarction in athymic nude mice. EPCs homed to the infarct region within 48 hours and, at 14 days, a marked increase was seen in the number of capillaries in the infarct and peri-infarct zones relating to the induction of vasculogenesis and angiogenesis. Moreover, a reduction in collagen deposition and cardiomyocyte apoptosis together with improvements in left ventricular performance were seen. Similar improvements in myocardial functional parameters have been shown in other models of myocardial infarction [56,57], and may relate partly to paracrine factors secreted by delivered cells [58].

Mesenchymal stem cells

MSCs represent a rare population of cells present in bone marrow stroma that do not express hematopoietic surface markers CD34, CD133, and CD45 [59]. They are 10-fold less abundant than hematopoietic stem cells and can readily differentiate into osteocytes, chondrocytes, and adipocytes. Studies show that MSCs can transdifferentiate into cardiomyocytes and vascular structures in vitro and in vivo, and secrete potent angiogenic cytokines [60,61]. Moreover, LV function and new capillary formation seem significantly increased after MSC transplantation [61]. Administering allogenic MSCs in a porcine model of myocardial injury produced several improvements in myocardial function parameters without evidence of rejection [62], because of lack of MHC-II and B-7 expression.

Resident cardiac stem cells

Accumulating evidence suggests the presence of cardiac stem cell populations within the heart capable of differentiating into cardiomyocytic or vascular lineage cells, representing a novel therapeutic target [63,64]. Moreover, it has been reported that cardiac stem cells can be clonally expanded in vitro from human myocardial biopsies. In this study, undifferentiated human cells also exhibited evidence of myocardial differentiation in immune-compromised mice [65].

Clinical studies of cell transplantation

Driven by the preclinical findings outlined previously, several clinical trials were initiated to evaluate safety and feasibility of cell delivery after acute myocardial infarction (Table 1). Table 1 shows published clinical trials of cell therapy for acute myocardial infarction. Most studies delivered unselected bone marrow mononuclear cells through intracoronary infusion. Overall, effect of cell therapy on left ventricular function seems modest in reported results.

Table 1
Trials of cell therapy in acute myocardial infarction

Study (Reference)	Cell type/number	No. of treated patients	No. of controls	Timing of cell delivery post-myocardial infarction (days)	Randomized	Delivery route	Results
Strauer et al [17]	$9–28 \times 10^6$ BMC	10	10 (standard therapy)	5–9	No	IC	Increased regional wall motion and perfusion; decreased infarct size
Fernandez-Avilés et al [66]	$11–90 \times 10^6$ BMC	20	13	10–15	No	IC	No significant functional improvement
Assmus et al [18]	$16 \pm 12 \times 10^6$ CPC; $213 \pm 75 \times 10^6$ BMC	30 (CPC group) 29 (BMC group)	59 historical	5	No	IC	Improved LVEF; decreased infarct size
Bartunek et al [68]	$12.6 \pm 2.2 \times 10^6$ CD133+ cells (57%–83% pure)	19	16 (standard therapy)	12	No	IC	Improved LVEF; decreased infarct size; increased in-stent restenosis
Chen et al [75]	$8–10 \times 10^9$ BMC	34	18 days (saline infusion)	18	Yes	IC	Increased LVEF; decreased infarct size

Wollert et al [69]; Meyer et al [70]	$24.6 \pm 9.4 \times 10^8$ BMC	30	30 (standard therapy)	5	Yes	IC	No significant LV improvement at 18 mo
Schächinger et al [73]	$236 \pm 174 \times 10^6$ BMC	101	103 (autologous serum and culture medium)	3–6	Yes	IC	Increased LVEF at 4 mo; improved clinical end point at 1 y
Lunde et al [72]	$87.1 \pm 47.7 \times 10^6$ BMC	50	50 (standard therapy)	6	Yes	IC	No significant LV improvement at 12 mo
Janssens et al [71]	$172 \pm 72 \times 10^6$ BMC	33	34 (autologous serum and normal saline)	1	Yes	IC	Reduced infarct size; no significant improvement in LVEF
Kang et al [74]	$1–2 \times 10^9$ GCSF-mobilized PBMC	25	25 (standard therapy)	10	Yes	IC	Increased LVEF; decreased LV volumes;no increase in restenosis

Abbreviations: BMC, bone marrow mononuclear cells; CPC, circulating progenitor cells; GCSF, granulocyte colony-stimulating factor; IC, intracoronary; LV, left ventricular; LVEF, left ventricular ejection fraction; PBMC, peripheral blood mononuclear cell.

In the first published clinical trial, Strauer and colleagues [17] recruited 10 patients for cell therapy and compared outcomes with another 10 who refused entry into the treatment arm. Bone marrow mononuclear cells were aspirated 1 week after percutaneous coronary revascularization of acute myocardial infarction. After overnight culture, cells were delivered through the reopened infarct artery under high-pressure infusion with an angioplasty balloon inflated proximally to prevent backflow of infused cells. The cell population contained only a small percentage of hematopoietic stem cells (0.65% ± 0.4% CD133+ and 2.1% ± 0.28% CD34+). Nonetheless, functional assessment at 3 months showed a significant decrease in infarct size and increase in infarct wall movement velocity in patients treated with cells compared with controls. In addition, radionuclide scintigraphy indicated improved cardiac perfusion in those undergoing cell therapy.

Fernandez-Avilés and colleagues [66] reported a clinical study of cell therapy in 20 patients and 13 nonrandomized controls. All underwent successful percutaneous revascularization of acute myocardial infarction. In the treatment group, autologous bone marrow–derived cells were harvested, cultured overnight, and delivered infused directly into infarct artery 13.5 ± 5.5 days after infarction. No adverse effects on microvascular function and myocardial injury were reported. No major cardiac events occurred up to 11 ± 5 months. Cardiac MRI at 6 months showed a decrease in end-systolic volume, improvement of regional and global LV function, and increased wall thickness in the infarct zone. The control group did not show any improvement in these parameters.

Investigators from the Transplantation of Progenitor Cells and Regeneration Enhancement in Acute Myocardial Infarction (TOPCARE-AMI) [18,67] randomized 59 patients after percutaneous revascularization of acute myocardial infarction to receive intracoronary infusion of bone marrow mononuclear cells or cultured peripheral blood mononuclear cells. Cells were infused into the open infarct artery 4 days after myocardial infarction. LV ejection fraction (LVEF) increased in treated patients from 51% to 58%, and increased significantly compared with historical non–cell-treated controls. Myocardial viability on FDG-PET evaluation, regional wall motion in the infarct area, and coronary flow reserve were also significantly enhanced. Fluorodeoxyglucose (FDG)-positron emission tomography (PET) scanning showed evidence of significantly improved myocardial viability at 4 months follow-up and significantly improved coronary flow reserve compared with historical controls.

In a clinical study of bone marrow CD133+ cell delivery after successful percutaneous reperfusion of acute myocardial infarction, Bartunek and colleagues [68] administered cells to 19 patients through intracoronary infusion 11.6 ± 1.4 days after infarction, and treated 16 controls with standard therapy. At 4 months follow-up, the treated group showed a significant increase in LVEF and reduction in fractional shortening measured with LV angiography and a significant decrease in the size of the original perfusion defect measured with technetium-99m sestamibi–single-photon emission computed tomography. However, seven cases of in-stent restenosis, two stent occlusions, and one de-novo lesion were seen at follow-up angiography in the cell-treated group. Two patients in the control group showed in-stent restenosis. Therefore, although evidence showed improved LV function related to CD133+ cell treatment, a safety concern remains about possible restenosis.

Once the safety and feasibility of this treatment in these smaller non-randomized studies were generally accepted, larger randomized controlled clinical studies of cell therapy after myocardial infarction were initiated. Five have been published and others are ongoing.

The Bone Marrow Transfer to Enhance ST Elevation Infarct Regeneration (BOOST) study is the first randomized control trial of unselected bone marrow mononuclear cells after acute myocardial infarction [69]. Cells were injected at 5 to 7 days in the infarct-related arteries of 30 patients. Compared with baseline investigation 3.5 ± 1.5 days after percutaneous coronary intervention (PCI), patients treated with cells showed an improvement in mean global LVEF of 6.7% compared with 0.7% in the non–cell-treated control groups at 6 months of follow-up ($P = .0026$). No differences in levels of restenosis or arrhythmia incidence were seen between the groups. Additional FDG-PET studies estimated engraftment of 14% to 39% of injected cells. In the 18-month follow-up to the BOOST study, the cell-therapy group showed a nonsignificant reduction in the composite clinical end point of death, myocardial infarction, and rehospitalization caused by heart failure. Although the study was underpowered for clinical end points, these findings at least provided additional evidence for safety. The improvement in mean global LVEF in the cell-therapy group was sustained at 5.9% [70]. However, mean ejection fractions in the control group also improved by 3.1%; the difference between the groups no longer reaching statistical significance. Analysis of the time course of LV functional improvements showed a significantly faster recovery of global ejection fraction in the cell-therapy group compared with controls, suggesting that a single dose of bone marrow cells may have accelerated postinfarction LV recovery in this study.

Janssens and colleagues [71] recently reported their results from a randomized, double-blind, placebo-controlled study in 67 patients from whom bone marrow was harvested 1 day after successful percutaneous coronary intervention for acute myocardial infarction. Cell or placebo preparations were injected in three fractions over 2 to 3 minutes using a perfusion catheter with three low-pressure stop-flow inflations in the stent. The cell-treated group showed significant reductions in MRI-generated myocardial infarct size and better recovery rates of regional systolic function after 4 months of follow-up, but no significant benefit in LVEF, myocardial perfusion, and cardiac metabolism on FDG-PET.

A similarly negative study was the recently reported Autologous Stem cell Transplantation in Acute Myocardial Infarction (ASTAMI) trial [72]. In this randomized study of patients who underwent successful PCI for anterior myocardial infarction, 47 received intracoronary bone marrow cells at a median of 6 days post–myocardial infarction, whereas those in the control group underwent no additional treatment. LV function was assessed with echocardiography, SPECT, and MRI. Using these imaging modalities, the cell-therapy group showed improvements in mean ejection fractions of 8.1%, 3.1%, and 1.2%, respectively, at 6 months follow-up. However, LV recovery was also seen in the control group, with ejection fractions increasing by 7.0%, 2.1%, and 4.3%, respectively. Both groups showed evidence of LV recovery, with the difference not statistically significant. These findings contrast with those of the Reinfusion of Enriched Progenitor Cells and Infarct Remodeling in Acute Myocardial Infarction (REPAIR-AMI) trial, which is the largest clinical cardiac cell-therapy study [73]. This double-blind, randomized, placebo-controlled trial involving 204 patients showed a significantly higher improvement in angiographically calculated LVEFs (5.5%) compared with placebo injection (3.0%) at 4 months. Subjects were administered autologous bone marrow cells suspended in medium (or medium alone as a control) through intracoronary infusion 3 to 7 days after undergoing successful PCI. Those who had lower baseline ejection fractions seemed to benefit more from cell therapy. Moreover, cell therapy was associated with a reduction in the prespecified clinical end point of death, myocardial infarction, and revascularization at 1 year.

In the Myocardial Regeneration and Angiogenesis in Myocardial Infarction with G-CSF and Intracoronary Stem Cell Infusion-3-DES (MAGIC Cell-3-DES) study, Kang and colleagues [74] randomized 96 patients to undergo intracoronary infusion of GCSF-mobilized peripheral blood stem cells (minimum 7 million CD34+ cells) within 14 days of percutaneous revascularization and after 14 days. Only the acute myocardial infarction group showed improvement in LVEF and remodeling, although coronary flow reserve improved significantly in both groups post–cell infusion. Most clinical studies have used unselected bone marrow cells for delivery. However, Chen and colleagues [75] randomized 69 patients post–primary angioplasty for acute myocardial infarction to undergo intracoronary MSC or saline infusion for a mean of 18 days after the event. At 6 months follow-up, significant reductions were seen in infarct size and left ventricular volumes compared with controls. LVEF increased by 14% in the treated group, suggesting that populations enriched for MSCs may have therapeutic potential.

Summary

Taken together, randomized clinical cell therapy studies suggest either no difference or a modest improvement in LV function related to cell therapy, suggesting at least that autologous bone marrow cell administration after acute myocardial infarction is not harmful. The REPAIR-AMI study, the largest of these trials, suggests a statistically significant

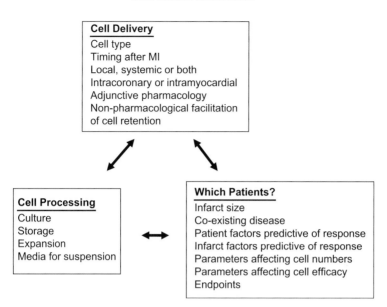

Fig. 2. Parameters to be considered for future clinical trial design. Multiple variables which may effect cell efficacy, engraftment, and clinical outcome, such as significant interplay between cell processing factors, cell delivery factors, and patient characteristics. Preclinical large animal studies may aid in clinical trial designs and are likely to help maximize mechanistic information obtainable.

improvement in a combined clinical end point at 1 year. However, the BOOST trial, which had the longest follow-up, suggested that early improvements in LV function related to cell therapy were later matched by the control group. No randomized studies were specifically designed or sufficiently powered to detect hard clinical end points. Some experts argue that large-scale clinical trials are now warranted [76]. However, given the number of clinical variables in the trials, multiple large-scale studies may be required (Fig. 2). Cell type, dose, and route of delivery may have a significant impact on cell engraftment and effect. Moreover, timing of cell delivery may be critical. Whether edema and inflammation early after myocardial infarction favors or discourages cell engraftment and effect is not clear. Ongoing animal studies may help optimize future clinical trial design in this regard. Continued basic and translational research may clarify the regenerative potential of human marrow and shed light on paracrine mechanisms attributed to cell delivery [77]. The small-scale clinical studies reviewed in this article may not have fulfilled the promise of the early animal studies and may have tempered initial enthusiasm for clinical myocardial cell therapy. Future larger studies, designed to maximize mechanistic insight while addressing critical clinical end points, may help clarify whether a role exists for autologous cell therapy in the treatment of acute myocardial infarction.

References

[1] 2004 Chartbook on cardiovascular lung and blood diseases. Bethesda, MD: National Heart, Lung, and Blood Institute. In: National Heart, Lung, and Blood Institute Morb Mortal; 2004:2–53.

[2] Soonpaa MH, Koh GY, Klug MG, et al. Formation of nascent intercalated disks between grafted fetal cardiomyocytes and host myocardium. Science 1994;264(5155): 98–101.

[3] Beltrami AP, Urbanek K, Kajstura J, et al. Evidence that human cardiac myocytes divide after myocardial infarction. N Engl J Med 2001;344(23):1750–7.

[4] Ferrari G, Cusella-De Angelis G, Coletta M, et al. Muscle regeneration by bone marrow-derived myogenic progenitors. Science 1998;279(5356):1528–30.

[5] Petersen BE, Bowen WC, Patrene KD, et al. Bone marrow as a potential source of hepatic oval cells. Science 1999;284(5417):1168–70.

[6] Alison MR, Poulsom R, Jeffery R, et al. Hepatocytes from non-hepatic adult stem cells. Nature 2000;406(6793):257.

[7] Brazelton TR, Rossi FM, Keshet GI, et al. From marrow to brain: expression of neuronal phenotypes in adult mice. Science 2000;290(5497):1775–9.

[8] Mezey E, Chandross KJ, Harta G, et al. Turning blood into brain: cells bearing neuronal antigens generated in vivo from bone marrow. Science 2000;290(5497):1779–82.

[9] Krause DS, Theise ND, Collector MI, et al. Multi-organ, multi-lineage engraftment by a single bone marrow-derived stem cell. Cell 2001;105(3):369–77.

[10] Jackson KA, Majka SM, Wang H, et al. Regeneration of ischemic cardiac muscle and vascular endothelium by adult stem cells. J Clin Invest 2001;107:1395–402.

[11] Orlic D, Kajstura J, Chimenti S, et al. Bone marrow cells regenerate infarcted myocardium. Nature 2001;410:701–5.

[12] Kale S, Karihaloo A, Clark PR, et al. Bone marrow stem cells contribute to repair of the ischemically injured renal tubule. J Clin Invest 2003;112(1):42–9.

[13] Ianus A, Holz GG, Theise ND, et al. In vivo derivation of glucose-competent pancreatic endocrine cells from bone marrow without evidence of cell fusion. J Clin Invest 2003;111(6): 843–50.

[14] Camargo FD, Green R, Capetanaki Y, et al. Single hematopoietic stem cells generate skeletal muscle through myeloid intermediates. Nat Med 2003;9(12):1520–7.

[15] Weimann JM, Johansson CB, Trejo A, et al. Stable reprogrammed heterokaryons form spontaneously in Purkinje neurons after bone marrow transplant. Nat Cell Biol 2003; 5(11):959–66.

[16] Quaini F, Urbanek K, Beltrami A, et al. Chimerism of the transplanted heart. N Engl J Med 2002;346:5–15.

[17] Strauer BE, Brehm M, Zeus T, et al. Repair of infarcted myocardium by autologous intracoronary mononuclear bone marrow cell transplantation in humans. Circulation 2002;106: 1913–8.

[18] Assmus B, Schachinger V, Teupe C, et al. Transplantation of progenitor cells and regeneration enhancement in acute myocardial infarction (TOPCARE). Circulation 2002;106: 3009–17.

[19] Stamm C, Westphal B, Kleine HD, et al. Autologous bone-marrow stem-cell transplantation for myocardial regeneration. Lancet 2003;361:45–6.

[20] Tse HF, Kwong YL, Chan JK, et al. Angiogenesis in ischaemic myocardium by intramyocardial autologous bone marrow mononuclear cell implantation. Lancet 2003;361(9351): 47–9.

[21] Murry CE, Soonpaa MH, Reinecke H, et al. Haematopoietic stem cells do not transdifferentiate into cardiac myocytes in myocardial infarcts. Nature 2004;428(6983):664–8.

[22] Laflamme MA, Myerson D, Saffitz JE, et al. Evidence for cardiomyocyte repopulation by extracardiac progenitors in transplanted human hearts. Circ Res 2002;90(6):634–40.

[23] Terada N, Hamazaki T, Oka M, et al. Bone marrow cells adopt the phenotype of other cells by spontaneous cell fusion. Nature 2002;416(6880):542–5.

[24] Ying QL, Nichols J, Evans EP, et al. Changing potency by spontaneous fusion. Nature 2002; 416(6880):545–8.

[25] Alvarez-Dolado M, Pardal R, Garcia-Verdugo JM, et al. Fusion of bone-marrow-derived cells with Purkinje neurons, cardiomyocytes and hepatocytes. Nature 2003;425(6961): 968–73.

[26] Wang X, Willenbring H, Akkari Y, et al. Cell fusion is the principal source of bone-marrow-derived hepatocytes. Nature 2003;422(6934):897–901.

[27] Camargo FD, Finegold M, Goodell MA. Hematopoietic myelomonocytic cells are the major source of hepatocyte fusion partners. J Clin Invest 2004;113(9):1266–70.

[28] Vassilopoulos G, Wang PR, Russell DW. Transplanted bone marrow regenerates liver by cell fusion. Nature 2003;422(6934):901–4.

[29] Nygren JM, Jovinge S, Breitbach M, et al. Bone marrow-derived hematopoietic cells generate cardiomyocytes at a low frequency through cell fusion, but not transdifferentiation. Nat Med 2004;10(5):494–501.

[30] Willenbring H, Bailey AS, Foster M, et al. Myelomonocytic cells are sufficient for therapeutic cell fusion in liver. Nat Med 2004;10(7):744–8.

[31] Hierlihy AM, Seale P, Lobe CG, et al. The post-natal heart contains a myocardial stem cell population. FEBS Lett 2002;530(1–3):239–43.

[32] Anversa P, Kajstura J, Leri A, et al. Life and death of cardiac stem cells: a paradigm shift in cardiac biology. Circulation 2006;113(11):1451–63.

[33] Jiang S, Walker L, Afentoulis M, et al. Transplanted human bone marrow contributes to vascular endothelium. Proc Natl Acad Sci U S A 2004;101(48):16891–6.

[34] Caplice NM, Bunch TJ, Stalboerger PG, et al. Smooth muscle cells in human coronary atherosclerosis can originate from cells administered at marrow transplantation. Proc Natl Acad Sci U S A 2003;100(8):4754–9.

[35] Simper D, Wang S, Deb A, et al. Endothelial progenitor cells are decreased in blood of cardiac allograft patients with vasculopathy and endothelial cells of noncardiac origin are enriched in transplant atherosclerosis. Circulation 2003;108(2):143–9.

[36] Orlic D, Kajstura J, Chimenti S, et al. Mobilized bone marrow cells repair the infarcted heart, improving function and survival. Proc Natl Acad Sci U S A 2001;98:10344–9.

[37] Murry CE, Field LJ, Menasche P. Cell-based cardiac repair: reflections at the 10-year point. Circulation 2005;112(20):3174–83.

[38] Hutcheson KA, Atkins BZ, Hueman MT, et al. Comparison of benefits on myocardial performance of cellular cardiomyoplasty with skeletal myoblasts and fibroblasts. Cell Transplant 2000;9(3):359–68.

[39] Horackova M, Arora R, Chen R, et al. Cell transplantation for treatment of acute myocardial infarction: unique capacity for repair by skeletal muscle satellite cells. Am J Physiol Heart Circ Physiol 2004;287(4):H1599–608.

[40] Ott HC, Bonaros N, Marksteiner R, et al. Combined transplantation of skeletal myoblasts and bone marrow stem cells for myocardial repair in rats. Eur J Cardiothorac Surg 2004; 25(4):627–34.

[41] Murry CE, Reinecke H, Pabon LM. Regeneration gaps: observations on stem cells and cardiac repair. J Am Coll Cardiol 2006;47(9):1777–85.

[42] Behfar A, Zingman LV, Hodgson DM, et al. Stem cell differentiation requires a paracrine pathway in the heart. FASEB J 2002;16(12):1558–66.

[43] Xu C, Police S, Rao N, et al. Characterization and enrichment of cardiomyocytes derived from human embryonic stem cells. Circ Res 2002;91(6):501–8.

[44] Chiu RC, Zibaitis A, Kao RL. Cellular cardiomyoplasty: myocardial regeneration with satellite cell implantation. Ann Thorac Surg 1995;60(1):12–8.

[45] Taylor DA, Atkins BZ, Hungspreugs P, et al. Regenerating functional myocardium: improved performance after skeletal myoblast transplantation. Nat Med 1998;4(8):929–33.

[46] Reinecke H, Poppa V, Murry CE. Skeletal muscle stem cells do not transdifferentiate into cardiomyocytes after cardiac grafting. J Mol Cell Cardiol 2002;34(2):241–9.

[47] Kamihata H, Matsubara H, Nishiue T, et al. Implantation of bone marrow mononuclear cells into ischemic myocardium enhances collateral perfusion and regional function via side supply of angioblasts, angiogenic ligands, and cytokines. Circulation 2001;104:1046–52.

[48] Harraz M, Jiao C, Hanlon HD, et al. CD34⁻ blood-derived human endothelial progenitors. Stem Cells 2001;19:304–12.

[49] Yoon CH, Hur J, Park KW, et al. Synergistic neovascularization by mixed transplantation of early endothelial progenitor cells and late outgrowth endothelial cells: the role of angiogenic cytokines and matrix metalloproteinases. Circulation 2005;112(11):1618–27.

[50] Gulati R, Simari RD. Cell therapy for angiogenesis: embracing diversity. Circulation 2005; 112(11):1522–4.

[51] Balsam LB, Wagers AJ, Christensen JL, et al. Haematopoietic stem cells adopt mature haematopoietic fates in ischaemic myocardium. Nature 2004;428(6983):668–73.

[52] Asahara T, Murohara T, Sullivan A, et al. Isolation of putative progenitor endothelial cells for angiogenesis. Science 1997;275:964–7.

[53] Lin Y, Weisdorf DJ, Solovey A, et al. Origins of circulating endothelial cells and endothelial outgrowth from blood. J Clin Invest 2000;105:71–7.

[54] Gulati R, Jevremovic D, Peterson TE, et al. Diverse origin and function of cells with endothelial phenotype obtained from adult human blood. Circ Res 2003;93(11):1023–5.

[55] Kocher AA, Schuster MD, Szabolcs MJ, et al. Neovascularization of ischemic myocardium by human bone-marrow-derived angioblasts prevents cardiomyocyte apoptosis, reduces remodeling and improves cardiac function. Nat Med 2001;7:412–30.

[56] Kawamoto A, Gwon H-C, Iwaguro H, et al. Therapeutic potential of ex vivo expanded endothelial progenitor cells for myocardial ischemia. Circulation 2001;103:634–7.

[57] Kawamoto A, Tkebuchava T, Yamaguchi J, et al. Intramyocardial transplantation of autologous endothelial progenitor cells for therapeutic neovascularization of myocardial ischemia. Circulation 2003;107(3):461–8.

[58] Rehman J, Li J, Orschell CM, et al. Peripheral blood "endothelial progenitor cells" are derived from monocyte/macrophages and secrete angiogenic growth factors. Circulation 2003; 107:1164–9.

[59] Pittenger MF, Martin BJ. Mesenchymal stem cells and their potential as cardiac therapeutics. Circ Res 2004;95(1):9–20.

[60] Makino S, Fukuda K, Miyoshi S, et al. Cardiomyocytes can be generated from marrow stromal cells in vitro. J Clin Invest 1999;103(5):697–705.

[61] Mangi A, Noiseux N, Kong D, et al. Mesenchymal stem cells modified with Akt prevent remodeling and restore performance of infarcted hearts. Nat Med 2003;9:1195–201.

[62] Amado LC, Saliaris AP, Schuleri KH, et al. Cardiac repair with intramyocardial injection of allogeneic mesenchymal stem cells after myocardial infarction. Proc Natl Acad Sci U S A 2005;102(32):11474–9.

[63] Beltrami AP, Barlucchi L, Torella D, et al. Adult cardiac stem cells are multipotent and support myocardial regeneration. Cell 2003;114(6):763–76.

[64] Oh H, Bradfute SB, Gallardo TD, et al. Cardiac progenitor cells from adult myocardium: homing, differentiation, and fusion after infarction. Proc Natl Acad Sci U S A 2003; 100(21):12313–8.

[65] Messina E, De Angelis L, Frati G, et al. Isolation and expansion of adult cardiac stem cells from human and murine heart. Circ Res 2004;95(9):911–21.

[66] Fernandez-Aviles F, San Roman JA, Garcia-Frade J, et al. Experimental and clinical regenerative capability of human bone marrow cells after myocardial infarction. Circ Res 2004; 95(7):742–8.

[67] Schachinger V, Assmus B, Britten MB, et al. Transplantation of progenitor cells and regeneration enhancement in acute myocardial infarction: final one-year results of the TOP-CARE-AMI Trial. J Am Coll Cardiol 2004;44(8):1690–9.

[68] Bartunek J, Vanderheyden M, Vandekerckhove B, et al. Intracoronary injection of CD133-positive enriched bone marrow progenitor cells promotes cardiac recovery after recent myocardial infarction: feasibility and safety. Circulation 2005;112(9 Suppl):I178–83.

[69] Wollert KC, Meyer GP, Lotz J, et al. Intracoronary autologous bone-marrow cell transfer after myocardial infarction: the BOOST randomised controlled clinical trial. Lancet 2004; 364(9429):141–8.

[70] Meyer GP, Wollert KC, Lotz J, et al. Intracoronary bone marrow cell transfer after myocardial infarction: eighteen months' follow-up data from the randomized, controlled BOOST (BOne marrOw transfer to enhance ST-elevation infarct regeneration) trial. Circulation 2006;113(10):1287–94.

[71] Janssens S, Dubois C, Bogaert J, et al. Autologous bone marrow-derived stem-cell transfer in patients with ST-segment elevation myocardial infarction: double-blind, randomised controlled trial. Lancet 2006;367(9505):113–21.

[72] Lunde K, Solheim S, Aakhus S, et al. Intracoronary injection of mononuclear bone marrow cells in acute myocardial infarction. N Engl J Med 2006;355(12):1199–209.

[73] Schachinger V, Erbs S, Elsasser A, et al. Intracoronary bone marrow-derived progenitor cells in acute myocardial infarction. N Engl J Med 2006;355(12):1210–21.

[74] Kang HJ, Lee HY, Na SH, et al. Differential effect of intracoronary infusion of mobilized peripheral blood stem cells by granulocyte colony-stimulating factor on left ventricular function and remodeling in patients with acute myocardial infarction versus old myocardial infarction: the MAGIC Cell-3-DES randomized, controlled trial. Circulation 2006;114(1 Suppl):I145–51.

[75] Chen SL, Fang WW, Ye F, et al. Effect on left ventricular function of intracoronary transplantation of autologous bone marrow mesenchymal stem cell in patients with acute myocardial infarction. Am J Cardiol 2004;94(1):92–5.

[76] Rosenzweig A. Cardiac cell therapy–mixed results from mixed cells. N Engl J Med 2006; 355(12):1274–7.

[77] Gnecchi M, He H, Liang OD, et al. Paracrine action accounts for marked protection of ischemic heart by Akt-modified mesenchymal stem cells. Nat Med 2005;11(4):367–8.

ELSEVIER
SAUNDERS

Med Clin N Am 91 (2007) 787–790

THE MEDICAL
CLINICS
OF NORTH AMERICA

What the Future Holds for the Diagnosis and Management of Patients with Acute Myocardial Infarction

David R. Holmes, Jr., MD, FACC, FSCAI

*Mayo Clinic, Cardiovascular Diseases and Internal Medicine,
200 First Street SW, Rochester, MN 55905, USA*

The care of patients with acute myocardial infarction has changed dramatically in concert with the expanding knowledge of the pathophysiology involved as well as the development of new pharmacologic and mechanical means of restoring flow. The field has been characterized by observational experiences leading to small pilot trials culminating in multiple "mega trials," which have involved multiple countries and thousands of patients and then finally to exhaustive evidence-based guidelines. Important issues remain to be resolved, many of which have been explored in this book.

System issues

Given the large number of patients hospitalized with acute myocardial infarction each year with the attendant morbidity and mortality involved, there are major societal implications. These implications have been magnified by the incredibly short time window during which reperfusion therapy has the greatest chance to improve outcome. It is now accepted that mechanical reperfusion, when performed in the experienced centers by expert physicians in a timely manner, is the preferred method of therapy. This is itself a major change in the field in the last decade, before which thrombolytic therapy was accepted as the treatment of choice. The issues now are how to make it available to the largest number of patients and achieve the shortest possible door-to-balloon time.

E-mail address: holmes.david@mayo.edu

medical.theclinics.com

Achievement of the shortest possible balloon time has become a quality of care indicator. Guidelines have identified a door-to-balloon time of ≤90 minutes as the goal. Increasing guidelines will use this as a metric to identify the quality of care, and in the relatively near future, this may be part of pay-for-performance measures.

Risk stratification and treatment of the highest-risk patients

Risk stratification is an increasingly important component of practice. Well-validated risk stratification approaches will facilitate evaluation of institutional and individual performance. Using these tools, evaluation of outliers defined as observed outcomes, which differ significantly from expected outcomes, will allow identification of system issues that can be compared with improved outcome; equally importantly, if observed outcomes are significantly better than expected using well-validated risk stratification schemes, then new strategies of care can be identified and developed that provide these superior outcomes.

Risk stratification is also a strong tool to match resource use with specific individual patient needs. For example, applying more intensive and advanced or expensive care that has increased risk might be selected in higher-risk patients and not routinely used in lower risk patients.

Finally, risk stratification is extremely important for patient and family counseling as part of the ongoing effort to include the patient in important decisions affecting their own care.

Myocardial salvage

The goal of reperfusion therapy is to restore full nutritive myocardial flow and salvage myocardium, thereby reducing morbidity and mortality. Tremendous resources—patient, physician, and industry alike—have been expended while trying to achieve this goal. The results of these energies have been mixed. Distal protection devices, while intuitively important, have not improved outcome in well-designed randomized trials. Whether this reflects inadequate design of or performance with these devices or reflects instead an erroneous intuitive assumption needs to be investigated further. Pharmaceutical approaches with a variety of agents such as compliment inhibitors or cell membrane stabilizers have similarly failed the test in large, randomized clinical trials. Again, whether this reflects lack of an effective agent or relates to the time-dependent necrosis that cannot be modified requires continued study.

Obviously, studying myocardial salvage requires the metrics to do so. Application of more advanced imaging technologies such as magnetic resonance imaging, which can more accurately detect the amount of irreversibly damaged myocardium or measure the amount of salvage, is essential.

Determining the extent of irreversible necrosis versus viable myocardium may also be very helpful in selecting the optimal treatment strategy.

Myocyte replacement therapy

Given the less than ideal results of salvaging ischemic myocardium, there is great interest in myocyte regeneration or replacement therapy. Early studies have documented modest improvement in left ventricular function with a variety of agents including skeletal myoblasts, circulating progenitor cells, and bone marrow–derived cells.

The mechanism of the modest improvement in left ventricular function is the subject of intense investigation. Whether this is truly the result of new physiologically functioning cells, of paracrine effects, or of some other mechanism is unclear. In addition, whether these efforts will be sustained remains to be determined. As part of this intense study, the specific cell type and number of cells required; the mode of therapy, eg, intramyocardial injection versus intracoronary injection; and finally the timing of therapy, eg, within the first few days or weeks after the index event also need to be evaluated.

As was true with the field of reperfusion injury, sophisticated methods at studying detailed regional left ventricular function and volume of distribution of infarcted segments will be required.

Prevention of myocardial infarction

The concept of vulnerability is an important one, because by identifying a plaque, a region, or a patient before the development of infarction has obvious great advantages. Initial interest was focused on the concept of a vulnerable plaque. This came from observations that in patients who have infarction, the lesion documented on coronary angiography before the infarction was often mild or moderate in severity. The issues of multiple vulnerable plaques, the time course of vulnerability, and the specificity of methods to identify a specific plaque raised questions as to the validity of the concept. Subsequently, interest has grown in identifying vulnerable regions, ie, those regions of the coronary bed that cause most infarctions in patient populations. Finally, the concept continues to evolve to include vulnerable patients using a variety of biomarkers or noninvasive imaging modalities. Validation of these concepts will require large-scale studies and then will require extensive evaluation and development of treatment strategies.

Identifying vulnerable patients, vulnerable lesions, or vulnerable plaque is of great interest. If this goal could be reached, intense preventative approaches could be applied. Attainment of this goal will require great advances in pivotal biomarkers, noninvasive and invasive cardiac imaging, and large-scale population-based studies to evaluate the natural history of the vulnerability. Finally, prevention—its risk-to-benefit ratio—will have to be documented in the patients at highest risk.

Evaluation and treatment of acute myocardial infarction has been a fertile field of investigation. These investigations have led to improved patient outcome. In some population-based studies within the last decade, there has been a 40% reduction in early and 1-year mortality. Continued investigation in the field would have led early investigators to conclude that patients might live long enough to make diagnosis as well as treatment possible.

ELSEVIER
SAUNDERS

THE MEDICAL
CLINICS
OF NORTH AMERICA

Med Clin N Am 91 (2007) 791–803

Index

Note: Page numbers of article titles are in **boldface** type.